Do You Have a
Beaumont Doctor?

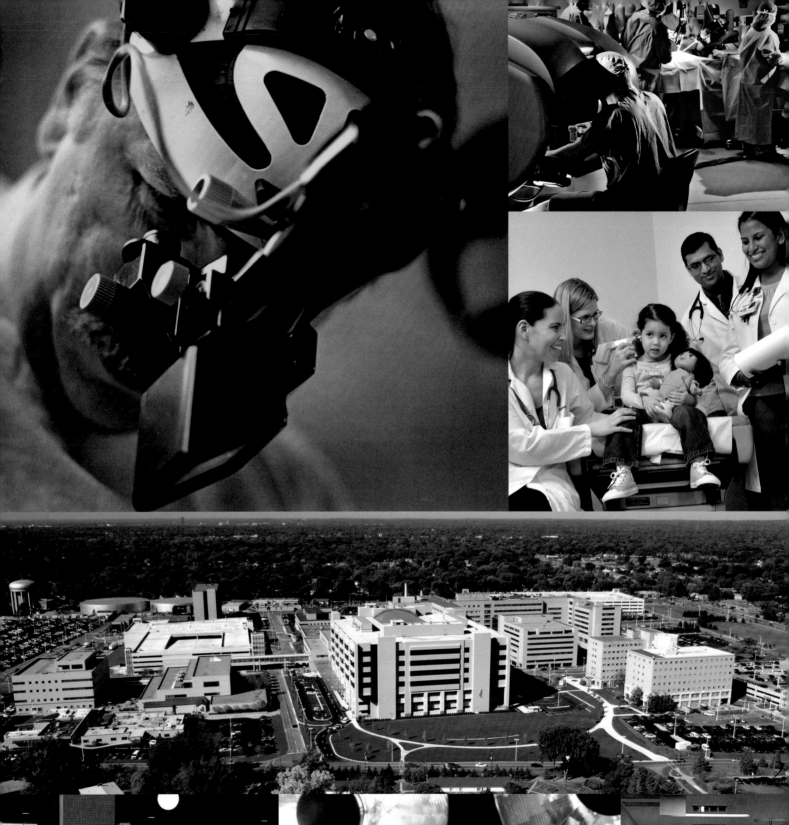
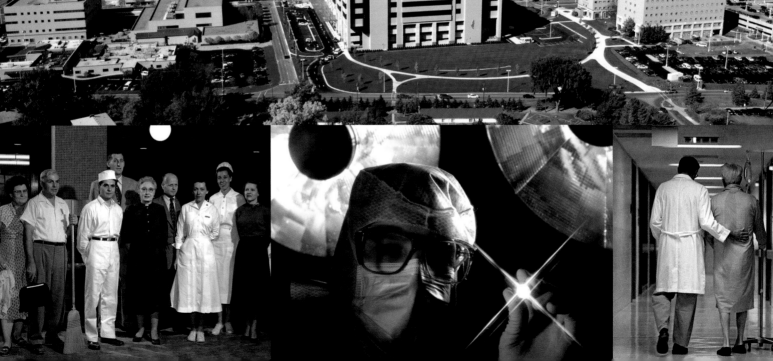

ANANIAS C. DIOKNO, M.D., and DIANE CAREY

Do You Have a
BEAUMONT
DOCTOR?

The Remarkable Story of Building One of America's
Most Successful Health Care Systems

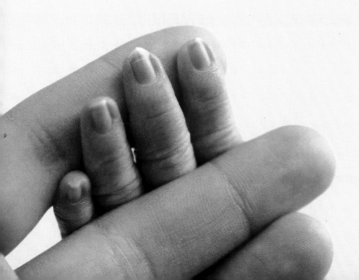

10 9 8 7 6 5 4 3 2 1

ISBN: 978-193239926-4

Huron River Press
PO Box 7797
Ann Arbor, MI 48107-7797
www.huronriverpress.com

Design: Savitski Design, Ann Arbor, Michigan
Printing: Oceanic Graphic Printing.
Printed in China

Library of Congress Cataloging-in-Publication Data

Diokno, Ananias C.
Do you have a Beaumont doctor? : the remarkable story of
building one of America's most successful health care systems /
by Ananias C. Diokno and Diane Carey.
       p. ; cm.
  ISBN 978-1-932399-26-4
  1. William Beaumont Hospitals (Mich.) 2. Hospitals–Michigan–
History. 3. Academic Medical Centers–Michigan–Interviews. 4.
Medical personnel–Michigan–Interviews. I. Carey, Diane. II. Title.
  [DNLM: 1. William Beaumont Hospitals (Mich.) 2. Hospitals–
history–Michigan–Interview. 3. Academic Medical Centers–
history–Michigan–Interview. 4. History, 20th Century–Michigan–
Interview. 5. Personnel, Hospital–history–Michigan–Interview.
WX 28 AM5]
  RA981.M5D56 2011
  362.1109774'38--dc23
                              2011013844

Our heartfelt appreciation goes to

Deborah Herveou, Kathleen Cesaro, Sherry Daniels,
Michele Barnard, Pamela Clarke, Margo Dees, Gayle Riley,
Maureen Nagle, and Elizabeth DeBeliso
for their tireless work and help in the assembly of this book.

Thank you!

Special thanks to Michael Killian,
Vice President of Marketing and Public Affairs,
for his expert editing.

WILLIAM BEAUMONT HOSPITAL

"I WANTED

BEAUMONT

TO BE A

SHINING LIGHT."

— Prem Khilanani, M.D.

ANANIAS C. DIOKNO, M.D., F.A.C.S.

Executive Vice-President and Chief Medical Officer, Beaumont Hospitals

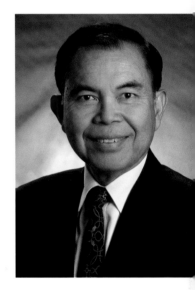

Why this book?

"William Beaumont Hospital is a major teaching facility that has 37 accredited residency and fellowship programs with over 400 residents and fellows. For undergraduate training, it accepts medical students from the University of Michigan, Wayne State University, and Michigan State University Schools of Medicine, as well as schools outside the state. Beaumont also has a nursing affiliation with Oakland University, including a top-ranked certified registered nurse-anesthetist school. In 2009, we joined with Oakland University to establish Oakland University William Beaumont School of Medicine.

"We say 'Beaumont Hospital,' but actually Beaumont is three hospitals with more than 14,000 full-time equivalent employees—the flagship quaternary health care hospital in Royal Oak, Michigan, which opened in 1955, the very cutting-edge community hospital in Troy, Michigan which opened in 1977, and our newest 2007 acquisition in Grosse Pointe, Michigan, formerly Bon Secours Hospital. All hospitals and ambulatory sites provide the highest quality compassionate care not only for our local population but also for patients coming from regional, national and international origin.

"This book is a good way to let the world know that the Beaumont health system is one of the great hospitals in the world to work for and that I would like us to be recognized for contributing much to the welfare of the people—patient care, safety, quality, teaching, training, and research. In one way or another, all of about 3,100 Beaumont doctors and all its employees contribute to the betterment of health care.

"I also believe it is important to recognize everyone who works hard to make the world better. This is also a way of recognizing those who are here and those who have passed away, those who have received awards, accomplished achievements, built departments, changed the way medicine is practiced, as well as those who quietly work hard and are left unrecognized.

"Perhaps this book will stimulate the interests of young people with medical aptitude, or to discover a medical aptitude they do not know they possess. Medical students may discover their fields of study or specialization within these covers, or whether they prefer private practice or employment as a hospital doctor. Patients and their families will be able to read about doctors, understand the journey they have to travel to be one, what makes a doctor choose a segment of medicine in which to practice, and let them glimpse into the private lives of doctors, both on and off the job.

"I hope this book will inspire those who are working in the myriad disciplines of medicine that anyone can work to be better, to accomplish more, and to be stimulated toward advancement."

The Spirit of Beaumont

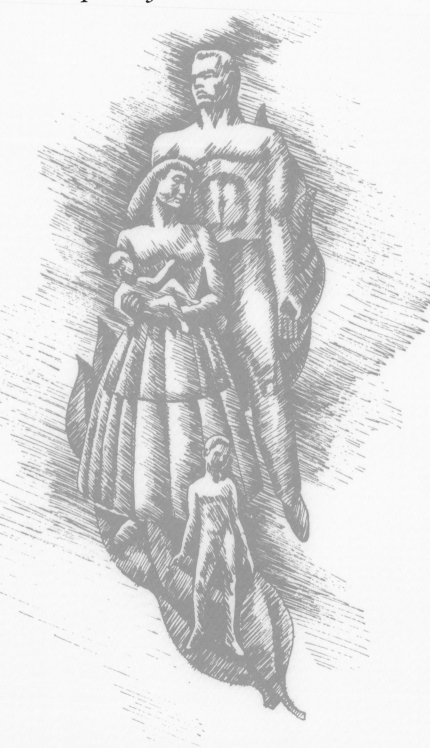

Where silence gripped darkness
And inertia filled space
When gloom bonded with doom
There evolved an echo with reverberation

Gaining momentum and resonance
Flanked by clouds and thundering
Striking the mountains
Overpowering the valleys
Awestruck, the people wondered
Was this dissolution
Creation
Or the Big Bang?

Through sleet and rain came the answer
I AM THE SPIRIT OF BEAUMONT
Tormented, sleepless, agonized
Yet hopeful, confident, energized
I shall never rest in peace till all the patients have
Able bodies, sound hearts
Alert minds, and restful souls.

Restore the sparkle in the eyes of children
Rejuvenate parents with hope and passion
Reinforce joy and dignity in the grandparents
Rebuild the community and the State
Through diligence and honesty alone
Integrity mingled with humanity
Respect, professionalism, empathy
Ethics, caliber and excellence
Service, humility and joy

Maintaining highest standards and quality
Through these I quench my desire
When the world is free of disease
Then only shall my soul rest in peace.

Forget not, I pervade all rooms
Omnipresent, omnipotent, omniscient
I scrutinize the "operations"
The Emergency Rooms and the ICU
My blessings to one and all
I am the guardian angel
I am the Spirit of Beaumont
The Spirit
of
Beaumont
Am
I

Prem Khilanani, M.D.

"The Family." An aluminum bas relief by Marshall Fredericks, adorned the east façade of the hospital. The sculpture was donated to the hospital in 1954 by Lola Jennings Erb, the first chairwoman of the hospital's Women's Service Committee, in memory of her late husband Lewis G. Erb, a civic and social leader. The subject was developed by Marshall Fredericks from a Biblical passage (Revelations 2:22): "…and the leaves of the tree were for the healing of the nations."

Humble Beginnings

How do hospitals get started? Haven't they "always been there?" Aren't they all venerated 200-year edifices? Hospitals don't actually begin somewhere, do they? They were just always there, forming our skylines as if stamped upon the atmosphere, rooted in ancient educational institutions where elder scholars once huddled in laboratories and classrooms. Only a Thomas Jefferson or a Sigmund Freud can actually reach out a hand and start a hospital. Right?

William Beaumont Hospital was started not by edicts thundering from above, but by an aggregation of concerned citizens who noticed that southeastern Michigan was in a furious growth stage, enjoying prosperity brought by the auto industry, and that there simply were not enough hospital beds to accommodate the community. The result was a surge of citizen action, a fund raising campaign, and a surge of new hospitals, including the "small community hospital" near the corner of Thirteen Mile Road and Woodward. The hospital may have started small, but its founding fathers and mothers had another idea. A much bigger idea.

The evolution of Beaumont Hospitals reflects our modern world since World War II. From a time when doctors came to farms for house calls, when many babies were born at home, when there was no cure for polio, Beaumont was able to be a place where mavericks could flourish. A great location, good doctors, and an administration and Board willing to say, 'Go do what you do best.' And the hospital bloomed. The organic problem with that is mavericks and strong-willed people want to do things their way, then continue doing things their way after the corporation gets bigger and needs to have people pulling together in the same direction.

While the health system strives to, and succeeds in, becoming a renowned medical entity in league with the national leaders, its doctors and officers remain devoted to caring for the individuals of the local community. The institution has developed a two-tiered administrative scaffold made of lay administrators on one hand, and an impressive roster of doctors who are also administrators, so the physicians of Beaumont can work with colleagues who understand their problems.

Beaumont was founded on, and has maintained, the principle of a private-practice medical staff. Private practitioners are entrepreneurs who run their own businesses in their private offices, then bring or send their patients in need of hospital services to Beaumont. These physicians have fueled Beaumont's astounding growth.

Campaign for 300-Bed Hospital Is Underway

H. H. Gardner, president of Birmingham National Bank and Ferndale National Bank, has accepted the chairmanship of the County Division in the So____ fund campaign

As county ____ tion composed ____ unteer workers ____ the campaign t____ dollars in the ____ County commu____ by the projecte____ pital, which wil____ ward and Thir____

The service a____ Berkley, Beverl____

DETROIT FREE PRESS—Monday, Dec. 22, 1947   3

NURSE SHORTAGE SEVERE

Hospital Situation in Detroit Critical

BY JAMES S. POOLER
Free Press Staff Writer

There is no pun intended when it is said the Detroit hospital situation today is unhealthy.

There is a shortage of 2,000 beds and 1,147 nurses. This means that even the available beds can't be fully used.

Hospitals are being crippled in the performance of their essential community services and many are reported going broke.

Because of the economic situation new hospitals aren't coming along fast. For instance, there was a concerted drive to raise $2,500,000 for a

Last of a Series

—is graduating its first class currently and that other classes will be graduated every 90 days.

These practical nurses will augment the present hospital forces and relieve the shortage which today has whole wings of hospitals closed.

Hospital costs have shot up and hospital directors complain that

A Patient's Voice

by Diane Carey

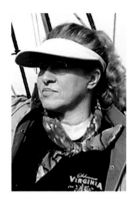

Diane Carey serving as Watch Leader on the Tall Ship *Half Moon*

"I came to Beaumont in search of surgical specialists. I needed both a hysterectomy and bladder surgery. I was delighted when Dr. Ananias Diokno, then the head of Urology, and Dr. John Sanborn, Obstetrics and Gynecology, arranged to coordinate their schedules and do everything I needed in one surgery, with one recovery.

"Imagine that! Imagine what it must take to merge the schedules of two busy specialists, just so I would have an easier surgical experience and only one recovery. I walked into the entrance to the building where I would have my surgery. Parking was right outside, and I was greeted by a volunteer coordinator, then taken to pre-op. No one talked about how huge the hospital really is; each employee and volunteer was involved in just this one building, and his or her own patients. Out of the thousands of patients treated at Beaumont hospitals every year, I was just one little person, yet I was treated as if I were the only concern of the hospital. I felt significant, and I guess that's because I really was.

"The Beaumont Hospitals are not the hospitals of my grandparents' time, where everything was in one building and a patient would be "Number 12" in a ward of white beds stretching into infinity. Beaumont is an enormous complex of specialized buildings and units, but each seems like a smaller hospital unto itself. There I was, walking into one part of the maze. Immediately I felt as if I were being treated an as individual, something medical services have learned to deliver and which Beaumont does especially well. I think they know the complex is huge and they want to counteract the factory-like sense of a giant operation.

"The coordination of my surgery was just right—amazing if you think about it, because it requires choreography between two departments and an army of support services—nursing, anesthesiology, surgical teams, office staff, recovery staff—yet they managed to make a complicated scenario seem simple from my perspective. These are specialists who are so busy that they don't have five extra minutes, yet my two surgeons and their surgical teams worked one after the other, right on time, as fluid as music. Just think about that.

"I was moved to a room in an area where the nurses were all trained in the recovery of my specific surgery—women's gynecology. They were well-trained in an assembly-line type operation, knowing exactly how to move me to my bed and settle me in, and I saw them do the same thing with the next patient and the next. While this sounds mechanical, somehow in practice it wasn't. The procedures had been honed by experience and were exactly what I needed, and what the other women needed, at every step.

"The Beaumont staff performed this flurry of activity and coordination behind the scenes, and still managed to make me believe it was all routine and simple. That illusion is part of the superior treatment I received—reducing tension and anxiety, making me feel at ease and special. I've had several surgeries and good experiences at other hospitals too, but I was truly impressed by the fluidity with which Beaumont delivered my most complex surgery, really two surgeries at once, and made the experience seem almost casual. Thanks to all of you at Beaumont for your good care of my body and my state of mind, all at the same time.

"My surgery at Beaumont was several years ago, and now I recognize that the service provided to me is the prototype of what many centers are just now establishing on a grand scale, now called a 'multi-disciplinary clinic'—a center of excellence where patients are seen and managed in the multiple disciplines that will take care of the entire patient in the most efficient and caring way.

"I'm thrilled to collaborate on this book about this wonderful place. I have many books with my name on them, but this book will mark a shining point in my career and my life. When the title pops into my mind—Do You Have a Beaumont Doctor?—I happily answer, 'Yes. I have two.'

"Beaumont is a remarkable complex, showing the phenomenal organic growth possible in a free economy, where ideas fledge energetically from fertile minds. Someday there's going to be a spaceport here."

The Many Identities of a Hospital

Hospitals, especially large multi-plex medical centers, are many things to many people. They are places to work, places to thrive, places to find answers, places to wait, places to find rescue, to heal, to hope, to be born and to die. A hospital's name will be interwoven with its community, and will become a household word around the block, and maybe around the world.

After the second World War, two groups of community citizens in south Oakland County, Michigan, each began working to found a hospital to serve the fast-growing suburban area north of metropolitan Detroit. A group in Bloomfield wanted to build the Bloomfield Medical Center near Adams and Square Lake Roads. The South Oakland Hospital Authority wanted to build Woodward General Hospital on Thirteen Mile Road, just west of Woodward Avenue. However, community leaders—and the Metropolitan Detroit Hospital Committee, which had funds for building—insisted upon one hospital, not two. The organizations soon merged into a new independent group: Oakland Hospital. There was still a considerable scuffle about where that hospital would be located. Ultimately, the 100-acre plot at Thirteen Mile and Woodward Avenue became the site.

Building began. Local philanthropists, entrepreneurs, businesses and corporations, the auto industry, civic groups and clubs, even moms and classrooms, gave money to building the hospital which was promised to be "ultra-modern," "more welcoming," and "on the cutting edge of medical science." The auto industries which made Michigan famous were also big givers. The hospital would be a private-sector victory, with everybody's fingerprints upon it.

However, there was one little sticking point. When a shipment of bricks meant for Oakland Hospital was delivered to the site of Oakwood Hospital in Dearborn, Michigan, the Oakland Hospital Board of Directors decided the hospital needed a new name.

They took the moment to think philosophically and practically about the name. What did they want the hospital to become? What would the name say about the hospital?

That's when a medical historian at the University of Michigan, Frederick Coller, M.D., suggested the name of a Michigan medical pioneer: Dr. William Beaumont.

Though not born in Michigan, Dr. Beaumont was posted at Fort Mackinac in 1822 where he made history by first saving and then experimenting upon a victim of a gunshot accident, he would eventually revolutionize medical science and found an entire field of practice—gastroenterology. He spent the bigger part of his career in various Great Lakes frontier posts, constantly experimenting with methods of treatment for the most common and debilitating diseases plaguing soldiers and pioneers, including women and children.

The new hospital would be near the old Mackinac Trail to northern Michigan, now Woodward Avenue. The name—William Beaumont Hospital—seemed to fit, even to link the new hospital to Michigan's history.

Beaumont was a pioneer and a researcher who understood that he had something special on his hands and unremittingly pursued more and more knowledge. That was the idea in the minds of the founding fathers of William Beaumont Hospital—to pursue excellence and to grow beyond obvious boundaries.

On October 31, 1954, Hospital Board President E. A. Tomlinson and the grandniece of Dr. Beaumont, Mrs. George Stokes, would stand at the laying of the cornerstone. The name of William Beaumont Hospital was an inspiration. It would allow the hospital to gain an international identity without being tied to a limited locale. Today the hospital is known around the world. Still a hospital for its nearby communities, William Beaumont Hospital is coming to fruition as a hospital for everybody, everywhere.

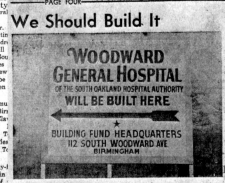

Woodward General Hospital Campaign Gathers Momentum

Projected New 300-Bed Hospital To Serve South Oakland Co. Communities

H. H. Gardner of Birmingham, president of Ferndale National Bank and Birmingham National Bank, has accepted the chairmanship of the land Hospital Authority paign for Woodward General pital.

As county chairman, Mr. ner will supervise a solicitin ganization composed of hundre volunteer workers who will on the campaign in the Sou Oakland County communities served by the projected new bed hospital, which will be at Woodward and Thirteen Road.

The service area commu are: Berkley, Beverly Hills, Birt ham, Bloomfield Hills, Cla Ferndale, Franklin, Hazel I Huntington Woods, Lathrup T site, Magnolia, Oak Park, Ples Ridge, Royal Oak, Royal Oak To hip and Troy Township.

"One hundred and sixty-f housand persons residing in ities and three townships of ection now are practically wi ut hospital facilities and depe a the heavily overtaxed hospi Detroit and Pontiac," said ardner.

PAGE FOUR — Tribune 1-15-47

We Should Build It

WOODWARD GENERAL HOSPITAL OF THE SOUTH OAKLAND HOSPITAL AUTHORITY **WILL BE BUILT HERE**

★

BUILDING FUND HEADQUARTERS 112 SOUTH WOODWARD AVE BIRMINGHAM

From this sign on Woodward near Thirteen-Mile road it is only a short walk to the site of the long-proposed Woodward General hospital.

A short walk—but a long ways to go nonetheless.

1 THE ADVERTISING CAMPAIGN
"DO YOU HAVE A BEAUMONT DOCTOR?"

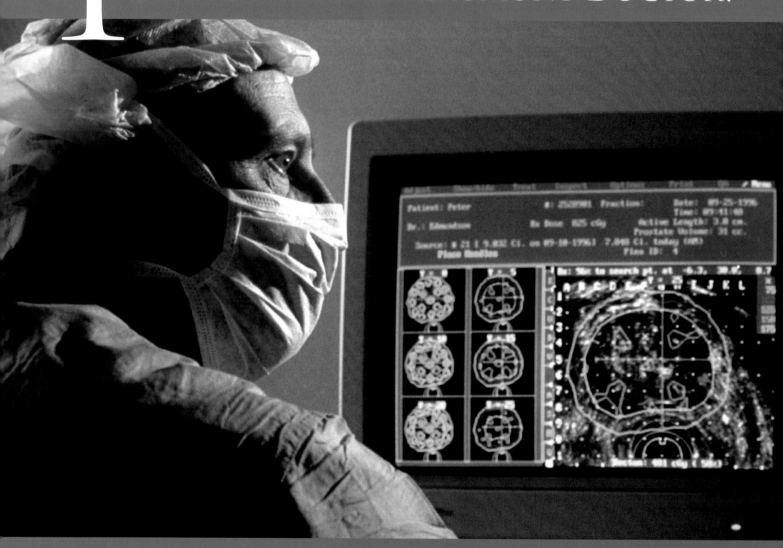

14

MICHAEL KILLIAN

Vice President, Marketing and Public Affairs,
Beaumont Hospitals

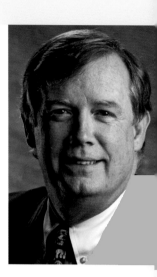

"In the mid-'80s, Beaumont was growing

quickly, adding specialists, but few knew all we offered. We had to communicate, and that meant trying something new. That meant advertise.

"In those days, it wasn't really acceptable for hospitals or doctors to actively advertise, but we decided we needed to do that. We formed a committee; the chairman of the committee was Board member J. P. McCarthy from WJR Radio. We selected the Campbell-Ewald Agency, which at the time was doing the Heartbeat of America campaign for Chevrolet. That was in '85. Our campaign lasted about two years. We felt we accomplished a lot, but our beds were full and we didn't continue the campaign.

"Along came the '90s. We were doing some targeted advertising. We were spending money, but the ads were not a campaign. We had an InterHealth program for travelers going overseas. Jeffrey Band, M.D., an epidemiologist from the Centers for Disease Control, ran that program here. We were developing ads for Lasik eye surgery; we were one of the first organizations to do laser surgery in the region. We brought in a group of advertising professionals, headed by Paige Curtis, to do this. Paige had learned her craft in New York, had worked on Breck and Prell shampoo commercials, Excedrin headache commercials, and had won 17 Clio's, the major international advertising award. Paige is married to a physician and at that time lived nearby.

"I started working with Paige. For our Lasik commercials, we came across a piece of music that sounded high-tech and urgent. We used it. People now think of it as a heartbeat, or as ominously referring to cancer. Professors at the Ross Business School at U of M

and other places call this 'sensation marketing.' What you hear and feel becomes part of the tapestry of the message.

"In 1998, we made a presentation to a strategic planning committee. I remember how the first radio commercial started:'

'Choosing a doctor seems like a simple thing.
'You ask around. Find one who takes your insurance. Someone who's close to home. Someone nice.

'That's all you care about, until someone in your family gets really sick.

'Suddenly, you wish you'd asked one more question: "Are you a Beaumont doctor?"

'Time after time, Beaumont has been rated the number one hospital in Southeast Michigan.

'We think the reason is a very simple one: Beaumont doctors.

'Do you have a Beaumont doctor?'

"And that's how it all started."

"We knew through market research that Beaumont doctors were in demand, and were the most preferred in the region. The reason for that was the work that had been done for many years by the medical leadership here who insisted upon high-quality medicine. I give them enormous credit. People preferred to come here.

"Paige was in a hair salon one day, listening to someone talking about her 'Beaumont doctor.' Paige thought about that and translated it into something very simple: 'Do you have a Beaumont doctor?'

THAT VOICE

"Paige knew a gentleman named Peter Thomas from earlier days in New York. He's now in his 80's and was then known in the advertising world as "the most trusted voice in America," and has done hundreds of documentaries and more than 60,000 commercials.

"We started to write a few commercials on the 'Do you have a Beaumont doctor?' theme.

"The first time we ran our commercial was April 12, 1999, the Monday after Easter week. From then until now, the music, the tone, and the message have been consistent with "tweaks" when needed. It not only works, but it's clear. Soon it'll be twelve years that we've stayed with this ad campaign, while other hospitals have gone through six or seven campaigns. People relate to the question, 'Do you have a Beaumont doctor?' When they think of that doctor/ patient relationship, they think of us. Our advertising is recognized as ours; ads from other hospitals are often recognized as ours too.

"We work to be scrupulous about not crossing the ethical barrier to say that Beaumont doctors are better than others. None of our scripts say that. We do discuss the preference for Beaumont doctors. We believe that the choice of doctors in the past has been rather fly-by-night. People would talk to their neighbors and ask, 'Who do you go to? Do you like your doctor?' We think choosing a doctor is a more serious choice. We're making it a serious choice."

FINDING THE "RIGHT" DOCTOR REALLY MATTERS

"A friend of mine who lives in another part of the state was diagnosed with breast cancer—very early, stage one, simple, small, treatable with a standard approach, which is partial mastectomy with radiation. With radiation, the standard of care is every day for six weeks. This woman has a business and had to travel. Every day for six weeks would be very difficult for her.

"This woman looked all over to find a way to avoid the six weeks of radiation so she could continue running her business, and she found Frank Vicini, M.D., our Chief of Oncology, a radiation oncologist, who actually invented and has done studies for years on a short-stay, targeted, high-dose radiation treatment. One treatment in the morning, one in the afternoon, and in five days you're done. This is a fabulous thing for women who are able to have the treatment. That's the importance of choosing the right doctor.

"So all these things fit together. We know that many people prefer Beaumont doctors for a number of reasons. Their reasons may be as simple as location, or that they think Beaumont has the latest technology, or they think, 'I know about Dr. Vicini. I know about Dr. Robbins, who did the surgery on the Red Wings when they were in the terrible auto accident in the late '90's.'
Our ads make people think. We try to be careful not to promise more than we can deliver. We have a system whereby every ad is reviewed by the chief of the service, the chief medical officer, and the legal officer before we put it on the air. We make sure we're saying the right things.'

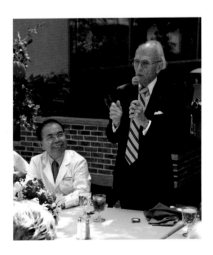

Mr. Peter Thomas (standing), the voice of "Do you have a Beaumont Doctor?" ad with Dr. Diokno looking on during his recent visit to Beaumont.

What is "A Beaumont Doctor?"

by Ananias C. Diokno, M.D.

Now that we know about the commercial "Do You Have a Beaumont Doctor?" the next logical questions is this: What is so special about Beaumont doctors? How does a doctor become a Beaumont doctor? In fact, the requirements are very stringent, and we're proud of that.

First, let's look at how one becomes a doctor. The conventional way is to take a four-year pre-med course in college, preparing a strong resume which includes a high grade-point average (GPA), high scores in the Medical College Admissions Test (MCAT), excellent letters of recommendation, some strong extra-curricular activities related to helping people, and a good interview.

Then, a portion of the applicants will be successful in getting admitted to a medical school for four years. Medical school teaches a wide general range of medical courses, including basic skills and provides some beginning experience in medical practice, then culminates in a Medical Doctor (M.D.) diploma or a Doctor of Osteopathy (D.O.) diploma.

An unconventional way is something called the Inteflex Program, a six-year program for high achievers, in which students are accepted after their senior year in high school to go directly into medical school, complete studies, and receive the M.D. Diploma after six years. Sometimes this is also combined with a Ph.D degree.

THE INTERN

Once the medical student has finished medical school and has a degree in medicine, but does not yet have a license to practice medicine without the supervision of a licensed doctor, he or she is referred to as an intern, and is considered to be a physician in training. In most training programs, the "intern" is blended with the specialty residency training program, which is the first year of training, also known as Post Graduate Year 1 (PGY-1). In most states a successful completion of a year of internship in an accredited program is a minimum requirement before being granted a license to practice medicine.

RESIDENCY

Once a student receives the M.D. or D.O. diploma, he or she can complete the licensing process in the state where he wishes to practice. However, a degree is not sufficient for practicing medicine. He must seek a residency training program for a specific focus. Residency programs average four to six years, but can be longer. The graduate may choose residency in any of several fields—internal medicine, pathology, radiology, pediatrics, obstetrics and gynecology, neurology, physical medicine and rehabilitation, family medicine, general surgery, anesthesiology, or many others. Following completion of residency, the new doctor must take the Board Certification exam in his field of specialty. Most of the Board certifications are offered two to three years after residency, because they examine not only knowledge, but outcomes of the first two years of practice in caring for patients.

There are some M.D. and D.O. Graduates who never get into a complete residency program. Either they don't make the cut, decide to quit for personal reasons, or cannot get positions. They may find research jobs or work in clinics, but by and large most doctors practicing in America have completed residency programs.

THE MATCH

How does one land a residency position? It is another hurdle that M.D. and D.O. Graduates must meet in a very competitive way, through a "matching" program. This program is managed by a private not-for-profit corporation, National Resident Matching Program (NRMP). They match 37,000 applicants to 25,000 residency positions. The match results are usually announced in March. There are specialty organizations in fields such as urology who conduct their own matches. Students write down their first several choices of places they wish to train, and medical facilities write down their first several choices of students. If a student's choice and a residency program's choice are the same, that student is "matched" to that place. Approximately 80% of students match into one of their top three choices,

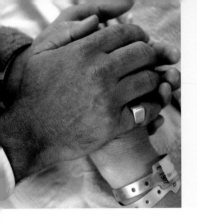

DONNA HOBAN, M.D., ON DOCTORS "Physicians spend so much time in school that they want to know they'll be able to do everything in medicine that they wanted to do, and make sure their patients have great care at the best facility where they'll have the best outcomes."

although a student may have as many as 15 programs on his or her list.

In the event that the student does not match, he or she will be notified two days in advance of the match day to participate in a "scramble." These unmatched graduates telephone unmatched residency programs in attempt to salvage their applications and land a position elsewhere, not necessarily their original choices.

The Match Day in March is a big day on many medical school campuses, because this is the day when medical students find out where they will be training and living for the next four to six years of their lives.

FELLOWSHIP

Once the residency is finished, a newly trained doctor has to find a place to work, either as a hospital employee or in private practice. He or she may join a group of doctors, with the option of becoming a partner after two years, more or less, or decide to do more training by entering into a fellowship program.

Fellowship is the next step to sub-specialization. After residency, a doctor may want to focus more narrowly on a field. For example, a doctor finishing a residency in internal medicine may decide to become a cardiologist. He will then have to seek a cardiology fellowship. Even within a sub-specialized cardiology fellowship, there is yet one more step to super-specialization by taking another fellowship in interventional cardiology, which means that a general cardiologist can perform cardiac catheterization, use of balloon dilators, and stent placement.

Another example would be a doctor who completes a five or six-year urology residency so he could become a urological surgeon. This surgeon

might then spend another two years as a fellow in urologic oncology, so he can sub-specialize in urologic cancers.

Whether the doctor goes into private practice or is employed by a hospital, he must apply for membership on the medical staff in the hospital where he wishes to practice. To be a member of the medical staff and receive privileges to practice in that hospital, the doctor must be "credentialed." The credentialing process is rigorous. The credentialing committee of the hospital will authenticate the doctor's degree, residency/fellowship record, personal record, intention to practice, history of malpractice, academic activities such as published papers or research, and review of requested privileges.

Now he is a doctor. Can he become a Beaumont doctor?

BECOMING A BEAUMONT DOCTOR

To be a Beaumont doctor, being an M.D. or a D.O. and having completed residency is not enough. The applicant must be above the 50th percentile of the qualifications of the current medical staff practicing in his or her specialty. Each department at Beaumont has its own manpower plan that defines what the 50th percentile is, and includes not only the medical school and residency program, but malpractice history, extra training, academic history, and much more. Of course, with each additional doctor accepted at Beaumont, the 50% percentile rises on the scale, therefore making even more strict requirements for the next applicants.

One requirement we enforce is that all Beaumont doctors must be Board-certified in their specialties. We will accept new graduates who are Board eligible, but we expect them to achieve Board certification in two to three years, otherwise their medical staff membership will not be renewed. Another preference, though not mandatory, is that a doctor has a fellowship or some equivalent experience such as having been a professor at a University or having a successful private practice for a specified period of time, thereby establishing strong credentials.

The requirements to become a Beaumont doctor are clearly very stringent. Not all doctors qualify. Our constant goal is to attract the best doctors, maintain a demonstrably superior staff, and deliver excellent medical care to our community, whom we can proudly ask, "Do you have a Beaumont doctor?"

Martin Tamler, M.D., (far right) Residency Program Director, Department of Physical Medicine and Rehabilitation teaching resident trainees.

LYNDA MISRA, D.O. ON THE MEDICAL COLLEGE ADMISSIONS TEST (MCAT)

"The Medical College Admissions Test is a standardized exam given to individuals planning to apply to medical school. All U.S. medical schools require this for admission. There are three categories on which candidates are tested: verbal, biological science, and physical science.

"The highest possible score in each category is 15 points. A perfect score on the MCAT is 45, I personally have only seen a 41. There is an essay portion as well which is graded with a letter J through T. The majority I have seen are graded as Q. I have seen some M's and N's.

"An example of an individual's score would be: BS–10, PS–9, V–10; Total 29Q. Average MCAT scores vary year to year, but range 25 or 26.

"The MCAT has been studied and been found to be a consistent predictor of United States Medical Licensing Examination I (USMLE) passing rates and overall success in medical school. USMLE are three exams I, II, III, taken after M2 (second year of medical school), after M3, and sometime during residency. Every student must pass these exams in order to be promoted to the next year and ultimately apply for a medical license.

"The MCAT and the applicant's GPA are the two most important metrics reviewed by medical school admissions teams."

LYNDA MISRA, D.O. is Associate Dean for Undergraduate Medical Education, Oakland University William Beaumont School of Medicine

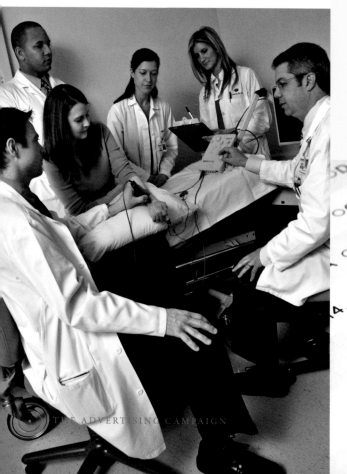

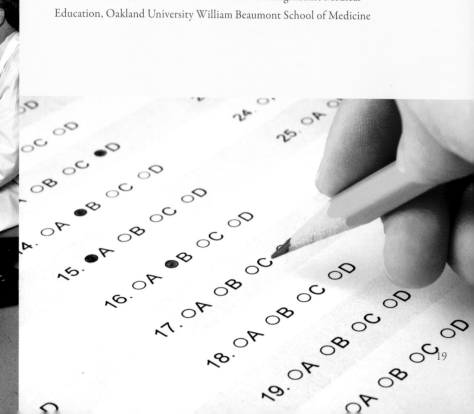

FEDERICO ARCARI, M.D.
Corporate Medical Director, 1987–1996

"I am privileged to have interviewed Dr. Arcari two weeks before his passing on, in the fall of 2009. He was one of my first interviews, and a charming welcome to Beaumont's history" — Diane Carey

"The past 50 years

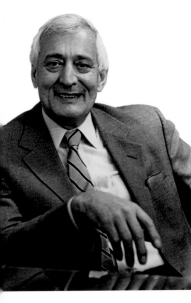

has been one of the most incredible 50 years in the history of medicine. It's as big as the changes involved in going to the moon.

"Fifty years ago, when I came here as a pediatric surgeon, there were only about forty-five pediatric surgeons in the whole country. I'm 80 now.

"I was a consultant in pediatric surgery at seven or eight hospitals, and then shortly after I went into practice, talk came up about establishing a new hospital—a 250-bed small general hospital. I joined the staff here in pediatric surgery in about 1964.

"As time went by, we established a pediatric surgery center here. It was my idea to set up pediatric surgery, even though it was unusual for a general hospital. As a result, they brought in a pediatric radiologist and a pediatric anesthesiologist. The difference between a radiologist for adults and a radiologist for children is vast. Children are not just little adults. There are different things to look for.

"Then we developed a pediatric intensive care unit, and so pediatric surgery grew up here. I watched this hospital grow and was always of the opinion that Beaumont's potential was without limits. There were no boundaries to it because of the attitude—the attitude of the Board, of the physicians and chiefs of departments, and those running the hospital, and all were determined they were going to have a first-class hospital."

AN EXTRAORDINARY STORY

"Beaumont was one of the first hospitals in the state that demanded its new members be Board-certified or certifiable in their specialties. Even university

hospitals didn't have that degree of demand on their potential physicians.

"Even now, I have to say that Beaumont hasn't reached its potential. It grew from 250 beds 60 years ago to 1100 beds, in the shadow of three major medical schools—University of Michigan, Michigan State and Wayne State—and Ford Hospital, from five OB-GYN residents to now getting medical students from all these institutions, to now having several hundred residents, interns and fellows, developed major fellowship programs, and all within the confines of a private hospital with a staff dedicated to teaching.

"It is an extraordinary story."

"At one time, I was Chief of Surgical Services here in Royal Oak and when they opened the Beaumont-Troy hospital, I was asked to go there and be the Medical Director, in that we were just opening a new hospital and we had to set some standards similar to what the Chief Medical Officer does here, in order to develop a staff and apply there what we had learned here. But that was twenty-five or thirty years ago. I was the first Medical Director at Troy. Then I came back to Royal Oak and became the Medical Director here. I've retired from all that, having been part of a great accomplishment."

"Fifty or sixty years ago, it was much easier to have an idea and go ahead with it. Today, there's so much red tape and government interference that I doubt the same success would be possible. In the capacity to enhance medical activity with research, the restrictions on research are considerable. Of course, there's some validity in having a state-wide evaluation of a circumstance that involves spending of money by the State and by the community. You don't want to duplicate efforts, or if you add 300 beds to 500 beds when you need 600 beds, that's a lot of waste of money. But as in most things, when the government gets involved, things get harder to accomplish.

"This institution was lucky in that regard. We didn't have limitations on our outlook. We had the kind of people and the conditions that were the result of an academic entrepreneurial environment. And they were an entertaining group to work with. I think we live in a different era now from a variety of points of view.

of these babies now. Or a baby's who's born with 25% of its intestine and we are able to create an intestine. Plastic surgery, changes in orthopaedic surgery with joint replacements, spinal column replacements—the changes since World War I, in this past 50 or 70 years, are enormous, fantastic.

"We now have bionics. We have laparoscopy. And now we're going into microscopic changes, even genetic changes that can be done before birth. Put a fresh hip in a 75-year-old—that's a major surgical onslaught on an individual, and we do it with regularity here.

"I don't think you'll find a parallel story to the growth of Beaumont in the United States at

The fact that Beaumont has achieved the status it has in this period of time is a tribute to those who went before and determined that this was going to be a first-class hospital.

"But the hospital itself has grown in all its specialties—internal medicine, surgery, orthopaedics, obstetrics, urology, pulmonology, cardiology, cardiac surgery, general surgery, eye surgery—all the surgical specialties, then all the medical specialties, then all the anesthesiologists, a school of anesthesia, each one pushing the other to excel. With their growing up here, they enhanced the capacity of the institution to train young doctors to such an extent that we went from small numbers, five or six interns, to a major teaching institution.

"Remember, most of these 'teachers' were in private practice and weren't paid to be teachers. They did the teaching in addition to their private practices because they enjoyed teaching and recognized it as appropriate. Part of the rules of the game is that you must be capable of passing on your knowledge to the younger people. At Beaumont there was a plethora of first-class, practicing, interested physicians who could provide a valid teaching experience for young people.

In my lifetime, cardiac surgery came into existence. Prior to that, there was no such thing. Various forms of thoracic surgery came into existence. The surgery of the newborn with a congenital abnormality was developed. Nobody thought you could save a newborn who was born without an esophagus. Well, we routinely take care

the present moment. The fact that Beaumont has achieved the status it has in this period of time is a tribute to those who went before and determined that this was going to be a first-class hospital. I credit the Board and staff, and the people whom the Board determined would be leading activists in the hospital, and the coterie of support they developed. None of this could have happened if the Board of Directors and the people they chose to run the hospital hadn't had this attitude about excellence.

"This hospital has not yet reached its potential."

Fund raising for the Hospital Fund included an exhibition golf match at Red Run Golf Club; those participating included Jimmy Demaret, Byron Nelson and Ben Hogan (2nd, 3rd and 6th from left respectively), three of the top U.S. professional golfers.

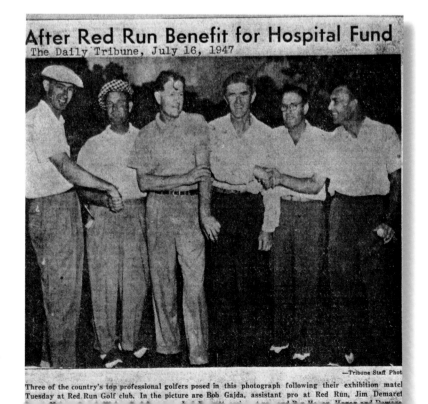

After Red Run Benefit for Hospital Fund
The Daily Tribune, July 16, 1947

—Tribune Staff Phot

Three of the country's top professional golfers posed in this photograph following their exhibition matc[h] Tuesday at Red Run Golf club. In the picture are Bob Gajda, assistant pro at Red Run, Jim Demaret

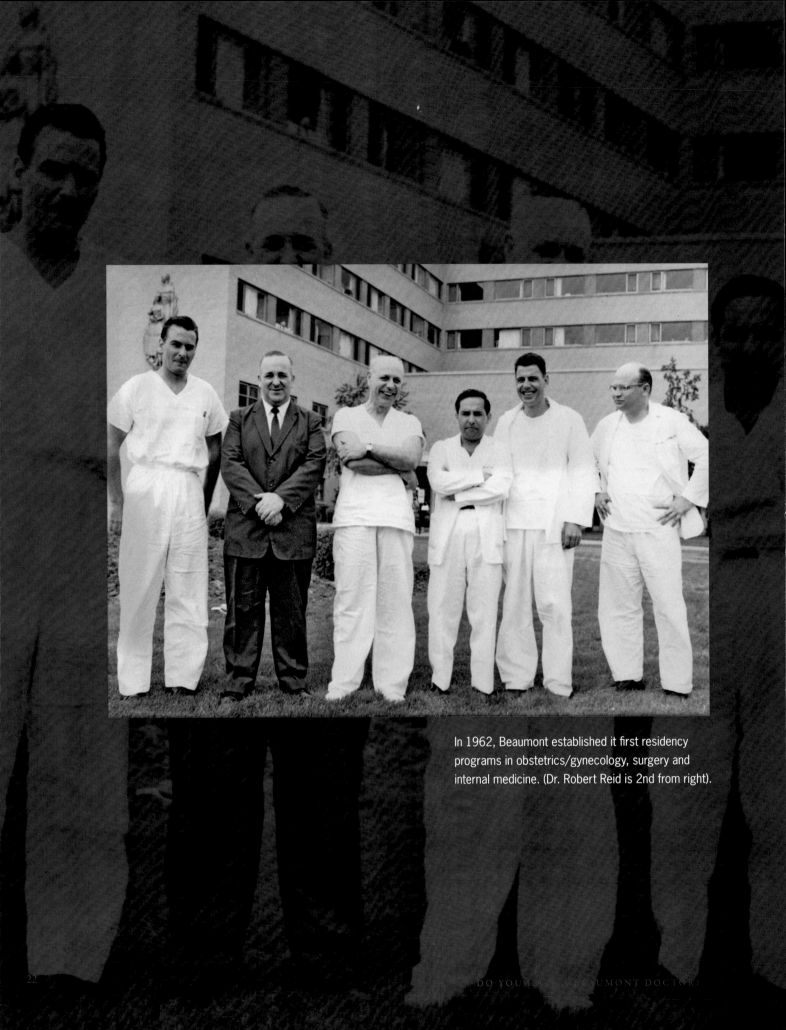

In 1962, Beaumont established it first residency programs in obstetrics/gynecology, surgery and internal medicine. (Dr. Robert Reid is 2nd from right).

"Everyone thought it was crazy to build a hospital way out here."

ROBERT REID, M.D.

Corporate Medical Director, 1997–2003
Beaumont's first intern

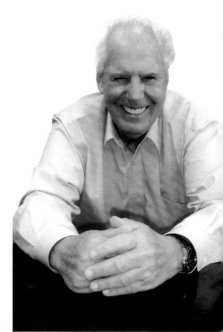

"I was born in the

upper Peninsula of Michigan during the Depression. In the beginning of World War II, my mom and dad moved to Royal Oak because jobs became available at the defense plants, and I grew up in Royal Oak. Most of the tanks that ended up in the war were made here in Michigan.

"I had no intention of going to college. I thought I was supposed to graduate from high school, then go into the military service—at the time they were still drafting—or get a job in a plant. But along came my English teacher, Eva Moore. I wasn't that good in composition or writing, but after class one day she called me to her desk and asked where I was going to college.

"Well, I was taken aback. I told her I was probably going into the Army. She told me, 'No, you're going to college.'

"She made all the arrangements for me to take exams and do the things you have to do to get into the University of Michigan with scholarships. The really sweet part of it for me was that I actually had Eva Moore and her friend Emma Doore as patients. I took care of them both well into their 90's.

"I really didn't know what being a doctor was all about, but I did like science and biology, and I loved medicine. When I came to Beaumont in 1958, I remember there wasn't much structural medical administration or teaching. They were just starting out. A fellow named Jerry Patterson & I graduated from U of M Medical School in 1958. We were the first two Matched interns at Beaumont. Jerry returned to U of M for a residency in dermatology and I remained at Beaumont for a residency in obstetrics and gynecology. The Match program is a national program for rotating internship. Three

months on medicine, three on surgery, three on pediatrics, with a few weeks of obstetrics thrown in. You put your name in the hat for the hospital where you were applying. You had to rank the institutions, and they ranked you. I ranked Beaumont Number One.

"I came to Beaumont expecting to spend one year here, then go back to U of M for my residency in obstetrics and gynecology. Well, fifty years later, I'm still hanging on to this place."

IF WE BUILD IT, THEY WILL COME

"The magnitude of Beaumont comes from its first Board members and physicians. They had a view of this place as becoming more than just a community hospital. My senior partner, Harold Longyear, who was one of the first Chiefs of Staff here, kept talking about 'the campus.' Remember, we were one building with 250 beds. He kept saying, 'the campus this, the campus that.' A lot of us were wondering what the crazy old man was talking about. Campuses were for colleges and universities, right? But he had the vision that this hospital could be more—keeping the priority of taking care of patients while also thinking about teaching, research, and really developing into something massive and encompassing.

STAYING POWER

"When I first came here, Jerry Patterson and I were the only interns who had graduated from American colleges. We were both in the Class of 1958. I stayed at Beaumont for my residency, and Jerry went back to U of M. All our fellow residents who came from Memorial Hospital in Detroit came from Italy, the

Campuses were for colleges and universities, right?
But he had the vision that this hospital could be more.

Philippines, Hungary, Greece—including one who
had just gotten out of Hungary as the Russian tanks
rolled into the town square. These were superb
individuals who were and are still practicing quality
medicine. They spoke with broken English, but when
I got to know them, I knew I had great teams around
me, great specialists who could help me if I got into
trouble. You can have the fanciest place in the world,
but if the people are incompetent or nasty, it's no fun
working there.

"Look at the longevity of the employees—
physicians, secretaries, nurses who have been in
this hospital for great lengths of time. I still see
people who've been here since I was in the residency
program. Longevity is a trademark of Beaumont,
and you don't get that unless you treat people well
and they treat you well. Most of the people are here
because they enjoy working at Beaumont and take
pride in working here, as I did as a physician. This is
one reason Beaumont has been voted as a 'Best Place
to Work in Health Care.'

"My forte was people. I love people. You can imagine,
after delivering women's kids, then delivering the
kids of the kids I'd delivered, then delivering the
grandchildren that over this time I formed very close
relationships with my patients. When you take care
of the patients, the kids, and the grandkids, it's very
enjoyable and more than just a job."

"If you're here long enough, you do just about
every job there is to do in the place. Back in the early
'80's, the Medical Director came up to me and said,
'I've got a little job I need you to do for me.'

"I said, 'Sure, whatever you want.'

"Then my daughter called me; she was a nurse on
the pediatric oncology floor here. She had called to
congratulate me.

"'What for?' I asked.

"'You're the new Associate Medical Director in
charge of Pediatrics!'"

YOU'RE "IT"

"I was an elected member-at-large, a Vice-Chief,
an Associate Medical Director, then I became the
Medical Director, then the Corporate Medical
Director, and nobody ever asked me whether I
wanted these jobs. They just said, 'Congratulations—
you're the next *whatever*.' At each of these changes
in position, I didn't do the usual things I would
normally do, like weighing the pros and cons. If it
was something they thought I could do well and they
wanted me to do it, I would be happy to do the job.
But that goes for almost anything they might ask
me to do. We have an organization that knows its
people.

"This is an unusual place. It's almost impossible
to walk down a corridor without somebody
recognizing you. Of course, my picture is up in the
delivery room, so it's hard to escape that! This is a fun
place to work."

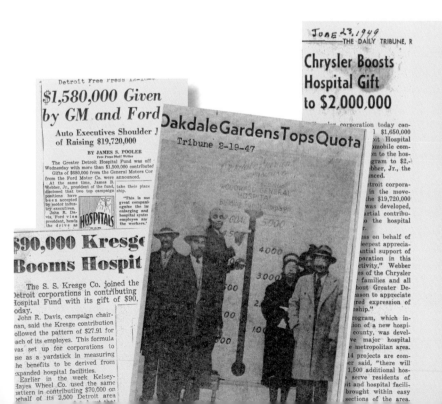

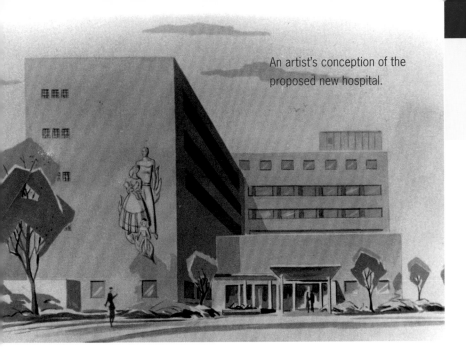

An artist's conception of the proposed new hospital.

THOMAS THOMPSON

Vice-President and Director, Beaumont Professional Services, 1966–2009

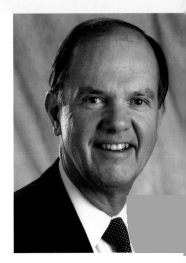

"A hundred and ten acres.

The founders of Beaumont had a vision back then that this would be more than just a community hospital. Their vision was the driving force. One of the earliest distinctions between a community hospital and Beaumont was the development of teaching programs and part-time salaried chiefs in all those departments—not just volunteers or elected members, but people whose jobs it was to develop the particular department. Fifty-some years ago, that was unique for a community hospital, and therefore it set Beaumont apart.

"As time went by, the departments got larger or more departments were added, more chiefs came on staff, and their stature in the medical community also rose. Beaumont established a full-time medical leadership, which distinguished it from other hospitals. Many hospitals have elected chiefs or elected department heads. From the very beginning, Beaumont didn't. They were all appointed by the Board, and the Board was careful in picking the right people."

"I just retired in April of 2009. I was the Vice President for Beaumont Professional Services, which is all the salaried physicians. We have roughly 550 of them.

"I've been at Beaumont for 42 years. I started in personnel and worked my way up through hospital administration, to medical administration. At that time, we were beginning to add more salaried physicians. We have a number of hospital-based departments that are staffed by salaried physicians, which is why we have such a large number.

"A private physician has his or her own practice, his own employees, he pays all his expenses—rent, employees, benefits, malpractice insurance, and anything leftover is his. The salaried physician has all those expenses covered by the employer, who pays the physician a salary and many times a bonus, and the employing organization keeps whatever is left.

Loretta Sharp tends to ducks on the family farm on the land that became the site of William Beaumont Hospital.

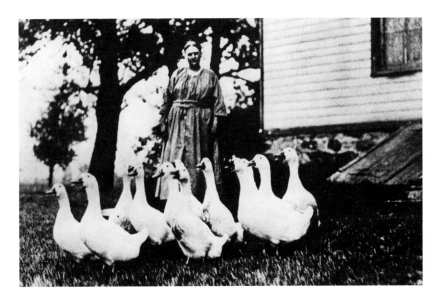

2 MAKING A HOSPITAL FROM SCRATCH

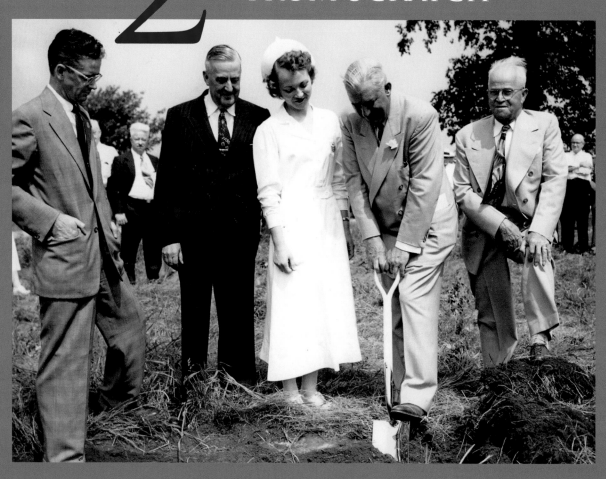

"The beauty of Beaumont is that it began without red tape and is unencumbered by tradition like many of the old-school places are. Beaumont can expand, and when they do, they do it in a state-of-the-art manner."

Harry Lichtwardt, M.D.
First Chair of Urology, Beaumont, Royal Oak,
Former Historian for the American Urological Association

Joining in the groundbreaking ceremony for the new William Beaumont Hospital on June 19, 1953 was (left to right) Mark Beach, executive director of the Greater Detroit Hospital Fund; Irving Babcock, board member; Colleen Cole, a student nurse; E.A. Tomlinson, board president; and H. Lloyd Clawson, board member.

Why Do Doctors Want to Practice at Beaumont?

by Ananias C. Diokno, M.D.

All doctors want to practice in safe environments, with high-quality support teams to ensure successful outcomes for their patients. In short, they want to know that the teams taking care of their patients, the environment and resources are top-notch.

Health care is a team sport. There is interdependence between doctors, doctors and nurses, nurses and nurses, doctors and hospital staff, including housekeepers, X-ray techs, and emergency room staffs.

Beaumont is the first hospital in Michigan to be designated as a Magnet hospital. Magnet status is awarded by the American Nurses' Credentialing Center, reflecting a hospital's nursing involvement, job satisfaction, communication with doctors and other health care professionals, a low turnover rate, involvement in teaching and research, and excellent patient outcomes.

Beaumont's mortality rate, adjusted for severity, is the lowest. Beaumont has the only Flash CT in Michigan, a machine that markedly reduces X-ray exposure to patients.

For 2009, all three Beaumont Hospitals ranked on the U.S. News and World Report "America's Best Hospitals" list. With eight departments ranked, Beaumont was one of only 33 hospitals out of a universe of over 4000 hospitals included in the USNWR ranking. Beaumont is a participant in over 800 clinical trials, allowing our patients the opportunity to participate in these unique and cutting-edge treatments. We hold special accreditation for our centers of excellence; an example is our breast cancer program and breast

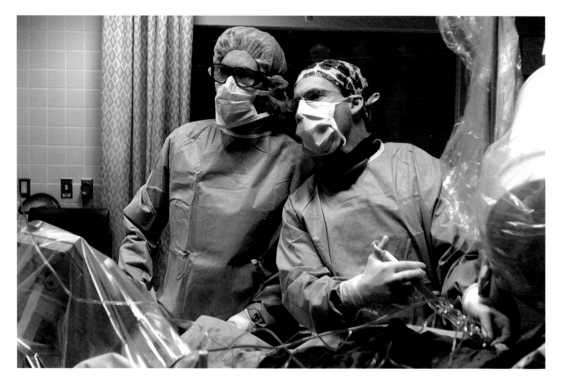

Cindy Grines, M.D., Program Director, Interventional Cardiology and Andrew J. West, M.D. former fellow, now practicing in San Antonio, Texas, performing an interventional cardiology procedure.

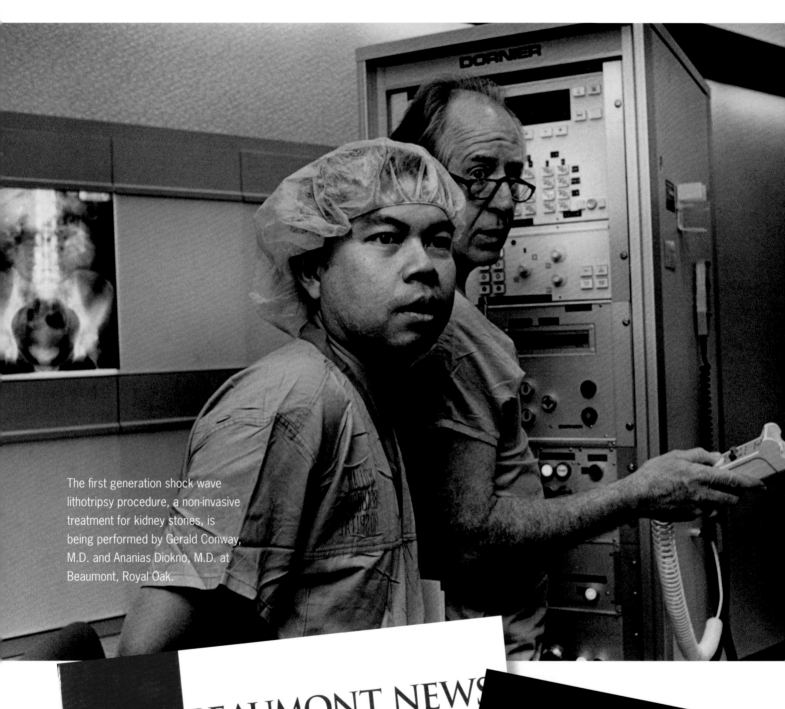

The first generation shock wave lithotripsy procedure, a non-invasive treatment for kidney stones, is being performed by Gerald Conway, M.D. and Ananias Diokno, M.D. at Beaumont, Royal Oak.

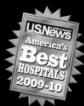

mammography program. Such a program must pass a very rigid inspection and review by national accrediting bodies before a seal of accreditation is granted. Another example is our bariatric program that is recognized by our insurance payors as a center of excellence.

Doctors are scientists, and scientists want to engage in discovery. According to many of our physicians, a recurring theme in their wanting to work at Beaumont is the support given to them by our administration and Board of Directors, to develop their own research, grow their departments, try new things, gain further education, and to do speaking engagements all over the world, so Beaumont's reputation is up-to-date and complete.

Another wonderful attribute of Beaumont is the culture of safety. All sentinel events, unexpected negative events or outcomes are reported to the Quality and Safety Director and ultimately to the Board of Directors, where it is presented and discussed in detail. Each event is reviewed thoroughly to discover why it happened and prevent its occurrence in the future. We do not stop at that, but rather develop the process of improvement based on our findings, and implement it throughout our health care system. By emphasizing the goal of learning from our errors and improving the system rather than emphasizing the "who-dun-it" and "gotcha" attitude, we have encouraged our health care providers to have the freedom to report sentinel events freely, without any fear of reprisal. The entire culture of Quality and Safety was championed to the highest level by none other than our Chairman of the Board, Thomas Denomme, who was given the 2010 Michigan Hospital Association Keystone Center for Patient Safety & Quality Leadership Award.

These accomplishments are not accidental. Our doctors, for the most part, are down-to-earth and willing to learn. The Beaumont culture has an embedded, unresting drive to improve and expand, all surrounding the goal of patient treatment on the highest levels of human accomplishment. It starts with people who want to work here not only because they want to practice in the medical field, but also because Beaumont wants them and makes the environment conducive to their work.

MARK KOLINS, M.D. ON BEAUMONT'S ATTRACTION FOR PATHOLOGISTS

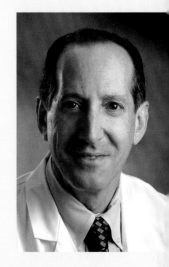

"William Beaumont Hospital has its roots as a community-based facility and remains a major resource for the community. Beaumont's role has evolved into a major national academic health center, spreading its roots to support even distant communities. Beaumont is a face of the community working, of caring and helping our neighbors. This integration of a community hospital and an academic medical center has attracted pathologists to Beaumont for many years. The high volume practice and experience has permitted our pathologists to serve as leaders regionally, nationally and internationally. People throughout the region benefit from the Beaumont academic physician leaders.

"The transition from a service hospital to an academic in-service institution is strongly present in pathology. Academic pathologists with national and international reputations in renal pathology, hematopathology, transfusion medicine, immunology, cytopathology, and microbiology have been recruited or they develop their reputations while at Beaumont. In the pathology world, this has put Beaumont on the map. For decades, every pathologist at Beaumont has been able to say where he or she practiced with instant recognition from colleagues from around the country. Many books and book chapters have been written by Beaumont pathologists, in addition to countless research projects. Dr. Jay Bernstein was internationally known in renal pathology well past his official retirement, and to this day Beaumont's excellence in renal pathology is sought through consultation. Pathologists have also been leaders within specialty organizations with presidencies of the American Society of Clinical Pathologists by Thomas Dutcher, M.D., and the American Association of Blood Banks by Richard Walker, M.D."

MARK KOLINS, M.D. is Professor and Chair of Pathology, Oakland University William Beaumont School of Medicine and Beaumont Hospitals

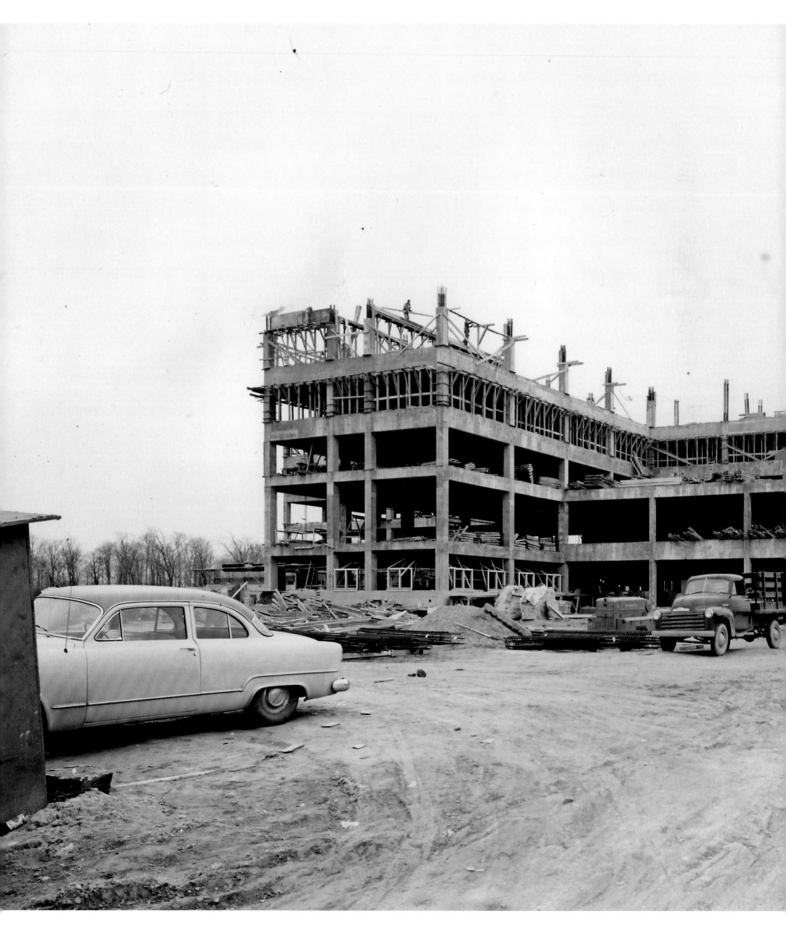

1953

The hospital construction project began on June 19, 1953, and the hospital opened on January 24, 1955.

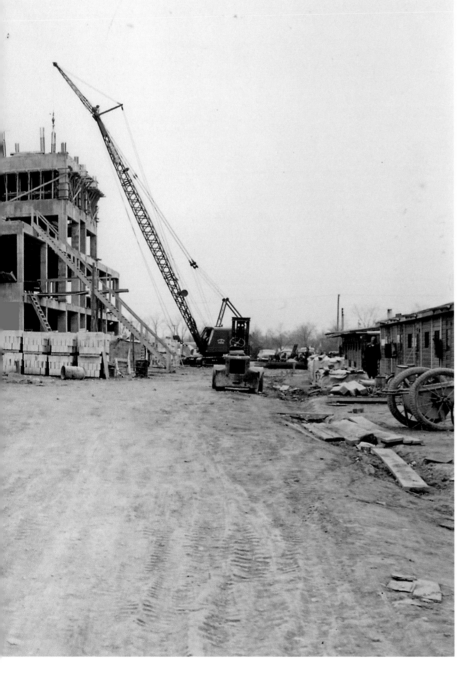

3 "BANG!"

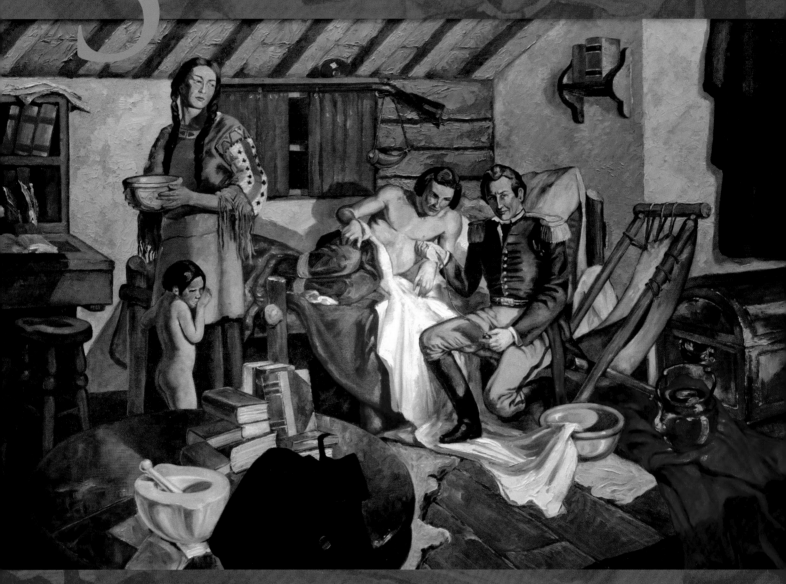

Dr. William Beaumont tending to the wound of Alexis St. Martin. This picture was donated to Beaumont by the well-respected medical illustrator, painter William Loechel of Troy, Michigan.

MACKINAC ISLAND, MICHIGAN. JUNE 1822

"I heard that shot. The loud, smoky bang

was unmistakably a gun discharge."

"Doctor! Doctor Beaumont!"

"My body tensed. Disaster, I thought. Someone's been shot. I must record this date in my journal. June 1822."

"Hastened to the scene, I was appalled to see a young fellow who should have been dead. Musket smoke shrouded the lad's collapsed body, his tattered linen shirt was blackened, and his eyes rolled in his head, as he clawed at the dirt floor, consumed by pain".

"I knelt beside my patient. 'How was he still alive?' The wound in his left abdomen was as large as the palm of my hand, with the skin blown wide open and showing its edges, deeper within showing the edges of the torn-open stomach. Smelling of duck shot and scorched clothing fragments, muscle tissue around the wound curled and cooked."

"I had seen ugly wounds like this, but only on the bodies of corpses. This was not a wound that could be survived."

"But the man was not yet dead, and I was an Army surgeon. Certain moral obligations bonded him to me. I explored the wound with my forefinger, which was able to fit into the hole in the stomach. I pressed the protruding lobe of lung. With my penknife I was able to clip off the ragged rib end, and pushed the lung back inside."

"'Put him on a cot. Take him to the Fort Hospital,' I said quietly. 'He will not see the sun rise.'"

"The victim was a French-Canadian voyageur in his twenties. His name was St. Martin. Now he was my patient."

"An hour after the accident, I attempted again to treat the appalling wound by clearing out fabric fragments, wadding, shot, and shards of rib, repositioning the lung and stomach as well as possible. I washed the area in muriate of ammonia, spirits and vinegar, then applied a poultice of flour, charcoal, yeast and hot water."

"The next morning, I found to my significant surprise that St. Martin was still breathing. His wound was a horror. The shot had struck a glancing blow from the oblique side, carrying away the skin and musculature, parts of the fifth and sixth ribs, damaging the lower part of the left lung, and causing perforations in the stomach and diaphragm."

"Twenty-four hours later, St. Martin developed pneumonia, fever, and a violent cough. I administered a cathartic, but anything he swallowed simply escaped through the hole. The fever continued ten days, long enough for St. Martin to become the talk of Mackinac Island, Mackinac City, and Fort Michilimackinac."

"St. Martin's stomach had not retreated to its normal position, no matter my efforts to push it back in. Instead, the edges of the stomach clung to the edges of the wound in the outer skin, and remarkably, inexplicably, began to heal. Not to close, but to heal—to form scars and to dry out and slough dead tissue. The stubbornly protruding parts of lung and stomach simply dried, flaked off, and left behind a tougher window frame, allowing me to apply a compress and strap that kept St. Martin's food inside his body."

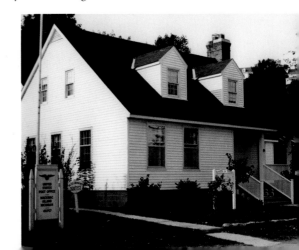

The site of Dr. Beaumont's clinic on Mackinac Island.

"For weeks I tampered with the wound. The brutally injured young man suffered through every trial. I experimented with varied dressings, poultices, lancing, bleeding, even attempts to close the lips of the wound. I created a plug made of lint, which served to keep food from falling out, but the plug also kept the outer wound from closing. St. Martin tumbled in and out of fevers, infections, abscesses and distress. Weeks spooled out and became months."

By September of 1824, St. Martin was in perfect health for a man with a port hole in his stomach. He chopped wood, toted water, and engaged in all manner of manual labor.

"I called myself 'doctor,' and had taken the apprenticeships to make the title legitimate, but never had I set foot in a medical school. There was only one in the United States, at the University of Pennsylvania. There were few hospitals other than military hospitals, and here in this remote settlement there was only myself. I read books on medical subjects, and in 1812 I enlisted as a surgeon's mate with the Sixth Infantry Regiment in Plattsburgh, New York. Every form of frontier illness plagued the soldiers from pneumonia to typhus."

"I worked very hard and took creative risks to make them live. My reputation was enhanced when they survived, even when the survival was as much mystery as medicine. St. Martin's wound developed into an aperture with leathery lips, and never closed. He would not let me close the wound with sutures. Perhaps he was frightened by some primitive belief which he never voiced to me."

"By the spring of 1823, his health had remarkably improved, though food still escaped if the dressings were removed. Unable to work any longer as a voyageur, he was declared a pauper and given some support by the Commissioners of Mackinac County. In April, I employed him as a handyman. This way I was able to continue treating and observing his wound."

"Word came from the Commission that St. Martin should be taken from the pauper role and returned by bateau to Canada. What madness! I protested that St. Martin would weaken, even expire, if he were subjected to such a trial of distance. To keep him near, I brought him into my home as our servant. Some unrevealed spark of curiosity simply would not let him go."

"By September of 1824, St. Martin was in perfect health for a man with a port hole in his stomach. When bound in a compress, he was able to consume and digest food. I could remove the compress and look directly through the gastric fistula into the stomach, and witness food and drink arriving through the esophageal ring. "

"This case afforded a most excellent opportunity of experimenting on the gastric fluids and the process of digestion. The procedure caused St. Martin no pain. I contacted Surgeon General Joseph Lovell, who encouraged physicians to send him notes on interesting cases. He believed that dietary discoveries were significant for the health of the Army, and encouraged me to experiment more systematically."

"I began a more ordered approach to investigation, keeping formal logs and learning from mistakes, suspending one item of food at a time into St. Martin's stomach, and food in varied conditions: raw fresh beef, raw cabbage, corned beef, stale bread,

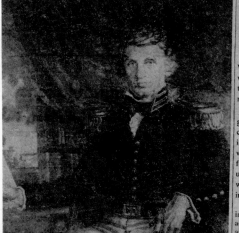

salted lean beef, raw salted fat pork, each in the measurement of an apothecary's ounce. I began at noon, then retrieved the items at one, two, or three o'clock. If I did not retrieve it before three o'clock, St. Martin experienced stomach distress, the stomach fluids became rancid, and I could see white pustules on the inner lining of the stomach. I did not realize until later that this was the physical manifestation of indigestion."

"With a gum-elastic siphon, I drew gastric juices into vials and experimented upon them outside of the human body. By suspending identical bits of meat into the vial and into St. Martin's stomach, I could study and compare in vitro digestion, warmed to 100 degrees in a pan of water, on a bed of sand, with digestion occurring in the human body. In a single day I accomplished more results than similar experiments had gained in four years. In February of 1825, I was unanimously elected an honorary member of the Medical Society of Michigan. I was pleased with myself and took pleasure in seeing my name printed in medical journals."

"I took a leave of sixty days to travel to Plattsburgh with my family, and that is when St. Martin took that chance to slip away. He did not fully comprehend the importance of his condition, the rarity of it, or the opportunity to science which it presented. I would not see him for another four years."

"In 1827, I contacted the American Fur Company in hope of finding St. Martin—and it worked. My interest in research reawakened. If I hoped to enhance my reputation and recognition in the societies of medicine, I would have to regain control."

"Posted in Prairie du Chien, Wisconsin, in December of 1829, I resumed my experiments. St. Martin arrived in a canoe, with a wife and two children. He demanded a contract, payment, medical care and a less tangible compensation, but likely the most important: respect."

"Together we engaged in fifty-six experiments involving digestion in various weather conditions, and after fasts of several hours, with gastric juice mixed with milk, and discovered that digestion could continue in gastric fluid outside the stomach. Two years later, exhausted, St. Martin once again returned to Canada, hoping to regain his living as a voyageur."

"Not until 1832 would I again entice him with money and whiskey to allow a further program of exacting experiments. In 1833, I would publish my treatise on gastric juices and digestion, revealing that gastric juice had the properties of a solvent, classifying which food items were more easily digested than others, the time needed for digestion of various foods, and concluding that gentle physical exercise encouraged digestion. I gained some renown and was able to gain the attention of admirable colleagues, ultimately to be awarded an honorary degree of Doctor of Medicine from the Columbian College in the city of Washington."

"The humble voyageur with an orifice in his stomach had crossed paths with an Army surgeon, and paddled us both into medical history."

By 1950, William Beaumont had become the first United States-born physician to be internationally recognized. He had initiated a new field of study: gastroenterology. Physiologists in Europe and elsewhere built upon his experiments and used his exacting log entries to further discover the mechanizations of the digestive tract. Dr. Beaumont enjoyed a successful career and died in 1853, knowing that his potential had been realized. St. Martin lived to be 80 years old and died in 1880, having fathered seventeen children. He had been born to a frontier life of obscurity and struggle, but that destiny had been tipped off course by an accidental gunshot and a persistent military doctor who had never gone to medical school. Together they initiated a new era in the science and practice of medicine.

Beaumont's notes relating to St. Martin's care.

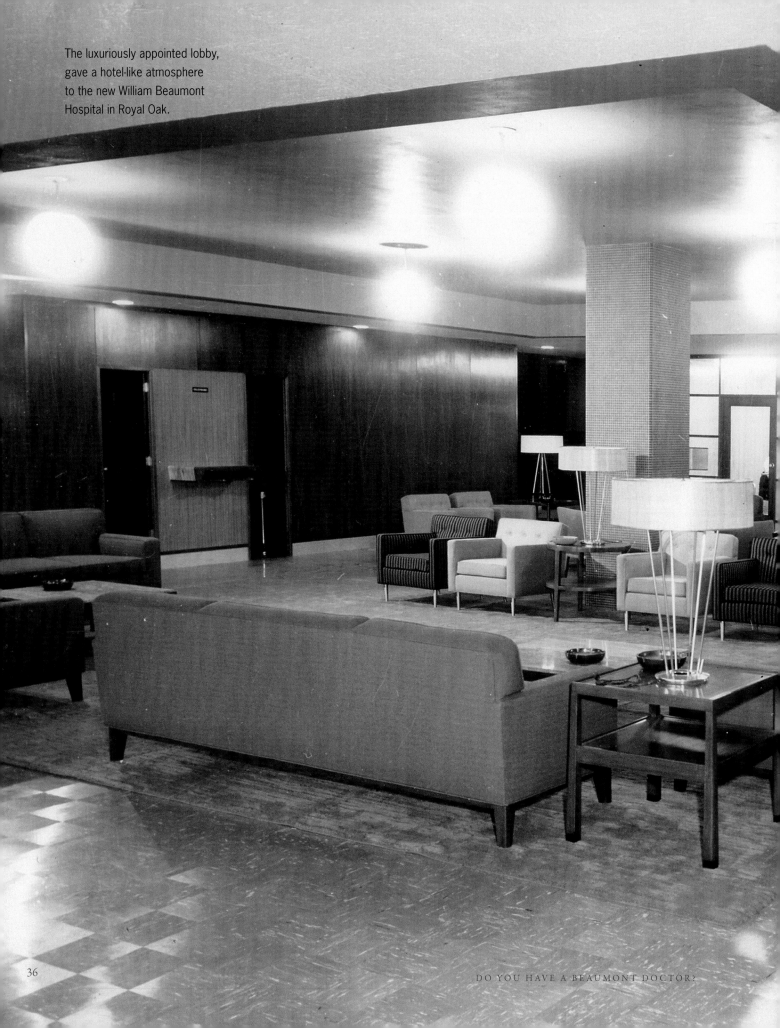

The luxuriously appointed lobby, gave a hotel-like atmosphere to the new William Beaumont Hospital in Royal Oak.

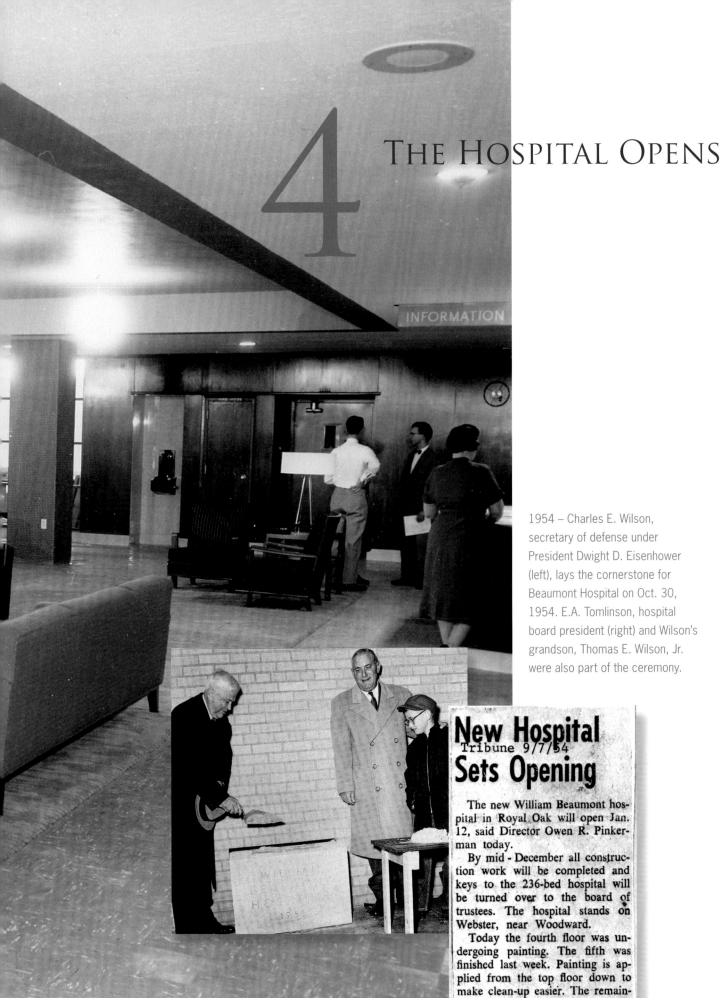

4 THE HOSPITAL OPENS

1954 – Charles E. Wilson, secretary of defense under President Dwight D. Eisenhower (left), lays the cornerstone for Beaumont Hospital on Oct. 30, 1954. E.A. Tomlinson, hospital board president (right) and Wilson's grandson, Thomas E. Wilson, Jr. were also part of the ceremony.

New Hospital Sets Opening

Tribune 9/7/54

The new William Beaumont hospital in Royal Oak will open Jan. 12, said Director Owen R. Pinkerman today.

By mid-December all construction work will be completed and keys to the 236-bed hospital will be turned over to the board of trustees. The hospital stands on Webster, near Woodward.

Today the fourth floor was undergoing painting. The fifth was finished last week. Painting is applied from the top floor down to make clean-up easier. The remaining floors have been plastered.

Open house for the public is

HARRY LICHTWARDT, M.D.

Chair, Department of Urology, 1955–1981
Medical Executive Board Member, Beaumont, Royal Oak,
  1956–1971

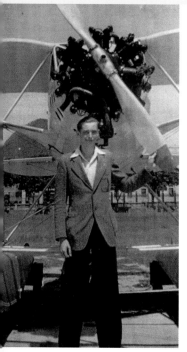

Harry Lichtwardt, M.D. founded the Department of Urology with its first graduate in 1969. Today, the department is ranked in the top 50 by the U.S. News and World Report.

"I have a long history with Beaumont,

starting actually a week before the hospital even opened. I had the privilege of admitting the first patient to Beaumont in 1955 a week before the official opening on January 24. The President of the Beaumont Board of Trustees, E. A. Tomlinson, was a patient of mine and had developed a ureteral calculus. I had planned to admit him to Highland Park General Hospital, but when Beaumont's Hospital Director, Owen Pinkerman, heard about this, he immediately called me and said, 'Beaumont is ready to go.'

"I checked with anesthesia and surgery, and they said they were just sitting around, waiting to get going. So we admitted Mr. Tomlinson that day. He ended up not needing surgery after all, but he was the first patient in the new 238-bed hospital.

"Our particular department was not a department at that time. It was the Division of Urology, and was under the Department of General Surgery. Initially we had just four urologists. In 1965 I felt we were far enough along in our abilities that we should have an accredited residency program to train new urologists. I contacted the Board of Urology. There were only six non-university affiliated urological programs out of 168, and the Board didn't think a non-affiliated program could do it. The program had a tough time, but we graduated our first resident in 1969.

"The Board of Urology had an annual accreditation examination of each of their approved programs. When we started, we were about 35 out of 168. Within ten years, we ranked number three overall.

"The program has grown and grown."

"When Medicare came into being, we had to begin to work the government way. I represented Beaumont on the Board of Directors of the Professional Standards Review Organization for Oakland County, and followed that with two years on the Board of Directors of the Michigan Peer Review Organization.

"Besides an active private practice, I also established a four-member partnership, Lichtwardt Urological Associates, P.C., which now numbers twenty urologists and is called Comprehensive Urology.

"I was the historian for the American Urological Association for ten years and co-author of *The Centennial History of the American Urological Association,* a two-volume book which was delivered to the membership in 2002. The book received an Excellent Award at the Chicago Book Show the year it was published. There's a copy in Beaumont's Medical Library."

"Urologists have all kinds of people, all ages, as patients in our practices. Urologists have to help people be at ease talking about personal things, and tend to be gregarious and like to get around with people. There have been more presidents of the American Medical Association that were urologists than any other specialty."

ALONG CAME THE WAR . . .

"I was born and raised in Rio de Janeiro, because my dad was from Detroit but was head of the YMCAs in Brazil. In Brazil I went to a girls' school for the first five years because it was the only good private school; they accepted boys up to the 8th grade. Then my dad switched me to the German school, and I spent the summer learning German and German script. For three years I did nothing but speak German and write German script.

"Then the Hitler Youth came in. They were very strong in Rio. I was the only 'Americaner' there, so Dad decided I'd better get out of the school. My senior year, I went to the American school that had just been opened the year before, and I graduated with the eight other students in the senior class. I've had quite a varied education, as you can see.

"I had dual citizenship in Brazil and the U.S. I couldn't avoid it. If you're born in Brazil, they consider you Brazilian. Well, everybody in Brazil

In 1988, Dr. Diokno established the Harry E. Lichtwardt Lectureship, which has been delivered by outstanding urologists annually in June during the residency graduation ceremonies at William Beaumont Hospital.

gets conscripted in the Army. Pan-American of Brazil had told me that if I got my flight training, they would take me on as one of their main pilots. I spent a year as a reservist and put in 200 hours flying. Then I came up to college at Oberlin College in Ohio, where my parents met. My mother was the first licensed woman driver in Cleveland. I went to Oberlin strictly to get my college out of the way, because to get into Randolph—Randolph, Texas, the West Point of the air—and Kelly Field, the final training that all of Randolph's people get, I had to have a college degree. By then it was 1938.

"Believe it or not, at that time you were only allowed to fly commercially until the age of 35, so my dad encouraged me to go into medicine.

"In 1939, between my junior and senior years in college, England declared war on Germany right about the time I decided maybe Dad was giving me good advice. My sister was two years ahead of me and had just been appointed the first fashion coordinator for Sears, Roebuck and Company. She was in St. Louis, and told me that if I could get into Washington University in St. Louis, she would put me up for two years' room and board. I graduated in December of 1943 and came back to Detroit for my internship, and the war was going on full-blast. I'd had all that military training in Brazil, and got into the U. S. Army as a medical officer."

"Easter Sunday, April 1st, is when we went into Okinawa. I watched the plane come in from Japan when they surrendered. They flew into Okinawa to make the agreement. When the announcement came out about the end of the war, we had more patients in the hospital than we'd had in months because everybody shot off everything they had, including off-shore. We had shrapnel and gunshot wounds—it was unbelievable.

"I had to get my passport brought up to date, so I went to the Ministry of War, which was where you would do that. They looked at my passport and my record, they said, 'You're a deserter.'

"I asked, 'Why?'"

"They said, 'You haven't reported in for six years.'

"That was the Brazilian Army. They considered me a deserter. So I called my dad, who knew General Davis, who was now the commanding general of American forces in Brazil. Davis sent over a colonel, and the colonel told them I'd been in combat with a nation allied to Brazil, which the U. S. was. The Brazilians decided to give me a promotion. Well, I didn't want a promotion; I wanted a passport immediately, which normally takes two or three weeks. We got one in two days.

"Then I got to meet General Davis. Early one morning he put me on one of his aircraft and flew me back to Florida. So Brazil thinks I'm still down there."

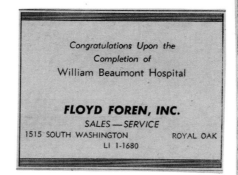
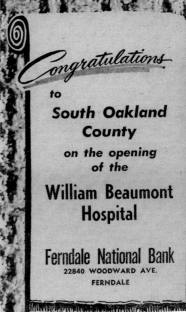

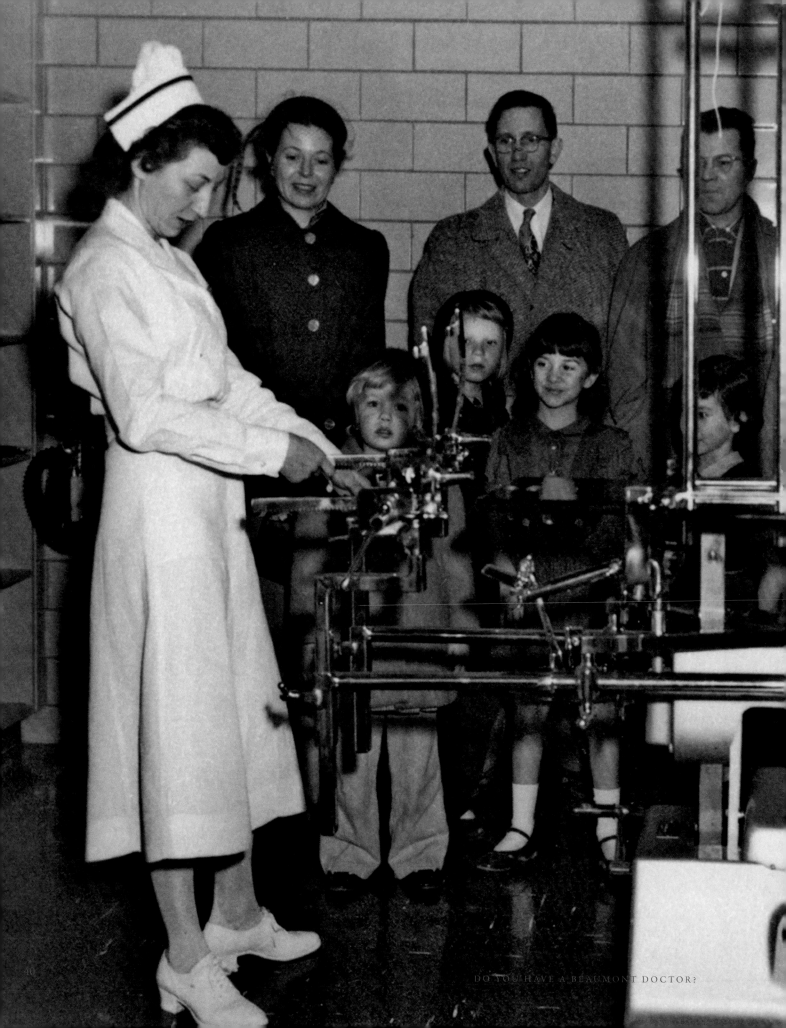

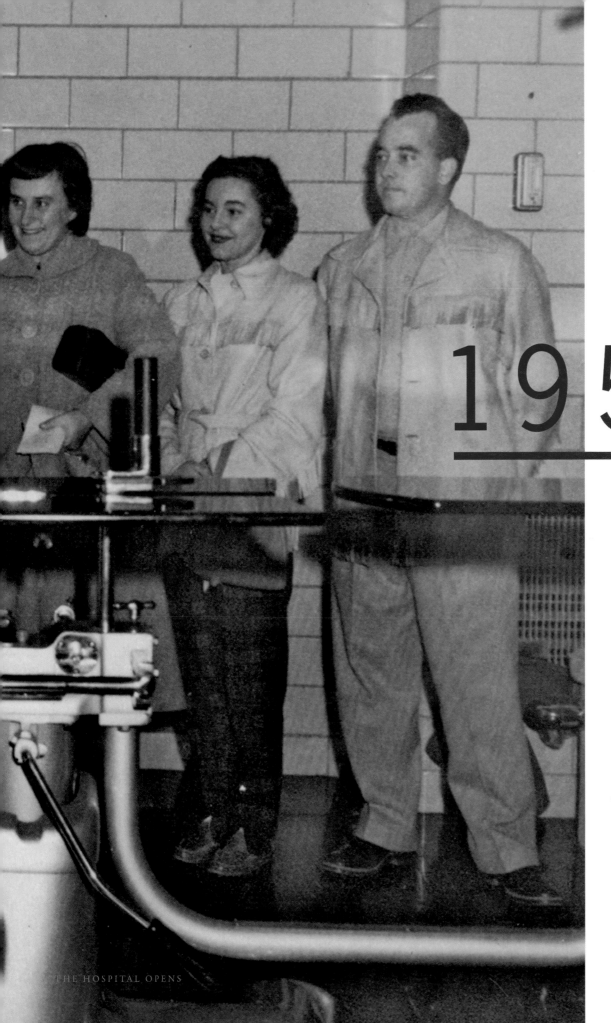

1956

Thousands of people attended the opening of William Beaumont Hospital and toured the new facility, viewing medical instruments which were cutting-edge for their time.

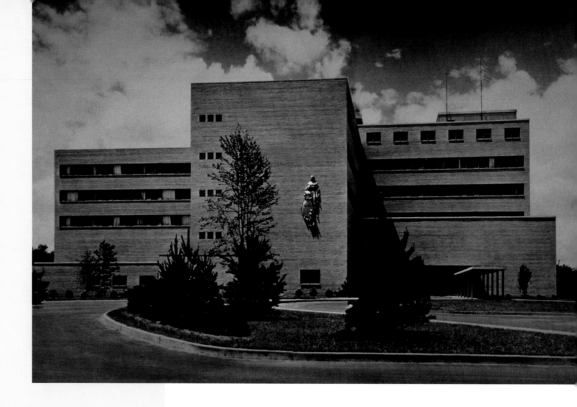

DEMENTIA

Her mind seemed but a hollowed gourd.
No substand there to coin a thought
Nor hold a simple fact---
Derebrum scarred in arid plots
Deprived of sanguine flow.
Her eyes, two puzzled lidded orbs,
Peered blank and imperceptively.
Her hair unkempt in oily strangs,
Half hiding a scaley furrowed brow
And nails too long and missing teeth
Were testament to witless self-neglect.
She views her world of strangers now
As captors in a hostile land,
Yet when I pulled her covers up
And patted twice her cheek,
She grasped and kissed my hand and smiled
Then lapsed into a snoring sleep.

E. J. Mueller, M. D.
1994

---FRIDAY, JANUARY 7, 1955---THE DAILY TRIBUNE, ROYAL OAK, MICH

Hospital That Generosity Built

Beaumont Dedicated Today

New SOC Hospital Opens Doors to Public for 2-Day Inspection

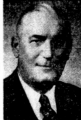

E. A. TOMLINSON

Recruits Wanted: Women Only

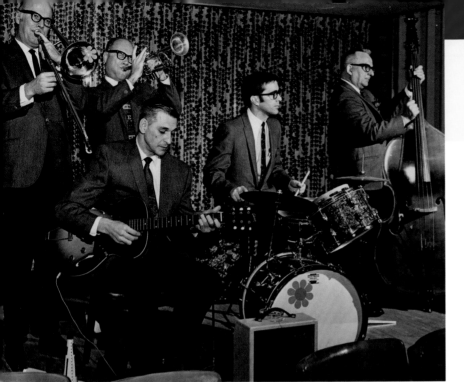

ELMER MUELLER, M.D.

Attending Staff, Department of Medicine
Beaumont, Royal Oak, 1956–2008

"The Heartbeats," originally called "The Lifesavers," a combo of Beaumont staff physicians, played lively tunes during employee and hospital functions. The aggregation consists of Dr. Thomas Grekin, on the vibes; Dr. Frederick Latimer, bass; Dr. Frederick Bryant, trumpet; Dr. Bill Bauer, drums, Dr. Bruce Bauer, saxophone, Dr. Adolph Bruni, guitar; and Dr. Elmer Mueller, accordion

"In 1953, I had completed four years

of residency, two in internal medicine and two in cardiology at Henry Ford Hospital in Detroit. I had a wonderful wife and three young daughters, and promptly accepted a position on the staff of a clinic in Champagne, Illinois, with thirty-two other physicians. I worked hard for two years, saw many patients, accumulated a lot of experience, and had two more daughters. The salary was inadequate, so I had to make a change.

"I was familiar with Michigan, and I like the state. I like the north woods particularly, because I've always been interested in nature and wildlife. I enjoy exploring caves in particular.

"A friend of mine was planning to leave Henry Ford for a new hospital on Thirteen Mile Road, which wasn't even completed yet. He suggested that we share office space. I left my family with my in-laws in Cincinnati, took my internal medicine Board certification in hand, and headed north. I had $1500 in the bank and a five-year-old Chevrolet.

"I felt immediately welcomed at William Beaumont Hospital. There were about 200 beds and a big field out back. We could go up to the fourth floor and look out southward, and literally count dozens of pheasants in the wild field behind the hospital. The location was excellent for future expansion, in the midst of the suburbs of Royal Oak,

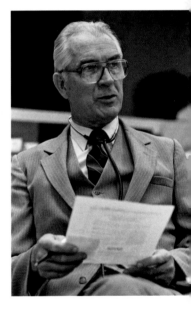

Birmingham and Bloomfield Hills, on a hundred-plus acres of flat, fallow farmland.

"We started to get residents here who were from all over—Japan, China, the Philippines, Germany, Hungary, the Middle East, Argentina, Haiti, Lithuania, Korea, and Yugoslavia. Some of them lived in apartments east of the hospital, where they were allowed to have vegetable gardens. Beaumont was a melting pot even then.

"I had no practice yet, and no office. While I was waiting for an office to open up, I sat in the lobby and read magazines, and every now and then one of the doctors would send me on a house call or refer me to a patient in the ER.

"Eventually I got my office, bought a house in Royal Oak, and retrieved my family. Beaumont's future glittered with promise. The medical administration and the Board of Trustees were always eager to accommodate the doctors' and patients' needs. Most of the young physicians elected to confine their hospital practices to Beaumont. I saw doctors walking down the hall, and maybe one would see a piece of paper on the floor, and he'd stoop and pick it up. They really treated the new hospital as if it were theirs.

"Yesterday I attempted to recall the names of the physician staff in the early days, and came up with

I WAS HERE

I was here.
You have my solemn word that I was here.
I made no waves – I left no mark.
No crypt with name and dates embossed,
Nor marble monument attests to this;
But believe me when I say that I was here.

Right where you stand, in an age that's past stood I.
I knew the name of every tree and shrub.
These stately pines and spruce are dear to me;
I planted them as seedlings – watched them grow;
They assimilate within their wood my dust.
Do you believe me when I say that I was here?

Can you see the birds perched hunchback on the wire?
They're Bluebirds – males have rusty chests,
The progeny of birds I knew and helped
With nesting boxes for them by the score.
In these berried shrubs I planted birds' winter fare.
If birds could talk, they'd tell you I was here.

A decade marks the years since I had left.
I willed my dust be broadcast o'er this land;
Dust dispersed will need no marking stone.
You're looking now upon my monument.
In its contoured green you'll sense my epitaph.
This planted verdure whispers, "He was here."

E. J. Mueller, M.D.
1993

A sampling of original employees form 1955.

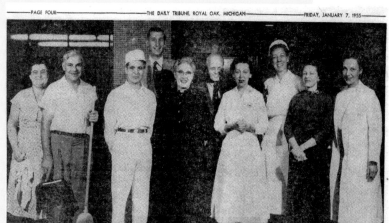

WAITING TO SERVE EACH PATIENT AT THE WILIAM BEAUMONT HOSPITAL are these 10 employes, each representing a different job. All play a part in services to the patient. There are about two employes for each of the hospital's 236 beds. Lined up in the lobby, above, are (left to right): Marie Adams, laundry; Albert James,

46 names without consulting a reference. When I attempted to recall the names in college or medical school, I came up with about 10. This attests to the close relationship of the early Beaumont staff and the impression they made on me."

CURB-STONE CONSULTATIONS

"We had what we called 'curb-stone consultations.' You'd be walking along and see a cardiologist and say, 'I saw this patient this morning and the EKG showed . . . so what do you think?' They were happy to give up the information. I remember a cardiologist, Dr. Renato Ramos, and I did these curb-stone consultations with him, and I'd give him a quarter.

"When we were young doctors, a group of us formed a band called 'The Heartbeats.' I played the accordion. One of the doctors passed away not too long ago—Dr. Arcari. At his funeral mass, a granddaughter played a solo on the tuba. It was beautiful—something by Puccini."

THE EARLY EMERGENCY ROOM

"In the early days of the hospital, the emergency room had only five or six small rooms and one large one. It was staffed by physicians who had left private practice. Specialized emergency physicians were non-existent in those days.

"There was an addition called 1-West, where we could admit patients if there weren't private or semi-private beds available in the hospital. There were two glassed-in wards, one for women, one for men, and a nurses' station.

"We had no cardiac care unit, no intensive care unit, no monitoring devices, nor any CPR team. There was no way to send an alarm if anything happened. If a patient needed to be monitored, we tried to get him into the alcove near the nurses' station, so the nurses could just look.

"I had a patient about 38 years old, whose name was Rita. She had five children. Her last child had just been born, and while she was pregnant she got rheumatic fever and developed heart trouble. She had a valve operation while she was pregnant, then delivered after that, but developed abnormal heart rhythm called 'atrial fibrillation.' It can be associated with clots forming in the heart and as a consequence strokes, or clots in other organs. The drug we used to correct that was called quinidine, and we gave this every two hours, then monitored her heart rate between doses, at five doses a day.

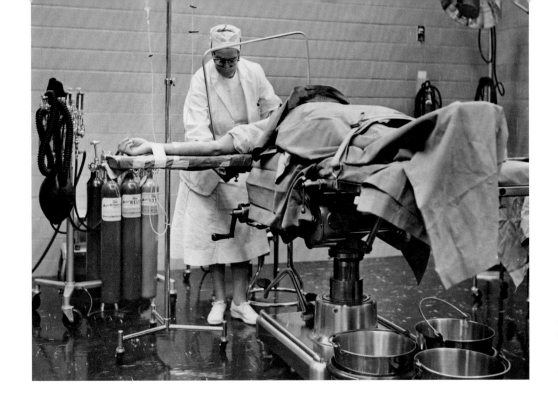

An operating room setup with the nurse anesthetist busy preparing the patient for anesthesia.

"Well, Rita didn't want to be on 1-West. She wanted a semi-private room, but I wanted her to be watched. The best I could do was put her in the glassed-in women's ward down in the ER. She wanted to be assured that the minute she converted to a regular rhythm, she would be discharged. Well, she got rid of her atrial fibrillation, but she still had ventricular premature beats, so I wouldn't let her go home. I kept saying, 'You have to stay at least another day.'

"One night around ten o'clock, another patient of mine was brought into the ER with a heart attack. I'd seen Rita twice that day, checking on her, but now I was in 1-West to see if we had a bed in the alcove for this coronary patient. When I arrived, some woman was knocking on the glass from inside the ward. I ignored her because we used to get a lot of people on drugs, kind of erratic, but she persisted. I finally went in there, to find that this woman was trying to alert me. Rita was in cardiac arrest.

"The beds were on wheels and they were high. I'm six-foot-five and still had difficulty giving Rita cardiac compressions. She was about 150 pounds and I had to lift her and get her down on the floor. I gave her CPR and I asked the lady who had alerted me to go for help, call Rita's husband and the priest over at Lady Queen of Martyrs.

"Well, I was pumping on Rita's chest, five minutes, seven minutes, ten ... with no response—when, after what seemed like an eternity, all of a sudden she woke up and said, 'What are you doing here?'

"If she'd been moved upstairs as she wanted, she would have died. It was good that I kept her in the ER against her wishes because of those premature beats—and just luck that I happened to be there at ten o'clock at night, and happened to pay attention to the woman knocking on the glass. Isn't that incredible?

"For about three months after this incident, I'd get a call once in a while at ten o'clock at night. I'd answer the phone, and Rita would just say, 'I just want to thank you.' And she'd hang up."

GRATIFYING YEARS

"I spent a total of 53 years on the staff of Beaumont. I retired a year and a half ago; my daughter, Kathleen Norton, M.D. eventually assumed my patients, and she now has three associates, Bradley Sabin, M.D., Jeffrey Klein, M.D., and Russell Hug, M.D.

"I marvel at the expansion of that brand new small hospital where I became a staff member 55 years ago. Even more remarkable is the increase in size, diversity, talent and quality of its staff, and of Beaumont's superb national reputation."

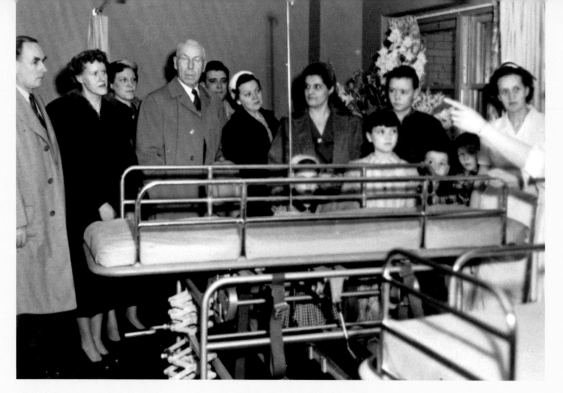

The open house festivities for the much-anticipated William Beaumont Hospital were successful beyond anyone's wildest dreams. An estimated 15,000 to 20,000 people flocked to the new hospital over the two-day event on January 8 and 9, 1955. Here, a group of local residents tours one of the ultra modern recovery rooms.

GROWING PAINS

When William Beaumont Hospital opened its doors, nearly 20,000 people toured the new medical facility in Southern Oakland County. The community had raised funds since 1943, seen the project through to completion, and on January 24, 1955, Dr. Harry Lichtwardt admitted the hospital's first patient—the President of the Board of Trustees, Edward A. Tomlinson. Dr. Lichtwardt almost admitted Mr. Tomlinson to another hospital, but Beaumont's Director, Owen Pinkerman, said the new hospital was ready to go with first-rate medical treatment.

Two days later, another milestone was passed when Beaumont's first baby was born. Little Michael Welsh, the son of Mr. and Mrs. Maurie Welsh of Birmingham, came into the world weighing 6 pounds, 7 ounces. Michael was a bit premature and was placed in an incubator, while gifts poured in from 15 South Oakland County merchants.

The hospital's expansion plan began within two years of the opening, because of demand and length of stay. Among the expanded areas were radiation, imaging, patient care floors, a Department of Pediatrics, and a Department of Physical Medicine and Rehabilitation.

E. A. Tomlinson died on May 27, 1958, from a sudden circulatory ailment.

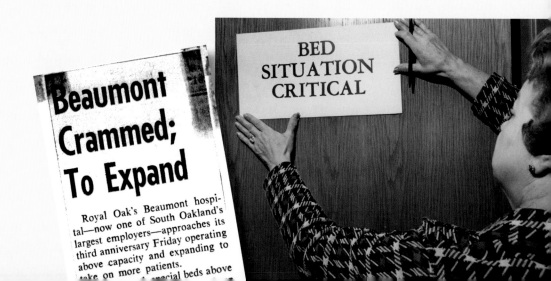

Beaumont Crammed; To Expand

Royal Oak's Beaumont hospital—now one of South Oakland's largest employers—approaches its third anniversary Friday operating above capacity and expanding to take on more patients.

BED SITUATION CRITICAL

RUBEN KURNETZ, M.D.

Director of Education
Chair, Department of Pediatrics,
Beaumont, Royal Oak, 1966–1986

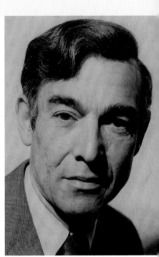

"I came to Beaumont in 1966.

I had been an instructor of pediatrics at Wayne State College of Medicine after completing my residency at Children's Hospital of Michigan. I was referred by Dr. Paul Wooley, Professor of Pediatrics, that someone was needed to develop a pediatric residency training program at William Beaumont Hospital, which was in its developmental period.

"I didn't want to go 'way out there,' but eventually Beaumont won me over. A year and a half later, I was asked to be the Chairman of the Department of Pediatrics and Director of the Residency Program. I remained in those positions for 20 years, until 1986.

"In 1979 I took a year's sabbatical and traveled to several medical centers to work and learn about how they practiced and taught pediatrics. I spent six months at Stanford, three months in Israel at three hospitals, one month at the Great Ormond Street Hospital in London, a month at the Karolinska Institute in Stockholm, Sweden—a magnificent place—and a month at Massachusetts General in Boston. The entire experience was one of the highlights of this old man's career and life.

"I brought back many of their approaches to teaching, patient support care, and physicians' concerns. The Great Ormond Street Hospital was a very old but stately building, and the level of care was magnificent. The pediatric ward was run by a nurse, not a physician. The nurse was in charge and informed the doctors when we were going to make our rounds, which patients we would see and which we wouldn't. It was all done with excellent patient care and outcomes.

"Israel was a different experience. I was used to the way things were done at Children's and in the program at Beaumont. The residents at Beaumont and CHM would remain with me until we completed patient rounds, but in Israel, if a parent wanted to ask some questions about his or her child, the resident would leave. By the time I finished rounds, very few were in attendance.

"There was no one running a pediatric service at Beaumont until I came. All the pedatricians were in private practice. I was the first physician hired by the hospital in pediatrics. I worked to improve pediatric care and attempted to expand the staff by asking the first pediatric surgeon to join, which caused great anguish for the surgery department, mostly for financial reasons.

"In the early years at Beaumont the pediatricians were all generalists. There were no sub-specialists and no intensive care unit. I didn't get an intensivist until the mid-1970's. I remember buying the first positive-pressure respirator for the nursery. It was a used model which we bought from the University of Michigan Department of Pediatrics, where the chairman was a former classmate of mine.

"I attempted to expand the subspecialist staff, but I couldn't find a neonatologist. I decided to go to New York to see my daughter, Lizzie, a publisher at Random House, and to visit Albert Einstein College of Medicine, where I had many friends, and Sinai Hospital in Manhattan. I wanted to find a neo-natologist whom I could hire. At Sinai, they thought I was from the sticks in Michigan—a hick. I spent the day participating on pediatric rounds, and they showed me a patient and said, 'You've never seen a patient like this.'

"It was a Jewish child with Gaucher's disease. I'd seen three patients like this. They were surprised that

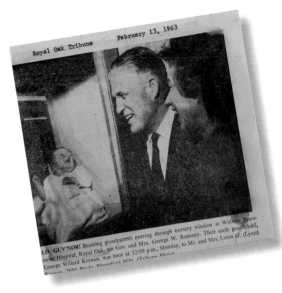

Governor and Mrs. George W. Romney enjoying their 6th grandchild, born at William Beaumont Hospital in February 1963.

Herman D. Scarney, M.D., Chief of Staff, 1959–1964. A well-known ophthalmologist who served in the U.S. Navy for 30 years and retired as rear admiral. His daughter, Shelley Ann Scarney, was Richard Nixon's secretary, married Patrick Buchanan, a former Presidential candidate.

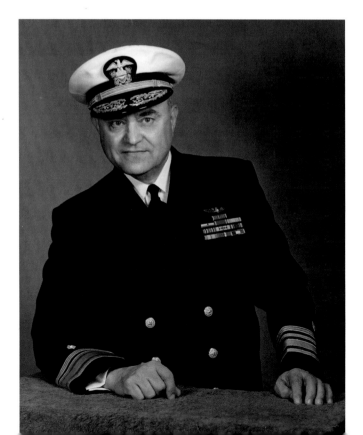

I wasn't such a backwoods hick after all. Since I had no success, I finally sent one of my residents away to be trained as a neonatologist."

UNFORGETABLE CASES

"There was one wonderful little girl whose folks owned a T-shirt company called 'Bull-Shirt.' She had a white cell abnormality and couldn't fight infections. She got recurrent infections and abscesses. When we finally sorted out the problem, we referred her to the University of Michigan, where work was being done on this specific problem and the end results were gratifying. Having contacts at other hospitals certainly paid off.

"Another patient was a little girl with osteomyelitis of the spine, caused by staphylococcus organism which was resistant to our available antibiotics. A friend of mine, Gunnar Sticklar, was working with anti-staphylococcus penicillin at the Mayo Clinic. I called and asked him to send me an adequate supply to treat this child. The results were excellent, and the little girl is now a practicing physician in Chicago.

"As I think back over the years, there were many challenging cases. I had a wonderful professional career, a good life, and raised three children, who are all gainfully employed."

NOT JUST LITTLE ADULTS

"The third day after I arrived at Beaumont, I caused great confusion when a child was admitted who had aspirated a peanut. This is not an uncommon occurrence. The child was breathing with only one lung. The in-house thoracic surgeon bronchoscoped the child, but had difficulty and couldn't get the peanut out. I got a little annoyed and asked to stop everything, which caused a flare of anger. I called Dr. Lyle Wagner, an ear, nose and throat doctor at Children's Hospital. I arranged for temporary surgical privileges, and he came from a formal affair, still wearing his tuxedo. In about three minutes, he removed the peanut. I was very satisfied, of course, and so were the parents. It took medicine a long time to figure out that children are not just small adults."

"Finally, leaving a pediatric as well as a med-peds residency program and the nucleus of a sub-specialty staff, I stepped down as chair of the department in 1986."

MYRON LABAN, M.D.

Professor of Physical Medicine and Rehabilitation, Oakland University
William Beaumont School of Medicine

Chair, Department of Physical Medicine and Rehabilitation, Beaumont,
Royal Oak, 1984–2000

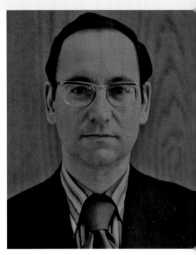

Dr. Laban in 1973.

"I'm a physiatrist. I'm a generalist

in my field. While more people are specializing, I do everything in my field.

"I joined the staff of Beaumont in 1967, after graduating from the University of Michigan in 1957 and medical school in 1961, and training at Ohio State University. OSU has, for the last 35 years, been the best residency program in Physical Medicine and Rehabilitation (PM&R) in the U.S. As a senior medical student at the U of M, I was awarded an international research prize, the Bernard Baruch Award. This honor fostered an appetite within me for research which has continued throughout my professional career.

"In 1967, my father suggested I visit William Beaumont Hospital, as well as the several academic programs that were recruiting me at the time. I wanted to remain in private practice and build a PM&R department at the same time, without being hired full-time by a hospital. I arrived at Beamont without an apointment, and met with Mr. Owen Pinkerman, the senior administrator at the time, who ran both the medical and administrative sides of the hospital with an iron fist. He told me he didn't want a Department of Physical Medicine and Rehabilitation. At the time, the Rehab Department had only two physical therapists and one aide, no occupational therapist, no speech pathologists, and no social workers. I told him that in order to have a first-class hospital, he would need a quality Department of Physical Medicine and Rehabilitation, and then I left with no intention of returning.

"I returned to San Franscisco to consider several offers from the University of California-Berkeley,

a neurosurgical group in Northern California, and jobs at the University of Minnesota, Ohio State University, and the Mayo Clinic. I planned on continuing my academic activity, but didn't want to do it full-time. Then I received a surprise phone call from Dr. Ivan Mader, the Chief of Medicine at Beaumont. He invited me to join his staff, even though I never had a formal interview. Because the physical therapists resisted having a physiatrist in charge of the PM&R department, I couldn't carry my specialty designation in PM&R. Instead, I was asked to join as a general medical specialist. I agreed."

"From the first day at Beaumont, I was as busy as I could be. By the end of my first year, I was medically responsible for the department, without compensation. I believed that, as the only physiatrist on the staff, it was my responsibility, and the administration eventually decided that PM&R could be an area of growth like radiology or cardiology, based on the increasing numbers of patients. With time, we grew from three physical therapists to a staff of 550, representing all the treatment specialties in rehabilitation. At last count we had 150 physical therapists, 52 occupational therapists, and the largest speech therapy department in the universe, employing the services of over 50 speech pathologists and other professionals, including rehabilitation nurses and social workers. We also developed a busy prosthetic and orthotic clinic, which is currently supervised by Dr. Martin Tamler. Beaumont is the only private hospital in the country that sponsors a residency training program in Physical Medicine and Rehabilitation. We currently have 16 residents. The current chair of the Department is Ron Taylor, M.D.

"We are one of the very few residency training programs that have two residents who have finished first among 700 or 800 physicians taking the yearly national Board exams. No other residency has had more than two number ones."

VESPER'S CURSE

"I'm proud of the research I've done over the years. For instance, we described a syndrome which I call 'Vesper's Curse.' It's an association between spinal stenosis, a narrowing of the spinal canal through which the spinal cord and spinal nerves pass, and the concurrent presence of cadiopulmonary disease. These patients are awakened at night with low back pain. I described the mechanism by which this occurs, and called it 'Vesper's Curse.' As a clinical syndrome, It is now commonly recognized nationally.

A LANDMARK CASE

Back in 1967, I was asked to see a young athlete whom the orthopaedic surgeon thought had a pinched nerve in his lower back which was not improving with physical therapy. One of our diagnostic tests is electromyography, which detects abnormal electrical potentials in muscle both at rest and with voluntary activity. Electrodiagnosis tells us whether there is nerve or muscle damage, where it is, and how severe it is. In this young man's case, we found an unusual pattern of electrical activity in which the nerves to the back muscles demonstrated severe damage. The adjacent leg was electrically normal and the neurological exam was also normal. Most often, nerve damage in the spine, as recognized by electromyography, is also present in the adjacent extremity. In this patient, that wasn't the case.

We are one of the very few residency training programs that have two residents who have finished first among 700 or 800 physicians taking the yearly national Board exams. No other residency has had more than two #1's.

"I had previously recognized this abnormal electrodiagnostic pattern in other patients with histories of cancer, or who were later found to have an undiagnosed malignancy. Tumors rarely disseminate to muscle, and this patient had no history of cancer.

"Then I got a call from the Chief of Pathology. The patient had suddenly died. An autopsy revealed widespread cancer. The primary lesion was in the bowel, but had spread throughout the body. There had been no clinical clues to its presence. Even the X-rays at that time were normal. Of course, CT scans and MRIs hadn't been invented yet.

"The Chief of Pathology wanted to know why I was the only one to even suspect cancer. I had suggested it after the electrodiagnotic exam, but nobody believed it. I had recognized it from the unusual pattern of electrodiagnostic testing. Subsequently, we identified several other cancer patients with this same abnormal pattern.

"I submitted a written report to the American Medical Association. An experienced electromyographer reviewed it and said, 'This doesn't happen!' The report was rejected. Even the Mayo Clinic gave me a hard time, denying the occurrence of this syndrome. Finally the report was published in our national professional journal, *The Archives of Physical Medicine and Rehabilitation*.

"We kept looking for patients with this odd pattern. When I came to Beaumont in 1967, we found a number of patients with a new onset of cancer, or a manifestation of recurrent cancer where the tumor metastasized to the muscle of the back. So we asked, 'Why is the back muscle unique? Why can cancer move into that muscle in particular?' Even with CT scanning, we still couldn't see the tumor in the mustle tissue, because the metastatic lesion was lost in the surrounding muscle.

"Then, one day we were asked to see a patient in the ER at Beaumont who had intractable lower back pain and had recently been discharged from Ford Hospital. There was no antecedent history of malignancy, but we did an electromyographic examination and concluded that he had a pattern that was consistent with metastatic cancer to the low back muscle—and then the patient died.

"Determined not to lose this opportunity, I arranged for a pathologist to do an autopsy. There in the muscles of the low back, we found tumor in the muscle as well as in the veins draining the muscles. We were also able to identify the pathway by which the tumor entered the low back, seemingly moving 'upstream' through a set of veins called the 'Batson's paravertebral veins' which drain these muscles. Batson's veins have no valves.

"Let's say a patient has breast cancer. A tumor can move from the breast through its venous drainage system, passing through the internal mammary veins into the portal system. A cough or sneeze, which increases intra-abdominal or intra-thoracic pressure, forced blood from the systemic portal system directly into Batson's valveless veins, to bathe the muscle of the back in tumor emboli. This discovery has aided in the early diagnosis of metastatic cancer.

"One of our surgical residents reviewed 5000 electromyograms performed at Beaumont and found that 1% of them demonstrated cancer in the low back. Nationally, 1% of all back pain is associated with metastatic cancer, which confirms the validity of this test. As MRI examination became available, we could readily confirm the presence of metastatic tumor in the paraspinal muscle.

"These two reports launched my national career. Since then, we have been fortunate to describe other clinical pearls now commonly recognized in medical practice. I've enjoyed the privilege of being President of the American Academy of Physical Medicine and Rehabilitation, serving as the only full-time private practitioner to hold the office. Each of my predecessors had been full-time academics. I've been privileged to receive several research awards in my field and have been honored with many academic and administrative awards and teaching honors in my field, and have also served as President of the Oakland County Medical Society."

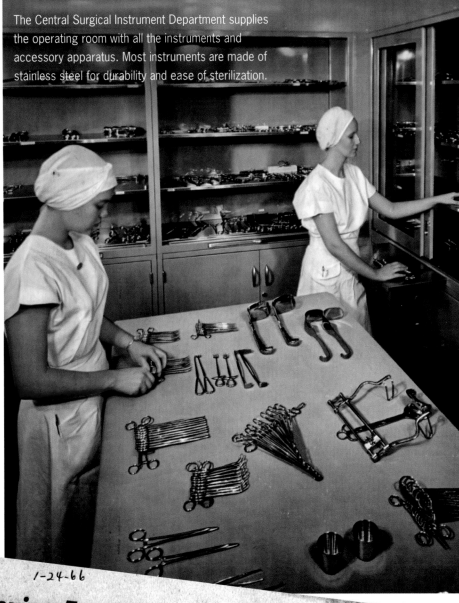

The Central Surgical Instrument Department supplies the operating room with all the instruments and accessory apparatus. Most instruments are made of stainless steel for durability and ease of sterilization.

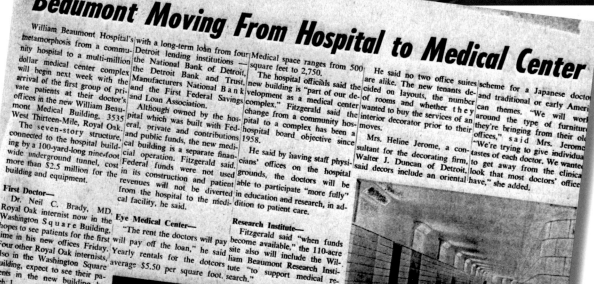

1-24-66

Beaumont Moving From Hospital to Medical Center

William Beaumont Hospital's metamorphosis from a community hospital to a multi-million dollar medical center complex will begin next week with the arrival of the first group of private patients at their doctor's offices in the new William Beaumont Medical Building, 3535 West Thirteen-Mile, Royal Oak.

The seven-story structure, connected to the hospital building by a 100-yard-long nine-foot wide underground tunnel, cost more than $2.5 million for the building and equipment.

First Doctor—

Dr. Neil C. Brady, MD, Royal Oak internist now in the Washington Square Building, hopes to see patients for the first time in his new offices Friday. Four other Royal Oak internists also in the Washington Square building, expect to see their patients in the new building by Feb. 1.

Seventy medical men—representing all areas of medicine from opthalomology to psychiatry—will move into the still unfinished structure between now and April 15. All are on the staff at William Beaumont Hospital, a rental stipulation set by hospital officials.

with a long-term loan from four Detroit lending institutions — the National Bank of Detroit, the Detroit Bank and Trust, Manufacturers National Bank and the First Federal Savings and Loan Association.

Although owned by the hospital which was built with Federal, private and contributions and public funds, the new medical building is a separate financial operation, Fitzgerald said. Federal funds were not used in its construction and patient revenues will not be diverted from the hospital to the medical facility, he said.

Eye Medical Center—

"The rent the doctors will pay will pay off the loan," he said. Yearly rentals for the doctors average $5.50 per square foot.

Medical space ranges from 500 square feet to 2,750.

The hospital officials said the new building is "part of our development as a medical center complex." Fitzgerald said the change from a community hospital to a complex has been a hospital board objective since 1958.

He said by having staff physicians' offices on the hospital grounds, the doctors will be able to participate "more fully" in education and research, in addition to patient care.

Research Institute—

Fitzgerald said "when funds become available," the 110-acre site also will include the William Beaumont Research Institute "to support medical research."

He said no two office suites are alike. The new tenants decided on layouts, the number of rooms and whether they wanted to buy the services of an interior decorator prior to their moves.

Mrs. Heline Jerome, a consultant for the decorating firm, Walter J. Duncan of Detroit, said decors include an oriental scheme for a Japanese doctor and traditional or early American themes. "We will work around the type of furniture they're bringing from their old offices," said Mrs. Jerome. "We're trying to give individual tastes of each doctor. We wanted to get away from the clinical look that most doctors' offices have," she added.

51

1966

The cruciformed or cross-shaped architecture allows all patient's rooms to have windows. Natural passage of day and night is helpful to hospital-bound patients. The architects, Ellerbe and Company, have fashioned a building which can be expanded easily to accommodate more and more patients—the planners envisioned new buildings and services on the spacious hospital grounds—a growing part of a growing community.

Below: The Honorable George Romney, Governor of Michigan participating in the cornerstone ceremony marking completion of the expansion program in 1966.

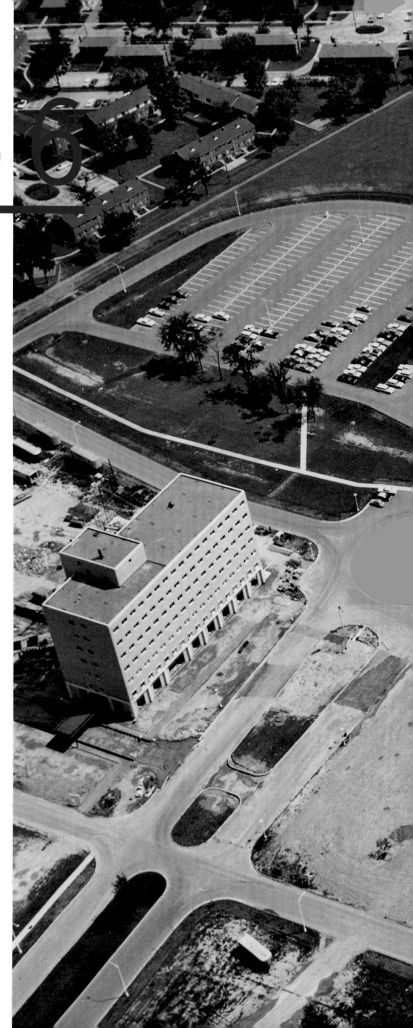

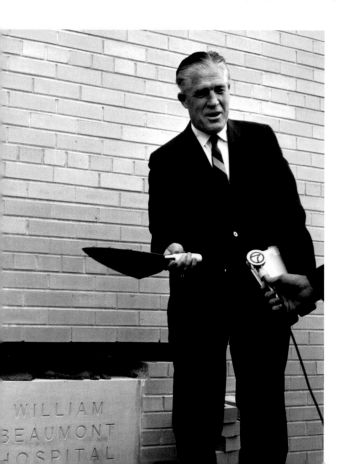

WILLIAM
BEAUMONT
HOSPITAL

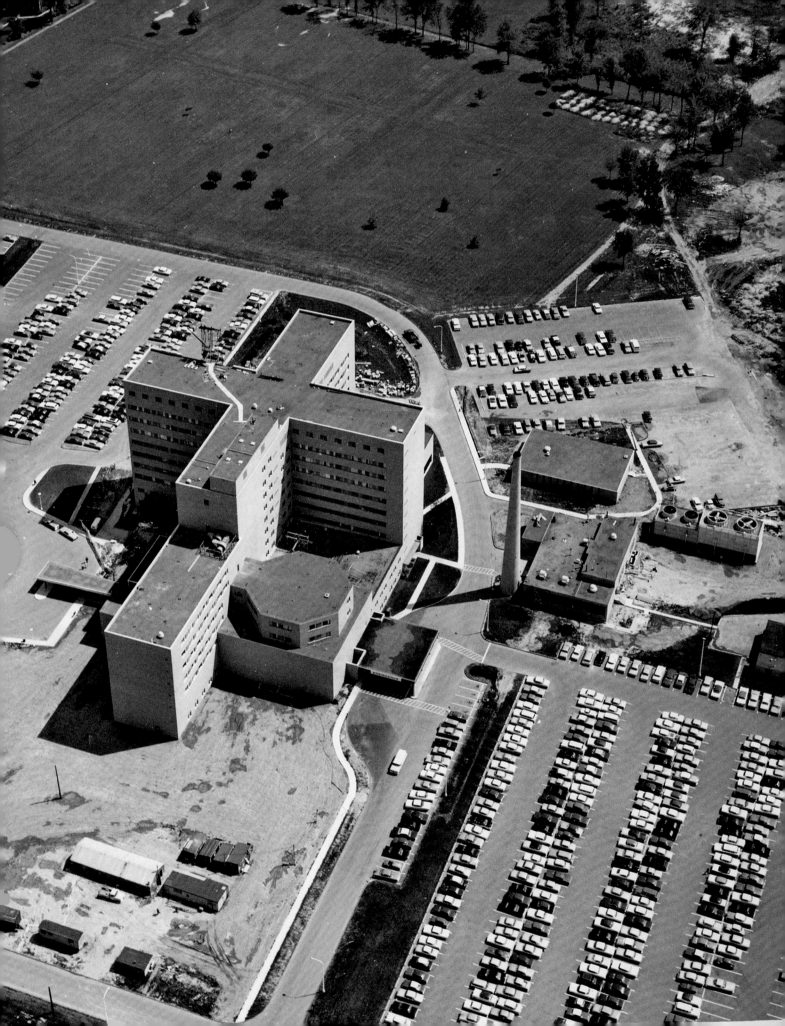

5 THE WORLD OF ADMINISTRATION

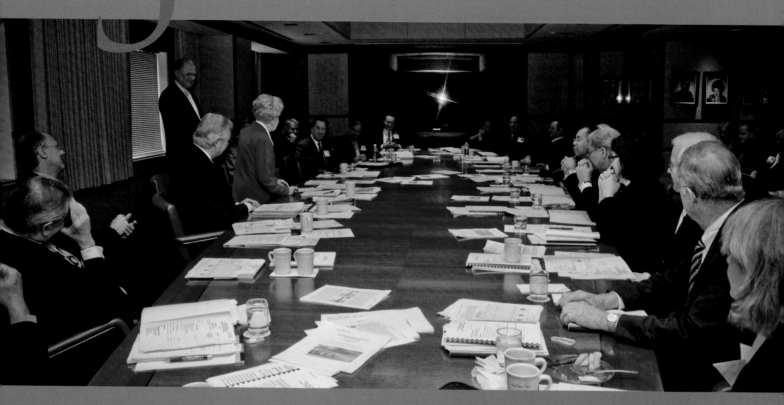

Beaumont Hospitals Board of Directors in session
presided by then Chairman Thomas Denomme
(standing) honoring Margaret Simmons (standing)
for her 50 years of volunteer work at Beaumont.

HAROLD BARKER, M.D.

First Chief of Staff, Beaumont, Royal Oak, 1954–1955

"Without doubt, (Dr. Barker is) one of the ablest surgeons in the Middle West."
— Dr. Frederick A. Coller, Chairman of Surgery, University of Michigan

Dr. Harold Barker graduated in 1916 from the medical school at the University of Michigan, where he stayed for his internship from 1921 to '22, residency from 1922 to '23 in anatomy and surgery, a fellowship the following year, and then joined the faculty in those subjects for three more years. In 1927 he moved to Pontiac and started a private practice at Pontiac St. Joseph and Pontiac General Hospital.

According to Dr. Frederick Coller, who was a famous doctor and Chairman of Surgery at the U of M, Dr. Barker was "a man of highest character and his personal and professional worth is universally recognized by his colleagues in surgery. He is fair, judicial and exhibits balanced thinking."

Dr. Coller would later be the man who would suggest that the new South Oakland Hospital be renamed "William Beaumont Hospital." He recommended Dr. Barker when the President of South Oakland Hospital, asked Dr. Coller about someone to be the first Chief of Staff. Destinies would cross again when Mr. Tomlinson became the first patient admitted to the new—and newly renamed—William Beaumont Hospital on January 24, 1955. Mr. Tomlinson was admitted by Dr. Harry Lichtwardt.

Dr. Harold Barker was what the Board of Trustees was seeking as a "triple threat"—a fine doctor, a teacher, and a researcher. He set an example of excellence and a high bar by guiding the fledgling hospital and its young physicians and surgeons in all phases of patient care. Beaumont's subsequent physician-leaders have held themselves to that strong example set by Dr. Barker from the beginning.

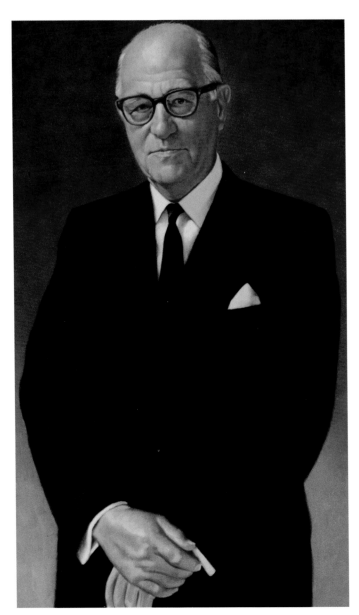

Harold Barker, M.D.

KENNETH E. MYERS
CEO of Beaumont Hospitals, 1969–1997

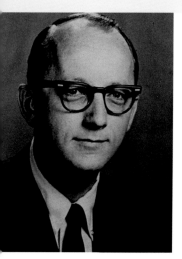

"Following graduation with an MBA,

I went to work for the Burroughs Corporation for nine years and left there in June of 1966 to join Touche Ross in their management consulting group here in Detroit. For my second assignment, they called me into the office downtown and asked, 'Ken, we want you to go out to a little hospital in Royal Oak that's run out of money. Do you know anything about hospitals?'

"I said, 'Well, I've had four children born in hospitals, but that's about all I know.'

"I hadn't thought about hospital administration at all. I was mainly interested in a business career. The Beaumont Board wanted to know how deep the financial hole was, how much they needed to borrow, and what the plan might be to pay it back. They gave me two weeks, with no margin for error. From a financial standpoint, I knew what to do, but I didn't know anything about hospital accounting.

"Those were different times, with a smaller hospital and different dollars. They had to borrow $500,000 on Wednesday to make Friday's payroll. The Board wanted a financial forecast, by month, for the next twelve months. We gave them a twelve-month financial projection showing how much they would need to borrow and when they could pay it back.

"Then they wanted to do a national search for a Chief Financial Officer. We presented three good candidates, and somehow I ended up being a fourth candidate. They brought me on board as 'Controller,' which now is the Chief Financial Officer. That was in 1966.

"Three years later, Owen Pinkerman, who had run the hospital since it was built, left to pursue another opportunity. The Board asked me to take over as CEO. That was a big-time career change for me . . . but I always had a desire to be the head of something. I was hoping it would be more than a one-person grocery store, but I never thought it would be a hospital. Then I got here and saw all the good that was being done and could be done with Beaumont's continuing growth and development, the change was easy."

"Once we stabilized the financial condition of the hospital, we looked at what Beaumont should be ten, twenty, thirty, forty years out. Fortunately we had a great Board of Directors. We knew we had a chance to grow and develop and become one of the best hospital systems in the country. The ultimate goal was to become one of the top three or four hospital systems of our kind in the country. We wanted to be a great community hospital, taking care of the people around us, while also becoming available to patients beyond our area. This could work as long as we kept one goal, one vision in mind: to provide the best medical care to those we serve, whether they come from our neighborhood or anywhere in the world. It's amazing in such a short period of time, how much has been accomplished from the mid-1950's until now.

"We had a strong philosophy of promotion from within, and it really has served us well over the years. That's why so many people have stayed for so long, because they knew that if they performed well, there would be a good opportunity for them. Many of our physicians and nurses have come up through the organization to become outstanding leaders at Beaumont."

A MAGNETIC PERSONALITY

"We finally got to the point in the late '70's when the hospital was big enough, with well enough developed clinical services, education and research programs that when we had an opening for which there wasn't someone in-house who qualified, we could attract the best physicians in the country to fill that opening.

"It was very challenging in the early years to attract those physicians. After all, most of them were already working in superior institutions. We had to be competitive and offer an exciting cutting-edge future, and be willing to give them quite a bit of freedom and support to draw them away from the venerated institutions where they were already ensconced.

"The common reaction was, 'Detroit? Why would I want to come to Detroit!' It was a difficult sell, but if we could just get them here our location and the quality of life in the Metro Detroit area was much better than they anticipated. When they saw what was happening in the community, our recruiting efforts were quite successful.

"Fortunately, most of those physicians have stayed. Dr. Diokno was one of what I call our 'major attractions.' He and many other excellent physicians became part of the attraction of Beaumont."

WHEN THE GOVERNMENT COMES TO HELP . . .

"Dealing with the government has always been difficult. In the 70's, when we wanted to expand, and were planning to add 300 beds, we couldn't obtain approval. The planning agency acknowledged that we had long waiting lists—for just normal medical procedures there was a six-week wait, and it was growing. They said there were empty beds in Detroit, and the people who wanted to come here should go elsewhere. The government wasn't refined enough to recognize that different hospital systems have different capabilities and limitations. They simply saw us as one massive service area. It was very difficult for us to expand, even on our own land.

"Eventually we found a way when the Certificate of Need program was instituted, which at least gave us a chance to make our case, and allowed us to get something done for which we saw a need. For us it was a breakthrough."

DR. ARCARI ON CERTIFICATES OF NEED

"A 'Certificate of Need' is a certificate provided by the state government after evaluation of your application to add a major aspect to the hospital, like a significant number of beds, a cancer unit, or spending $100 million on a new technique in radiation therapy, and so on. The hospital has to apply for that, the state evaluates the 'need' in the location where you intend to do the work, and determines whether there's validity and it's justifiable in the sense of quality, costs, and access.

Do we need this piece of equipment or are there enough of them? If we have enough, then Oakland County and the state shouldn't be spending this kind of money on unnecessary equipment. If they approve, the hospital gets its Certificate of Need, which is the permission to go ahead. If they don't, then it can't. It's like a building permit, taking into account the medical environment in that locality."

DENNIS HERRICK

Senior Vice-President and Chief Financial Officer,
Beaumont Hospitals

"There's that old saying: 'No margin,

no mission.'"

"Beaumont is a private 501-C3 not-for-profit institution. Its Board of Directors is made up of representatives from the community. Being a 501-C3, we have certain obligations and relationships to charitable care, particularly of anybody who presents at the Emergency Center. It's an important part of the mission.

"Medical education is very active at Beaumont for residents. Those residencies train a significant number of doctors, even though up till now we haven't had a medical school or been attached to a university. I think that's been one strong differentiator. We're a significant enterprise, recognized across the country, sprouting from a little community hospital and growing very quickly to become much more than that. Beaumont has been terrific for clinical care, but also terrific in medical education."

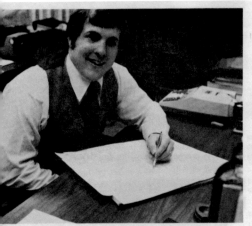

ok who's happy! He's Dennis Herrick, proud to be a CPA that means he has just been certified by the state as a blic accountant. Mr. Herrick has been a reimbursement alyst in Financial Analysis since April 14, 1975. He lives Berkley.

"I've been with Beaumont thirty-plus years, which has been a wonderful ride, and obviously I've had lots of mentors here. There was a strong financial inclination from the Board and from its leadership, making a platform and discipline to have a strong balance sheet, and focusing on operating performance. We have to balance what we ought to be doing with the community with financial viability."

"Some people believe that health care might move to a concept of integration in which entities such as Beaumont also become part of the insurance delivery mechanism. We did that a few years ago,

not terribly successfully. We didn't own the plan all ourselves. We were with several of our competing hospitals. There was an insurance product on the market called 'Select Care,' and we were a part-owner. It's not a conflict of interest, but instead is integrated health care. Henry Ford Health System owns the Health Alliance Plan. In many markets you'll find others, like the Kaiser Health System, a well-known large system on the West Coast that has stretched across the country; they own hospitals, ambulatory centers, and much of their medical staff are employed, and they also have a health plan. It's the ultimate in integrations. It ties everything together in relationship to the flow of funds, outcomes, and quality.

"When you look at Beaumont and this tremendous clinical base, with both private physicians and employed staff, we may create something like an 'accountable care organization,' which is the physicians and the hospitals joining together to become a conduit for insurance companies, government, or whomever, to funnel payments in to us and to then basically accept the risk of taking care of patients. Some of the payments would flow based on outcomes and quality, which is somewhat missing today in the system. That's one of the challenges in the health care business today. People are recognizing that most of the reimbursement systems are 'the more you do, the more you get paid.' That's not necessarily what's best when measured against outcomes and cost of care. Those are some of the things we may be facing as far as what we should be to meet the future.

"It's challenging, and one of the debates is the 'big bang' of change, the pace of how health delivery will change in the future."

NICKOLAS A. VITALE

Senior Vice President, Financial Operations,
Beaumont Hospitals

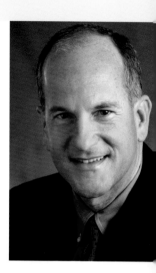

"The key here at Beaumont has been an approach to being strong financially, but also to invest back into the community. We've always felt there was an appropriate balance to how much money we retain as cash on hand as opposed to putting that money back into the community. Early on, the Board of Directors decided that we're here for the community and want to be a place that attracts that private medical staff of wonderful people who want to take care of patients, and that the community can help support us through philanthropy. We've always been aggressive in investing our operating cash back into the enterprise to provide a very pleasing place for physicians to practice, and to be at the vanguard of technology. We buy the best technological equipment—PET scanners, CT scanners, cath labs, the Biobank, the simulators, imaging equipment---a whole slew of machines that are very important to physicians who want to practice with the right tool sets at hand."

THE BLOSSOMING OF BEAUMONT

"I'd like to stress the secret of the growth of this institution. It had its origin in 1955, so it's relatively young in comparison to major medical centers that go back long before 1955. We're taught that without a margin we can't have a mission; an institution like this has to be financially viable to attract the kinds of folks who want to practice here and feel they're tied to a successful enterprise, and for philanthropy to be attracted. The blossoming of Beaumont happens because of the focus not just on the finance side, but on clinical excellence, on being the best we can be for high-quality patient care, patient safety and patient satisfaction.

"There is great pride, loyalty and commitment to this institution from those of us who work here. I found a home here, found opportunity and the chance to grow with the organization, as have many others. Because of the blossoming and tremendous growth, many of us have had the privilege of moving up a career path. Very few people find the benefit of staying with the same employer for such a long time, for a whole career."

Nickolas A. Vitale, became senior vice president of financial operations in March 2007, after being vice president of finance, Beaumont Hospital, Troy since Jan. 1, 2005. Has been in healthcare finance since 1980.

Vitale received his B.B.A. and M.B.A. at Western Michigan University and Wayne State University in 1980 and 1988, respectively.

He has held various financial administrative positions in the healthcare industry including:

- Controller, Rehabilitation Institute of Michigan, 1985
- Vice President and Chief Financial Officer, Children's Hospital of Michigan, 1988
- Vice President and Controller, The Detroit Medical Center, 1998
- Executive Vice President and Chief Financial Officer, The Detroit Medical Center, 1999
- Vice President and Chief Financial Officer, Bon Secours Cottage Health Services, 2003

Vitale has served on a number of Community Boards in various capacities including: Wayne Community Living Services, The Birmingham, Y.M.C.A., the Ronald McDonald House of Greater Detroit, the Boys and Girls Club of Troy, MI and the U of M Club of Greater Detroit. More recently Nick was the Board Chair of the American Diabetes Association, (ADA), of Michigan and was the ADA National Finance Committee Chair and a National ADA Board Member. He is currently the Chair of Board of Visitors for the Applebaum School of Pharmacy and Health Science at Wayne State University.

Vitale is a fellow in the Healthcare Financial Management Association and a fellow in the American College of Healthcare Executives.

"As a financial officer, I am confident that Beaumont will weather the current financial challenges facing our System because Beaumont has a very strong and respected medical staff and medical staff leadership including extremely well known physician specialists. Our quality, safety and service are well recognized in the community and the loyalty of our patient base is quite high. The administrative leadership team is very well respected and cited in most of our rating reviews as an asset to the organization. Lastly, our Board of Directors, led by the current Chairman, Steve Howard, are extremely engaged and active in assisting management, where needed, to ensure attention is being placed on the most important issues.

While a bit stressed, our balance sheet remains strong and our ability to generate high levels of operating cash flow margin continues to be very strong with results typically at the "AA" rated medians or higher. Beaumont captures the greatest market share in its primary service area and is consistently named as the preferred health care system by our patients. Our new school of medicine with Oakland University will serve to enhance this view."

TED D. WASSON

President and Chief Executive Officer 1997–2005
Executive Vice President and Chief Operating Officer, 1984–1997
Executive Vice President and Corporate Hospital Director, 1980–1984
Director, Beaumont, Royal Oak, 1976–1980

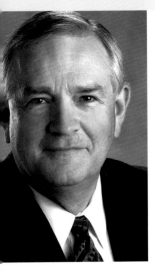

"I started at Beaumont Hospital as a

resident in hospital administration. I'm not a doctor. I went to Michigan State University as an undergraduate in hotel, restaurant and institutional management followed by a Masters degree in Hospital Administration from the University of Michigan. As an undergraduate degree requirement, I worked summers in hotels and restaurants and decided that wasn't what I wanted to do with my life. The only things left were prison or hospital management...I decided to try hospitals.

"My wife and I moved into Belle Court with a ten day old little girl. That was is 1962. I stayed for 43 years. I was lucky to be a part of Beaumont during a time of phenomenal growth. We just seemed to blossom at the right time. It was go, go, go. I don't know whether any of us ever envisioned that Beaumont would become what it is today although we always felt it would be more than just a community hospital. A major reason for this success is incredible tenure. People come here for a year or two and stay for decades.

"As a part of my residency program as an administrator in training, I rotated through all the departments. I worked as a housekeeper, an orderly, in the kitchen, in the maintenance department and the business offices, etc. It was a once-in-a-lifetime opportunity to be working at every level of a very complex organization and asking people what they did, how they like their jobs and what they would change about their jobs if they could."

'The original construction money going back to the 1950's came from the Metropolitan Detroit Building Fund. Actually, Beaumont was debt-free the day it opened, which was a wonderful thing. After that came borrowing determined by how much debt load we could carry through patient revenues and philanthropy. Until 12 or 15 years ago philanthropy

was a relatively minor part of Beaumont's history, but by then it became obvious that we couldn't sustain ourselves through operations and patient revenue only. Philanthropy is now a vital part of Beaumont. Access to capital is tough.

"Although the American health care system has many problems, I still believe it is far superior to a national health service. In a speech to the Michigan Hospital Association, former Prime Minister Brian Mulroney said, 'Our system would never work in your country because Americans want everything and they want it now! Furthermore, our system works only because we share a border with the United States and you are our relief valve for critical services on a timely basis.' However, Canadian patients are welcomed in US hospitals because their rate of reimbursement far exceeds that of US insurers who pay only a small fraction of what patients see on the explanation of benefits forms."

THE FREEDOM TO BUILD

"We couldn't build fast enough . One of the bigger problems that kept me up at night was that we didn't have enough beds for all the patients who wanted to come here. We took our capacity to over 900 beds, built the North Tower and opened Troy.

"Beaumont's surge of growth was remarkable, driven by a seemingly insatiable demand and an overwhelming desire to fulfill our destiny as foreseen by the founding fathers in the early 50's. The Boards of Directors have always trusted, believed in and supported the management team. For many years there wasn't a CEO in place. If there was a CEO, it was the Chairman of the Board. In the early 80's the organization had become so complex that it was decided to officially put an executive CEO in place."

THOMAS R. MCASKIN

Vice President, Chief Legal Officer,
Beaumont Hospitals, 1999–2011

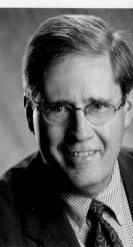

EXECUTIVE DECISIONS

"Even when we had hard times, when there was tension, it wasn't malicious, we were all just trying to make the place better. There are a lot of egos involved in an institution of this size and quality. We might have different ideas about how to make Beaumont better, but we generally didn't hold it against each other. Medical Staff issues and hospital issues are often at odds with each other. That's just part of the business. Managing those conflicts becomes the CEO's task. The pie is only so big.

"In the final analysis it is the *people* of Beaumont who have made this hospital one of the very finest in the world. As a Joint Commission of Accreditation inspector said in the late 90's, 'Never have I seen so many extraordinarily talented overachievers assembled in one institution. You people are unique!'"

In-house legal counsel at Beaumont dates back to when Kenneth McGregor, joined Beaumont's Administrative team as House Counsel, in 1967. Mr. McGregor was eventually joined by William McNeil and was later succeeded by William G. Lerchen, as General Counsel. In 1983, Mr. Lerchen hired Thomas R. McAskin to serve as Assistant General Counsel. In 1985, Mr. McAskin was appointed as Director of the newly created Office of Legal Affairs.

In May, 1987, Malcolm J. Sutherland was appointed as Beaumont's Vice President and General Counsel. Mr. Sutherland served through December, 1999. Mr. McAskin was named Vice President, Chief Legal Officer in December, 1999 and continued in that capacity until January, 2011. Gordon J. Walker is currently serving as the interim Vice President and Chief Legal Officer. Additional in-house counsel that have been part of the team, over the years, include Robert Zack, Sharon Finnie, Eric Hunt, Dawn Harimoto, Gloria Jelinek, Karen Luther, Amy Rosenberg, Beth Derwin, Terese Farhat, Gordon Walker, Valerie Rup and Ian Wilson.

Mr. Sutherland, among many other contributions, developed the concept of a self-insurance program for high risk surgeons, at a time when professional liability insurance was not available or its cost was excessive. The Physician Malpractice Responsibility Program (PMRP) began in 1989 and continues today.

Mr. McAskin saw the benefit of utilizing experienced Beaumont nurses as trained legal assistants. As legal assistants, these Beaumont nurses work with physician defendants and experts, physician and nurse treaters and directly with outside defense counsel. The first legal assistant, Jan Forge, was hired in 1983. Since that time, legal assistants, now known as Legal Nurse Consultants, have been Beth Harper, Diane Lysak, Eva Blow, Gail Melrose, Terri (Erdman) Brooks, Allison Frontera, Kris Pennycook, Margie Hamilton and Debbie Jagow.

Another novel concept was initiated by Legal Affairs in 1985, as requested by Beaumont's Chief of Surgery, John Glover, M.D., which addressed the needs of residents. Beaumont offers its residents the opportunity to observe and participate in various aspects of risk management and the legal system, as these relate to the practice of medicine. A "Legal Affairs Elective" was developed in response to a perceived lack of education, recognition and understanding of risk management concepts and the legal system. Residents observe malpractice trials, depositions and mediations/hearings. In addition, residents review and summarize medical records relevant to malpractice litigation; attend various hospital committee meetings; review and discuss litigation files; assist in answering interrogatories; read assigned materials and attend lectures; and, prepare a written evaluation of the Elective.

Results: Through December, 2010, 814 residents have participated in the Legal Affairs Elective. All extoll its benefits and encourage their colleagues to participate. Most residents indicated that the experience would alter their practice, especially in two areas: 1) changes in communication with patients, physicians, and nursing personnel, and 2) improved clarity in the medical record.

The functions of the Office of Legal Affairs have evolved over the years and the Office offers a full spectrum of legal services.

KEN MATZICK

Chief Executive Officer of Beaumont Hospitals, 2005–2010
Executive Vice-President and Chief Operating Officer, 1997–2005
Director, Beaumont, Royal Oak, 1983–1997
Director, Beaumont, Troy, 1976–1983

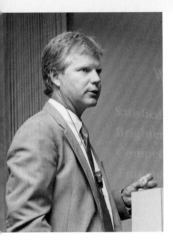

"I've been with the organization

forty-plus years now, since 1969. Every time I got antsy and wanted more responsibility, an opportunity would pop up within the company to challenge me. I have an M.A. in hospital administration and my undergraduate studies were in pre-med. I'm not a doctor, but the pre-med helped. My first position in the field was at Morristown Memorial Hospital in Morristown, New Jersey for about two and a half years, then I wanted more responsibility and found Beaumont. The rest is 40 years of history."

A TEACHING HOSPITAL

"The fact that we've had unparalleled growth in that period of time has attracted top-quality doctors and professional staff. Beaumont is flourishing and that goes back to the folks who founded the hospital and the Board leadership at that time. They wanted to differentiate Beaumont from any other community hospital and recognized that one way to do it was to become a teaching hospital.

"In those days, they described their vision as a 'medical center.' They didn't necessarily know exactly what that meant, but they wanted to be more than just a community hospital. In the very early days, they pursued residencies and a teaching mission. They realized that attracting good faculty meant they needed to offer good research opportunities as well. Beaumont quickly became a magnet for high-achievers."

"NO MARGIN, NO MISSION."

"At the core, hospitals are safety nets for the community. The hospital is the first place people

go to in an emergency—pandemic, natural disaster, tornado, hurricane—so serving the community is part of the mission. Hospitals, by law, are not allowed to differentiate between paying and non-paying patients. A physician can choose whether or not he treats Medicaid patients, the uninsured, and so on, but the hospital is required to take all.

"On the other hand, 'no margin, no mission.' If we don't figure out how to make money and work with doctors to help the hospital have a financial margin, then there's no hospital at all. Sometimes the general public has trouble understanding that. It can be confusing because there's a whole new language in our industry. 'Non-profit' doesn't mean 'no margin.' 'Non-profit' is a tax status established by the Internal Revenue Service that enables us and obligates us to meet community service needs, including charity care, educational programs, health screenings, and other services that need to be done in sufficient quantity to justify our tax exemption. Those services have to exceed what otherwise would be our normal tax obligation and we have to be able to demonstrate that. So we must create mechanisms to support the community."

THE PATIENT, THE DOCTOR, AND THE BOTTOM LINE

"When doctors want to keep treating a patient, but the costs are getting out of hand, what brings the doctors and the administration together is the one thing we have in common: the patient. If we always do what's best for the patient, we learn to manage the money. Today, we practice evidence-based medicine; if the evidence says this is the right thing to do for the patient, that's what we do.

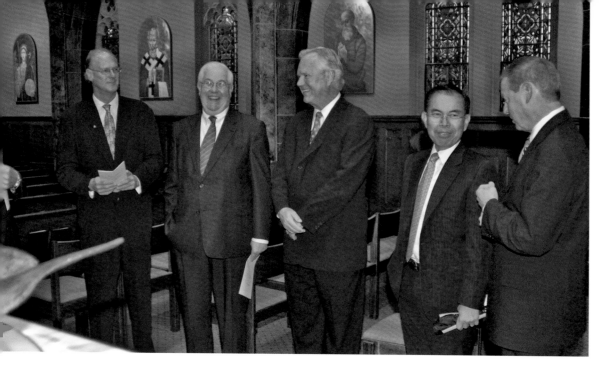

From left to right: Steve Howard & John Hartwig, (Members of the Board of Directors), Ken Matzick, CEO, Ananias Diokno, M.D., CMO and Gene Michalski, COO, preparing to celebrate the official transfer of Bon Secours Hospital to Beaumont Hospitals.

Ken Matzick was the driving force behind Beaumont's acquisition of what is now Beaumont, Grosse Pointe.

"If by that method we lose money, it's up to the management to figure out how we can offset that loss. We have no choice but to treat all patients and want them to get the best care, so it's a balancing act. We create mechanisms to resolve these differences, and they are very real issues. There are arguments to be made that, regardless of cost, we need to do certain things. On the other hand, if the outcome can be achieved with less cost and consumption of resources, then we need to do that.

"Different family wishes, cultures, religions, ethnic traditions, all fold into the decisions We have to honor those needs. We have over forty interpreters for language and cultural sensitivity. There are cultures in which no man other than the husband is allowed to touch a woman. For medical diagnoses, we have to find a female doctor. We've done some breakthrough work with picture books to overcome language barriers and help patients understand procedures they might be facing.

"With the treatment of someone who is going to die, we leave it to the doctors and the families to decide how far to take treatment. The hospital administration has to be prepared to honor the family's wishes, but just because we can do something doesn't mean we should.

"The doctor's pen is the most expensive piece of technology. We don't do anything unless there's a doctor's order. If you're going to be admitted, the doctor admits you. If you get an X-ray, the doctor ordered it. If you get a prescription, the doctor ordered it. The end-of-life choices are a combination of the doctor's voice, the family's voice, and the patient's voice—if he or she had a living will or other advanced directives.

"On the other hand, in Michigan, a family member might fly in from somewhere and short-circuit the patient's desires. When it's personal, when it's you, and you're not a doctor, you're going to react in a personal way. Then the doctor and the hospital's support staff, social workers and counselors will meet with the family and help to work the way down this difficult road."

THE UNSOLVED PROBLEM

"An example of a problem that hasn't yet been solved is the misalignment of incentives for all players in health care. There are incentives that work against each other. For instance, doctors are paid piece-work while hospitals are paid a fixed amount for the whole case. When a doctor orders something for an in-patient, it may represent revenue for him or her, but it is a cost to the hospital. For some doctors, every day the patient is here the doctor gets a fee while the hospital gets a fixed fee for the entire stay. So the hospital's incentive is to move the patient out, while the doctor's incentive is to keep the patient in. That conflict remains.

"For patients who need a continuum of care—a nursing home or home health care—those are paid differently. In order to qualify for Medicare to be admitted into a nursing home, the patient has to be hospitalized for three days, but the medical condition may not require a three-day hospital stay. It would be cheaper for the patient to go straight to

1966 – Michigan Governor George Romney dedicates an $11 million expansion, tripling Beaumont's size from five stories to 10. That same year, the medical office building opened, the School of Radiologic Technology was established, and the Research Institute was founded.

the nursing home, but the federal government, in its infinite wisdom, is costing itself money to keep that person in the hospital when what he really needs is nursing home level care.

"Health care is a major business in the United States, the second largest employer, second to the government. The business community periodically calls to get our opinion on one thing or another, and they'll ask me what keeps me up at night. I tell them, "Congress keeps me up at night." Congress, essentially 500-plus people in Washington, is trying to legislate solutions to the most complex business problems that exist. All the management gurus in all the schools that have studied health care agree that it's the most complex industry and a hospital is the most complex organization that you can find in the world. To think that Congress can legislate a one-size-fits-all solution to a complex business problem

just doesn't make sense. They don't understand the complexity, and their solutions are always political. Political solutions always favor somebody, whether it's the chair of a committee, or the party in power, or some pork-barrel deal or other, and every few years the players change, so everything else changes.

"It seems that anything the government does adds complexity. Complexity lends itself to corruption. It creates lots of opportunities and work for lawyers, consultants, politicians, and thieves.

"In our hospitals, we must first and always stay focused on what's best for the patient. I have a tremendously challenging job, which makes it a very satisfying job. We have to solve complex problems, and we're never done. The complexity of the problems can be frustrating and stimulating at the same time. I've never had the same day twice."

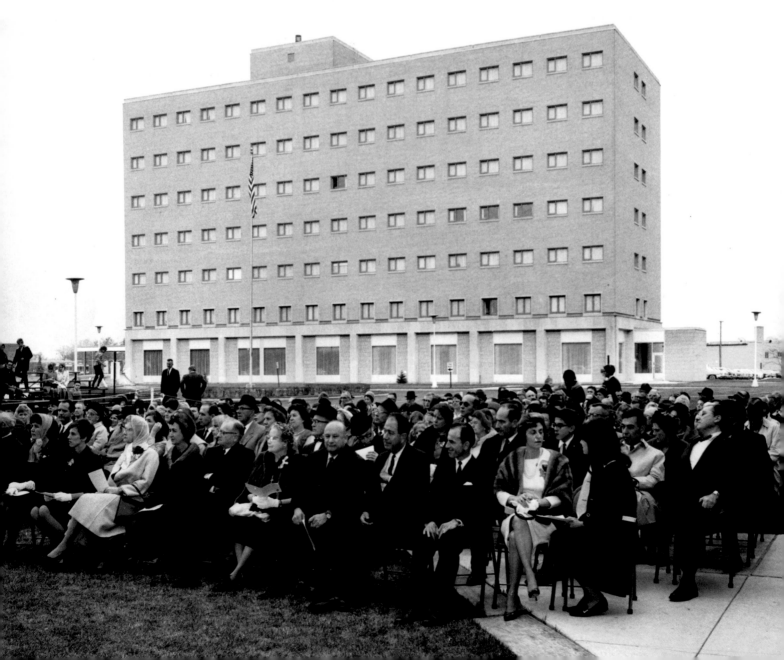

GENE MICHALSKI

Chief Executive Officer, 2010–present
Executive Vice-President and
Chief Operating Officer of Beaumont Hospitals, 2005–2010
Director, Beaumont, Troy, 1997–2005

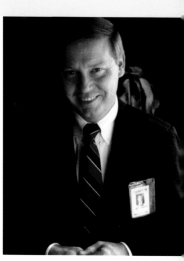

"I started as a phlebotomist in 1971,

drawing blood on the afternoon shift at the Royal Oak hospital as a part time job. I was working on a Master's Degree in physiology at the time at Wayne State University. A colleague in one of my physiology classes was the supervisor on the afternoon shift and told me there was a position open. A job at Beaumont could help pay for my college education. One of my first mentors, a very bright lady by the name of Hazel Stoerck, happened to be the chief tech for Beaumont in the laboratory at Royal Oak, and worked for the Chief of Pathology, Dr. Julius Rutzky. Hazel told me I could move from phlebotomist to lab tech junior, then lab tech senior, and they gradually taught me more of the individual laboratory areas—hemotology, chemistry, urinalysis, and so on. As I took more physiology classes, they matched me up in parallel with lab medicine collateral with what I was doing at Wayne.

"One day Hazel said, 'When you finish your Master's Degree, let me know. There may be other opportunities here for you.'

"When I finished my M.S.—I was doing research with sharks on blood clotting factors—Hazel went to Dr. Rutzky and said she'd like to promote me to a co-supervisory role on the afternoon shift, along with a lady by the name of Ruth Balks. I gradually assumed more and more responsibility until one day I was given the full afternoon supervisor's job.

"About a year and a half later, Hazel said, 'They're building a hospital somewhere out in Troy, and they've appointed Dr. Paul Goodman as the pathologist for that hospital. Why don't you go throw your hat into the ring?' So I called Dr. Goodman and approached him about the Chief Tech job. He said, 'Let's get to know each other.'

"He was very shrewd. He said, 'Here are the kinds of services we're thinking about. Come back in two weeks and tell me what you think a hospital of this kind, with this kind of patient mix, would want to have in terms of laboratory medicine.'

"So I did. Then he said, 'Given that list of blood tests, what would you have to meet the needs of this hospital and this population? What kinds of equipment would you get?'

"So I put together a plan, working with all the division chiefs at Royal Oak about the types of equipment that would be needed at a hospital like Beaumont, Troy.

"He said, 'Why don't you devise a staffing plan?'

"By the end of six months, we had also put together the plan for the lab. Dr. Goodman then told me I would have to meet the new hospital director for Troy, who was Ken Matzick. By now it was 1976.

"So, enter Mr. Matzick. Labcoat in hand, I went to meet him, and was offered the opportunity to head the lab at Troy. I was one of the first people hired for Troy. We brought the labs from two smaller hospitals in Warren and Ardmore, which were closed and consolidated as part of a Certificate of Need for opening a new hospital in Troy.

"There wasn't much out there at the time. The new building and everything were built on a swamp. As Ken brought his team together, all new people, we got to know each other by setting up our departments, then we'd all go out to the Alibi Lounge for lunch, because we had no lunch room yet.

"The Troy hospital opened in May of 1977. I was in the Chief Tech position for about a year. The lab was brought up to College of American Pathologists certification within a year—which was very unusual for a new lab—and about a year and a half after that, Ken asked whether I'd be interested in becoming the Administrative Assistant. He was creating that role because he was managing the lab personally at that time and was looking for someone to take over some of the administrative tasks. I had received an offer from Dr. Rutzky to come to Royal Oak as the Chief Tech. Dr. Rutzky got approval to bring me back at the same time as Ken Matzick was offering me the position of Administrative Assistant at Troy. I could see that laboratory medicine alone wasn't going to meet my goals. I chose the career decision and went into administration.

We launched the hospital's first joint-venture ambulatory care center, out at North Macomb, included a joint-venture surgery center and syndicated a joint-venture medical building. Doctors could now own a piece of the medical building.

"Ken suggested furthering my education as part of stepping into the administrative role. I had to take many prerequisites because my undergraduate work had been in the sciences. I went back to Wayne State to get an MBA. A year later, Ken promoted me to Assistant Director.

"My initial responsibility was to build the Medical Building, develop the departments, syndicate the building, meaning to fill it up by leasing it to private doctors' offices.

"In the 1980's, I got a call from an executive recruiter about a job as Chief Operating Officer for a small hospital system in Lansing. Sure enough, they made me an offer on a Friday. I got home that night and Andrea said there was a message from Ken Matzick, and I should call no matter how late. Ken asked, 'Did they make you an offer and did you accept?'

"The answer was 'Yes' and 'Not yet.'

"'Meet me in Birmingham for breakfast. I want to talk to you.'

"At breakfast, Ken went on. 'I'm glad you didn't accept, because I'd like you to come with me to Royal Oak as Administrative Director. I'm the new CEO of Beaumont, Royal Oak.'"

"This was about 1982. I worked for Ken about ten years as Associate Director, Senior Associate Director, with progressively more responsibility, taking on much of the planning and building responsibilities. The projects at that time were a new South Hospital, an addition for obstetrics, a new entrance, a connector bridge to a parking deck, a critical care tower, a second medical building, expansion of the medical administration building—in other words, big steps in building a major hospital complex from the ground up.

"In 1991, when most of that was in play, I got another call from another executive recruiter about a position as the Executive Vice President and Chief Operating Officer of St. Frances Hospital in Evanston, Illinois. It was part of a 10-hospital system that was owned by the Sisters of St. Frances out of Mishawaka, Indiana.

"Eventually they offered me the job. It was a tough decision. I asked Ken not to make me a counter offer, but I knew he would. He offered more money and a bigger title, but essentially the same job. I chose the much more difficult decision—to go to Chicago. I left Beaumont after twenty years. I became one of the few who have ever left Beaumont, and later returned."

A MINI-BEAUMONT

"I didn't think about it at the time, but some people consider it a strength to have a diversified background in terms of job experiences, and organizational and cultural experiences. That turned out to be a good experience for me and probably was one of the reasons I'm in this position today.

"Evanston was a mini-Beaumont. It had a nursing home, several ambulatory care centers, home health services, and a number of teaching programs. It was a system within a system, with all the elements of the continuum of care: out-patient testing, hospital work, recovery, follow-up, ambulatory care, and back to the doctor's office. It had the complete care experience, but was very small.

"They had no salaried medical administration. At Beaumont, we have a full-time salaried Chief Medical Officer and many full and part-time medical directors who report to him. That's a parallel organization to the hospital side, where I have many lay people reporting to me. We have counterparts running all the way throughout the organization. The St. Frances model is a private-practice elected medical staff leadership model. The doctors elect a Chief of Staff, who is not salaried by the hospital. He or she is either a volunteer or the medical staff pays the salary. They change every two years, unlike ours.

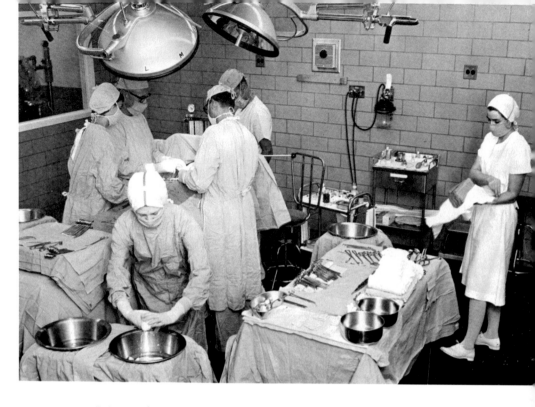

"Interestingly, I was in a planning session at the corporate office about three years into my tenure, when I had said, 'Have the sisters ever considered selling some of their holdings, concentrating their mission in Indiana?'

"You could've heard a pin drop. But that's what they ended up doing, including St. Frances.

"In my fourth year, I was actually involved in the transition of St. Frances Hospital to Resurrection, which purchased St. Frances of Evanston. I was on the acquired side of an acquisition rather than acquiring. They asked me to stay on as CEO, but by then I had received a call from the folks back up here that Ken Myers was going to retire. They asked, 'Are you interested in coming home?' So the timing was good for me to come back."

GENE RETURNS TO BEAUMONT

"When I returned to Beaumont, I wanted to grow the hospital. I didn't want to come back as the Director of Troy, but Ken said it wasn't the Troy I had left. There was a nursing home partnership to manage, and a home health agency, and I would be in charge of ambulatory services, which needed a lot of work. I told Ken I would come back if he would give me the freedom to grow the hospital and these other services.

"Five years almost to the day, I came back to the Troy hospital. I had gone away to work as CEO within a multi-hospital system, and came back just as Beaumont was blossoming into a multi-hospital system. I never thought it would make a difference, but my Catholic experience in Chicago would become helpful. Beaumont would later acquire Bon Secours Hospital in Grosse Pointe, Michigan, a Catholic hospital, and this time I was on the acquiring side. And guess what—Bon Secours had a hospital, a home health company, a nursing home— it was a mini-St. Frances of Evanston.

"Evanston as a very nice older suburb on the shore of Lake Michigan, north of Chicago. Grosse Pointe is an affluent community on the shore of Lake St. Clair, in a suburb of Detroit. Very similar demographics, and similar hospitals in how they were managed. For me, history was repeating itself.

"The Troy hospital at that time was 189 beds. It's now 454. It'll top 500 shortly. We've increased by more than 2 ½ times. We launched the hospital's first joint-venture ambulatory care center, out at North Macomb, included a joint-venture surgery center, and syndicated a joint-venture medical building. Doctors could now own a piece of the medical building. This was a 'first' for Beaumont—to invite doctors to have an ownership interest in a Beaumont building. And now we have five nursing homes.

"I substantially expanded the Troy hospital from a basic community hospital to an emerging tertiary care facility with open heart surgery, radiation therapy, MRI's, CT scanners, and which now has robotic surgery.

"The Chicago experience and the expansion of the Troy hospital helped prepare me when Ken Matzick went to the CEO role, and when a year after that he asked me to become Chief Operating Officer of Beaumont Hospitals. I've been at Troy twice, Royal Oak twice, about fifteen years each. The Royal Oak hospital is one of the biggest in the country, with 1069 beds. It's a very big baby to feed.

"My story seems to be part of a pattern as Beaumont grew—finding the right person, teaching, investing, mentoring, and plugging that person in, then helping him or her grow in experience and career status. A lot of us grew up with Beaumont, along with others who helped pull us up."

LORRAINE BOUDREAU
Assistant to the President and CEO

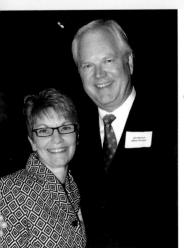

Lorraine Boudreau has been an assistant to the presidents of Beaumont Hospitals (here pictured with Ken Matzick) since 2000.

"I've been in this position for ten years,

so I've worked for three president/CEO's—Ted Wasson for five years, Ken Matzick for five years, and now for the new CEO Gene Michalski. I had worked for Ken Matzick and Gene Michalski in the Royal Oak Directors Office, currently known as Hospital and Medical Administration.

Working for various individuals is somewhat like starting a new job. The duties remain somewhat the same, but personalities and individual leadership styles differ, so there is an adjustment. However, having worked with Ken Matzick and Gene Michalski previously has helped in each transition. Additionally, the focus of each CEO I have supported has been the same—the patient.

From my perspective, the mid 1980s began a system-wide growth that has been ongoing—the North Tower expansion, Heart Center addition, Research Building, Child Care Center, the new South Hospital (now known as the South Tower), additional parking decks, acquisition of Grosse Pointe, establishment of the Ambulatory Division, and so on. Change is continual and seems to be necessary.

Obviously, the CEO has responsibility for the entire organization, which allows me the opportunity to interact with the various divisions and many departments. The CEO reports directly to the Board; thus, a primary function of my position is to support the Board and all if its duties and functions. The current Board is comprised of 19 independent directors—community members from varied backgrounds, a number of whom have been associated with the auto industry. Additional duties of the CEO include being active in local, state-wide and national organizations related to the health care industry (e.g., Detroit Regional Chamber, Michigan Health and Hospital Association, American Hospital

Association, attending local community events and fund-raising events sponsored by the Beaumont Foundation). The CEO position is definitely not a 9-to-5 job.

As the newly appointed CEO, Gene Michalski worked tirelessly to prepare for this position—interviewing Board members, Foundation Board members, Trustees, and staff physicians to gather input as to what is good about Beaumont and what needs to change. He has a vision and has crafted a plan he refers to as the "Four Ps"—People, Plan, Practice and Purpose, with, again, the most important "P"—People, represented by patients—our reason for being here. We're just coming out of an economic crisis never before experienced by this organization. Mr. Michalski's goal is to bring people together to work toward one common result. He recognizes the importance of communication and he is attending various regularly held meetings, system-wide, to address physicians, managers, and nursing staff to share his vision and message and to gain additional input. He spends his lunch time in the employee cafeteria talking with patient family members and/or fellow employees to gain their perspective and he follows through on any concerns that are shared with him. He is a natural with people, who truly cares.

I've been very fortunate throughout my 38-year career at Beaumont, particularly in my time in "Administration." All of the individuals I've worked for (with) have been approachable, even-tempered—genuine, down-to-earth people.

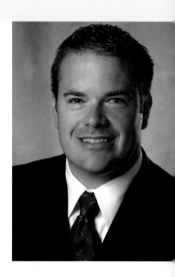

SHANE M. CERONE

Senior Vice President, President
Beaumont, Royal Oak

Shane M. Cerone is President of Beaumont Hospital, Royal Oak. He joined Beaumont, Royal Oak in 2008 as the hospital's senior vice president and chief operating officer. In 2009, Cerone succeeded hospital director John Labriola, who retired after 40 years of service with Beaumont.

Before joining Beaumont, Mr. Cerone spent 13 years at the University of Iowa Hospitals and Clinics, a 763-bed facility. While at the UIHC and the Iowa Carver College of Medicine, he held many leadership roles. From 2007 to 2009, he was the associate hospital director and reported to the chief executive officer. He is also an adjunct assistant professor in health management with the University of Iowa College of Public Health.

He holds a bachelor's degree in biology from Nebraska Wesleyan University and a master's degree in health administration from the University of Iowa.

In 2009, Crain's Detroit Business named him to their "40 under 40" listing. It honors the best and brightest in Southeast Michigan who have made their marks in business before age 40. He is a member of the American College of Healthcare Executives, American Hospital Association and the Association of American Medical Colleges.

Mr. Cerone envisions that in 2016, Beaumont Hospital–Royal Oak will be one of the nation's leading teaching hospitals and referral centers, ranking in the top 10th percentile nationally in quality, safety, service, employee engagement, efficiency and cost. "Patients, families and staff will feel a palpable difference in the care and the 'caring' they receive. More than a great place to work, the cornerstone of Beaumont's culture will be pride of ownership where all staff are skilled and dedicated to continuous improvement on a daily basis. This state will be achieved using Beaumont's adaptation of the Toyota Production System model and built upon the enterprising spirit of a large private medical staff model in partnership with Beaumont's core employed medical staff. Beaumont will excel in managing the patient's transition through the care system, and be known for outstanding communication with the patient and family that makes the patient experience outstanding and reliable. This culture will be instilled in the undergraduate, graduate and continuing medical education curricula, further serving our local, regional, and national community by preparing physicians and other clinicians with the skills required to provide exceptional care and to excel in the new health care system."

6 THE LADIES AND GENTLEMEN OF THE LAMP: BEAUMONT NURSES

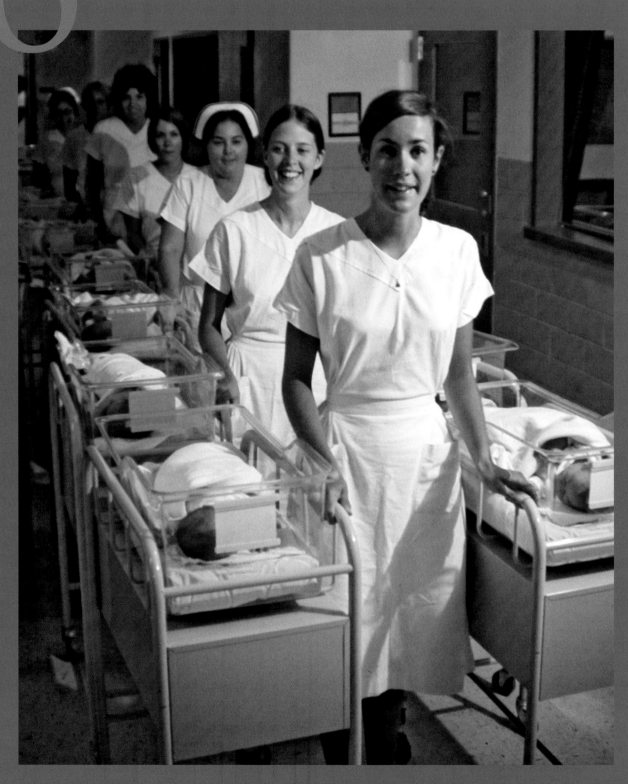

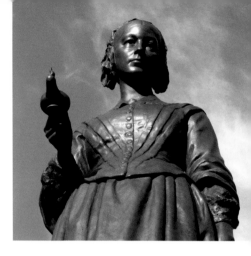

A fictional interview with

FLORENCE NIGHTINGALE
Mother Of Professional Nursing

Some time in the 1860's:

"Nursing is said to be a high calling, an honorable calling. But in what does that honor lie? In working hard during training to learn to do all things perfectly. The honor does not lie in putting on Nursing like your uniform. Honor lies in loving perfection, consistency, and in working hard for it . . . in being ready to work patiently, ready not to say, 'How clever I am,' but 'I am not yet worthy, and I will live to deserve to be called a Trained Nurse.

"I have no particular gifts. And I can honestly assure any young lady that if she will but try to walk, she will soon be able to run the appointed course. But then she must learn to walk first, and when she runs, she must run with patience. Most people don't even try to walk. But I would also say to all young ladies who are called to any particular vocation, qualify yourself as a man does for his work. Don't think you can undertake it otherwise.

"In the year 1820, I was born in the city of Florence in Italy, and named after that city. My parents were of the privileged class, my father being a landowner—William Nightingale of Embly Park, Hampshire, England, where we had dozens of gardeners and servants to do work for us. My father was my childhood companion. He taught me to speak Latin, Greek, French, Italian and German. Though I was a girl in the lacy age of Queen Victoria, he also taught me history and mathematics, and we engaged in discussions of philosophy.

"My mother, Fanny, was strict in the most upright English way, a firm Unitarian who dominated our household and held as her life's mandate to marry myself and my older sister off to elite young men of promise, and to create children in the Queen's example—ten or twelve of them, to populate the manors of the Realm just as the Queen populated the thrones of Europe.

"I met the Queen when I was 16, presented to her formally, doomed to become one of the lounging, dependent, pampered caged birds of the Empire. This, I knew, was not for me. At the age of 17, I felt a calling to a higher purpose—a purpose other than creating a family.

"The family? It is too narrow a field for the development of an immortal spirit, be that spirit male or female. The family uses people, not for what they are, not for what they are intended to be, but for what it wants for—its own uses. It thinks of

> *Lo! in that house of misery*
> *A lady with a lamp I see*
> *Pass through the glimmering gloom,*
> *And flit from room to room.*
>
> Henry Wadsworth Longfellow, 1857

them not as what God has made them, but as the something which it has arranged that they shall be.

"I have a moral—an active nature which requires satisfaction that I would not find in the life with a husband. I could be satisfied to spend a life with him in combing our different powers to some great object. I could not satisfy this nature by spending a life with him in making society and arranging domestic things.

"Thus driven, holding to my creed that a person must be single-minded and undistracted in order to concentrate upon a purpose, I rejected many suitors. At the age of 24, I declared my intent to become a nurse. My mother and sister were scandalized. Affluent young women should be wives and mothers of society, while nursing was restricted to servants and women of the bottle and the street.

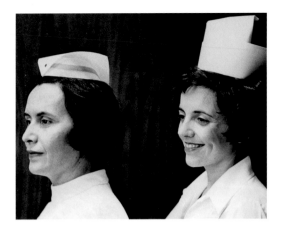

Nursing caps hold a place in nursing history as part of the professional uniform. Due to concerns of the cap's being a carrier of bacteria and with the increasing number of men in the nursing profession, the nurse's cap has gone away and has been replaced by nursing scrubs.

"While my family floated from opera to cotillion, I educated myself about nursing and mathematics, and I traveled. Europe, Greece, Egypt, the Nile . . . I wrote letters to my sister, enhancing my literary skills. While visiting a Lutheran community on the Rhein, I found a better reason to write; I observed the care of the sick and poor by a pastor and a deaconness, and began to studiously record their methods. Rather than writing about travel, I would write about nursing. Of course!

"In August of 1853, I became superintendent of the Institute for the Care for Sick Gentlewomen in London. That same year, Russia invaded Turkey, an act of distant aggression which would turn my little life on a new path. In 1854 news came from the war in the Crimea that British wounded were being kept in squalid conditions, without the comfort of a motherly hand.

"But the British Army rejected the services of women. Women were not supposed to engage in medical concerns. While this seems on its face a men's plot to hold women away from professional life, in fact it was men's way of shielding women, whom chivalry charged them to protect, from the gory underbelly of life and death, especially on the battlefield. Indeed, most women held the same opinion.

"Then the *London Times* published an account of our suffering sons, and the Army relented. I obtained permission to take my trained staff of 38 nurses on the 500-mile journey across the Black Sea to the British camp in Scutari. We set off for the Crimea.

"There, we found the most ghastly countenances. British soldiers lay crumpled and unwashed, still wearing uniforms starched with dried blood and dirt, receiving not even the elementaries of medical succor. The sanitation was appalling—there was none at all. During my first winter there, more than 4000 soldiers died, nine in ten without a battle wound. Cholera, malaria, dysentery, typhus, and other diseases of filth, crowding and poorly working sewers—those were our enemies."

THE LADY WITH THE LAMP

"In the quiet and coolness of night, I made my rounds. Guided by my Turkish fluted-paper lantern, I could work better and more efficiently at night, check my patients while they slept, feel their brows and look at their dressings, then silently move to the next bed, the next ward. Of course, they were not always asleep, but night made them drowsy and placid. I could pat their hands or touch their cheeks, smile or make a little joke, and they would sink back into their fevers knowing that at least one soul was on watch and they were not alone with their troubled dreams.

"Eventually our work drew the eyes of the public in England. The British government sent the Sanitary Commission to flush the sewers and improve ventilation. Blessedly, the unremitting death rate began to shrink. I was often given credit for this improvement, but I reject that accolade. Sanitary living conditions should be the most basic of human situations, and the most important. It should not be 'special' for hospitals or households to be clean.

"I collected evidence of my findings. While I was still in the Crimea, a fund was established in my name—the Nightingale Fund for Training of Nurses. After the war, I engaged many travels, but with a purpose. I visited hospitals and spas, recording methods and descriptions of wards, diets, health conditions, and details of patient care and sanitation.

"By 1859, I published my findings in the book 'Notes on Nursing'. The Nightingale Fund had grown enough for me to establish the Nightingale Training School at St. Thomas' Hospital, the world's first secular school for nurses, and my book would become the template for its curriculae. Every day, sanitary knowledge, or the knowledge of nursing, or in other words of how to put the (human) constitution in such a state as that it will have no disease, or that it can recover from disease, takes a higher place. It is recognized as the knowledge which everyone ought to have—distinct from medical knowledge—which only a profession can have."

Parts of the above interview were paraphrased from Florence Nightingale's writings and letters.

Florence Nightingale died in her sleep at the age of 90, in the year 1910. Her mathematical talents made her a pioneer in statistical studies and graphics, such as use of the pie chart; she invented the Nightingale Rose Diagram, to compare and illustrate data of mortality in a military hospital. She was the first female member of the Royal Statistical Society, and an honorary member of the American Statistical Association.

Her work and publications provided guidelines for nursing and the organization of field hospitals and treatment in the American Civil War. She rejected the drowsy lifestyle of Victorian noblewomen, but also did not support the goals of other women to become doctors or engage in the forefront of political change, and she disapproved of women's speaking in public. Instead, she used quiet influence to change legislation and attitudes toward women's aspirations to have professions, especially in the minds of women themselves. She believed women were enobled by having careers, but that women in the medical field should not be doctors. Instead, they should become excellent trained nurses, serving and nurturing at the bedside. For her, nursing was the higher calling.

DR. RICHARD HERBERT ON NURSES AT TROY:

"The nurses really bear the brunt of the responsibilities for medical care on their shoulders. If not for the strong nursing staff at Troy, the hospital wouldn't have been nearly as successful."

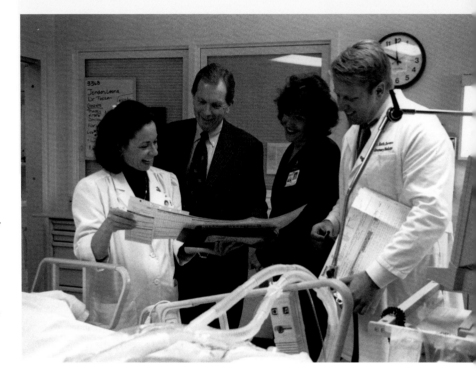

DOROTHY HANNA, R.N.

Registered Nurse
Assistant Hospital Director, 1988–1995
Beaumont, Royal Oak

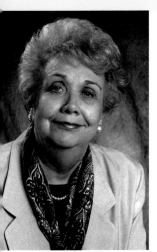

"I came to Beaumont in 1967 as a

nursing supervisor. I'm retired now, but I still keep my eye on things here. I had taught nursing at Henry Ford Hospital and had worked there for seventeen years, and had been a supervisor. I was at Henry Ford during the riots of 1967 and that was a real experience, I can tell you.

"Beaumont was expanding from 250 beds to 700. I picked up emergency, psychiatry, medical surgery, critical care, and pediatrics. Nurses were the jacks of all trades. Nurses cover everything and coordinate activity from all other departments at the patient's bedside. The doctors, the labs, the radiology—we all work as a team, but the nurses really do coordinate all that. The staff at the bedside really are the people who give an organization its reputation. That will never change. You can come into the 21st Century, but the patient is still the center of all we do.

"In 1972, we were looking at building the Troy hospital and were also looking at our North Tower. Nurses really did help design the patient care areas at both Troy and the North Tower. I'm a proponent of the idea that the people who work at the bedside and within departments should be involved in planning the flow of the patient care areas.

"For instance, the bathrooms, how are the toilets and showers going to be positioned? From housekeeping to the pharmacy, radiology to physicians, we worked as a team. When Dr. Diokno came, I was an Assistant Hospital Administrator and we were designing the lithotripsy room. The equipment came from Germany, so we had to work in terms of budgeting and work with the Certificates of Need through the Michigan State Department. And, of course, we had to work within

fire department codes, building codes, and so on. Everyone had a chance to elect representatives, like the head nurses, who were going to be accountable for the new areas. I'm sure they all got tired of my telling them this, but I kept saying, "You have to keep your eye on the core business. Our core business is the patient and the family."

NO ONE TURNED AWAY

"I think we were one of the first hospitals to work with interior designers, to have lower lighting, music, richer colors and artwork, and we even put an aquarium in our ER waiting room.

"We never turned patients away from our ER, ever. Everyone was treated regardless of his or her ability to pay or lack of insurance. There's a difference between not having health *insurance* and not getting health *care*. The media and many politicians have deliberately used 'care' when they mean 'insurance,' but that's not fair to the medical community. No one can be turned away from an emergency room.

"I won't even go into some of the things we've seen. Suburban hospitals often don't get credit as much as inner-city hospitals. They think we're some kind of country club. We really didn't get the recognition from the Michigan Nurses Association or the Detroit Nurses Association who thought that since we were out in the suburbs, we weren't nursing. I did not take kindly to that."

EVERY CONCERN, EVERY PATIENT

"I always told the staff that we had to take care of every concern a patient had. From maintenance to housekeeping, every employee is part of our team, because we're all dependent upon one another.

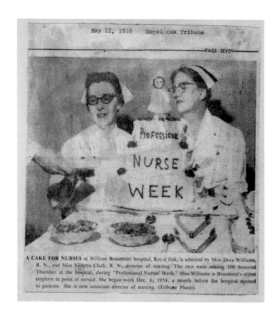

A CAKE FOR NURSES at William Beaumont hospital, Royal Oak, is admired by Miss Dora Williams, R. N., and Miss Violetta Clark, R. N., director of nursing. The two were among 106 honored Thursday at the hospital, during "Professional Nurses' Week." Miss Williams is Beaumont's oldest employe in point of service. She began work Dec. 6, 1954, a month before the hospital opened to patients. She is now associate director of nursing. (Tribune Photo).

"It's old-fashioned, but we treat people as we would like to be treated. If a patient says, 'Nurse, you're giving me the wrong medicine,' no one should be so arrogant as to say, 'I'm the nurse, so take what I give you.' Patients don't check their brains at the admitting office.

"We always had a full staff throughout the hospital, seven days a week, 365 days of the year. Whenever I was in, I always went to all the departments to make sure everything was operational during off-hours, and I always made a point of talking to the staff, so they knew somebody was hearing them. Meetings in the Board room are fine, but I'm here for one purpose and that purpose is the patient.

"I have an investment here even though I'm retired. Having been both on the floors and in administration, I understand how difficult it is to put together a budget and I know where the financial people are coming from. I used to say to them, 'Come and make rounds with me. I'd like you to take a look. Let me show you what I'm talking about. The view from the other side of the pillow is very different from what you do every day.'"

ANANIAS C. DIOKNO, M.D.
ON BEAUMONT'S NURSES

"Beaumont would not be successful without outstanding nurses and outstanding health care providers other than nurses. This is a team business. Doctors alone will not be successful if they don't have nurses and technicians beside them. We make sure we have as good nurses as we have doctors; actually they are as respected by our patients as our doctors are. In fact, sometimes they are more trusted than doctors, because nurses do most of the direct patient care.

"Since nurses are with the patients, they are the ones who are executing our plans, who connect with us, who tell us what's going on. We want them to be the best. We were the first Magnet hospital in the State of Michigan.

"The Magnet Designation is given by the American Nurses Association in the United States. They develop criteria the hospital must pass in order to be designated 'Magnet,' which is the highest award that the hospital can get in terms of demonstrating the best nursing service. Not only the delivery of patient care, but also in terms of whether the nurses are continuing to improve their performance, continuing to investigate and discover knowledge in education and research, helping one another in terms of training and teaching, and providing an all-around service. There is a very stringent accreditation committee that comes and reviews the hospital. Beaumont, Royal Oak was the first one in the State of Michigan. Beaumont, Troy recently received the designation, so we are very proud of that."

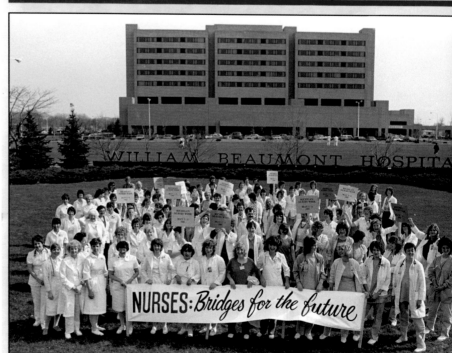

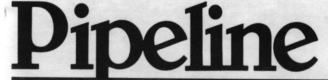

Pipeline

May 6, 1985

WILLIAM BEAUMONT HOSPITA

NURSES: *Bridges for the future*

Over 100 nurses from throughout the hospital discover that more really is the merrier as they gather to celebra Michigan Nurses Week, May 5 to 11. (photo by Elizabeth DeBeliso)

Celebrate Nurse Week!

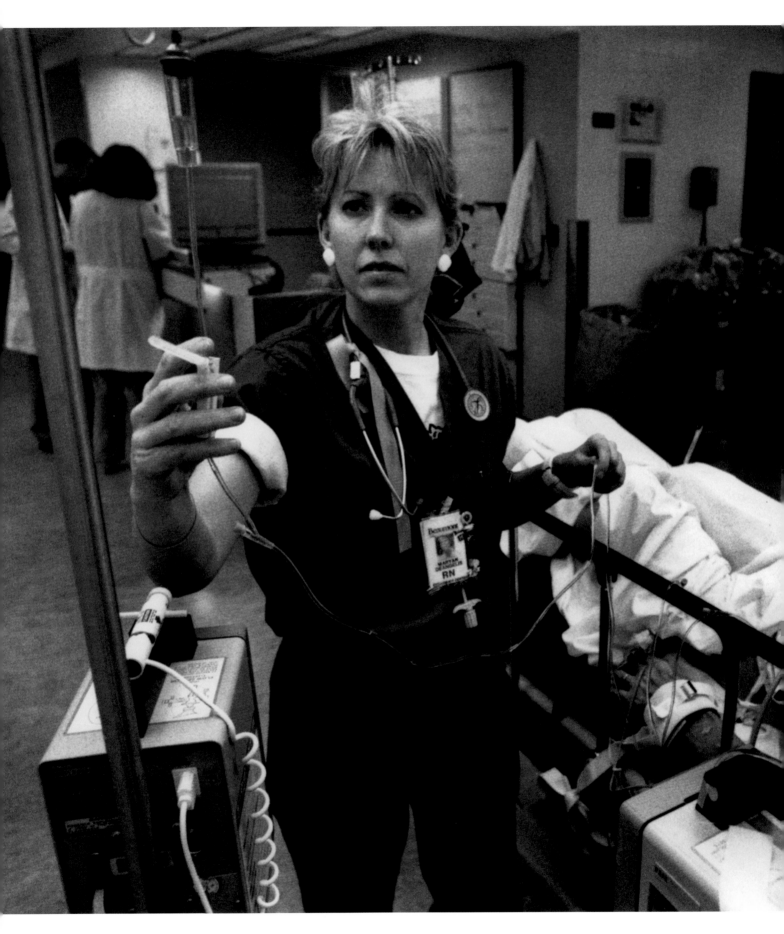

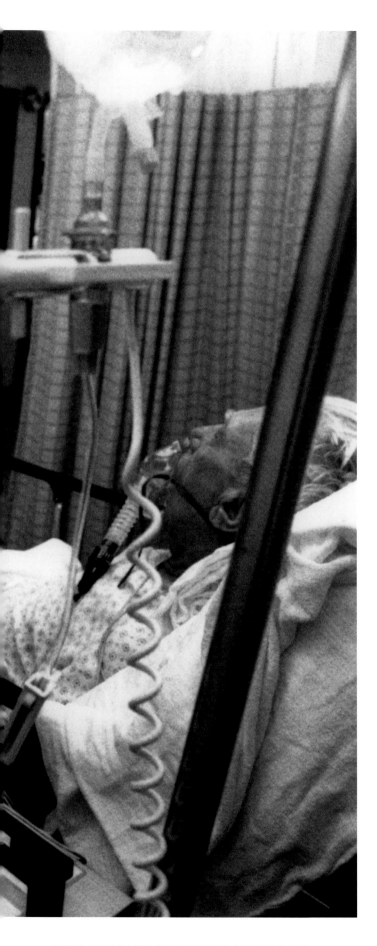

The mission of nursing

at Beaumont Hospitals is to maintain excellence in professional nursing practice, service, quality and research while promoting the needs of patients and the communities we serve. It is the vision of nursing to strive for excellence. Nurses are well rooted in the efforts of a safe environment for patients and staff. In the current health care climate nurses have expanded opportunities. The future of nursing will be greatly influenced on the nurse's ability to practice to the full extent of their education and training, achievement of higher levels of education and training, and full partnerships with physicians and other health care professional in redesigning health care.

KAY BEAUREGARD, R.N., M.S.A.
Interim Chief Nurse Officer
Vice President, Quality and Patient Safety
Beaumont, Royal Oak

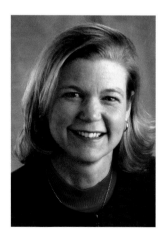

VAL GOKENBACH, D.M., R.N., R.W.J.F.

Vice-President and Chief Nurse Executive, 2006–2010
Beaumont, Royal Oak

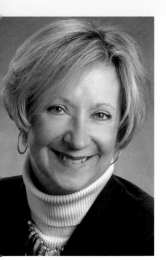

"Nursing is not what it used to be.

The Royal Oak Chief Nurse Executive is responsible for the whole nursing division at the Royal Oak Hospital, and the many ancillary departments that somewhat interface with nursing. The staff is big, at about 3,500. Nursing alone has a budget of about $350 million. Troy and Grosse Pointe Chief Nurse Executives although separate from Royal Oak work together corporately for policies and procedures for any big systems, like the EPIC installation goal line. There is a very good working relationship between the three divisions.

What does a nurse have to be in our big wired society? Nurses have to be almost space-age computer professionals They also handle emotional content, the physiological content, and are responsible for everything in the unit.

"Younger doctors know how to handle computers and electronic medical records because they've had computers since they were six, but the older docs just don't, so nurses have to be safety nets. For older doctors, the people working for them can be four generations away, so they have the silent generation, the baby-boomers, the generation-Xers, and the milliennium babies that are growing up right now.

"We brought the nurses along before the doctors with the Electronic Medical Records when we saw what a big installation it was going to be. First the billing and registration process went live, then the nurses, then the physicians, and now the ambulatory network and surgical services will go last."

"Nurses have always been a safety net and the advocate for the patient just by virtue of our career dedication—to take care of patients. Physicians will visit the patients, but it's a very short period of time through the course of the day, and once the physician goes, the nursing staff stays with the patient for the rest of the day and night. Nurses rescue the patients if there are changes in medical conditions. Nurses are responsible to find discrepancies in orders, medications and diet. The nurses make sure the patients are ready for procedures and that those procedures are done well and that the patients are cared for well after the procedures."

MAGNET-IZED

"There's a lot of excitement working at Beaumont. We've always tried to be on the cutting edge and to move forward. The nursing at Royal Oak is a Magnet organization, and Troy is now Magnet. The Royal Oak division was the first Magnet hospital in Michigan, which happened in 2004. We were the 100th Magnet hospital in the country, so Magnet came out here for a big celebration. Then we were successfully redesignated in 2008, and expect to redisignate again in 2012.

"Magnet is an accreditation that a hospital gets through the American Association for Credentialing and the American Nurses Association for Credentialing. They developed a way to evaluate nurses so quality nursing organizations could be identified and recognized. It's the gold star of nursing organizations. They assess things like collaboration, empowerment, research, and how the nurses think about the hospital. When Magnet comes in they don't talk to me; they talk to the staff. And they come in around the clock—midnight, breakfast, lunch, and dinner. So we're very excited about being a Magnet organization.

"The physicians are part of that, because of collaboration. Nurses have to collaborate well, or Magnet will pick up on that. Nobody can be the grumpy nurse down the hall."

A GREAT PLACE TO BE A NURSE

"Here at Beaumont, we've always had a very low turnover rate in comparison to the national average. I'm proud of that.

"When I started in nursing, my first love was critical care. I worked in critical care units and open-heart units. In those days, a patient would come in for preparations and stay three days for the prep, then have surgery, and stay another week. Now, people are prepping at home, coming in for surgery, and often going home the same day. The people staying in hospitals are really very sick. People in the ICUs are desperately ill.

"I think we're going to need more of a pipeline for nursing. How are we going to achieve that? There is a great deal of discussion out in the nursing community. Should nurses and nursing students go for two-year degrees, three-year degrees, or could we facilitate a four-year degree where we can get people through faster? There are also people coming into nursing as their second degrees. People in arts, journalism, music can't find jobs, so they go back to school in second-degree programs designed specifically for people who already have undergraduate degrees. They pick up the types of classes they need—the sciences if they didn't get those. They go into a strict two-year program and within two years you have another degree. I find that the second-degree students are excellent learners. They're more mature, more committed, and driven."

REACHING OUT

"We really try to reach out to the community. We're linking up with radio personality and author Mitch Albom, and helping him with his clinic. He has a free clinic in Highland Park called SAY, 'Super All Year' clinic. It's named that because Mitch wanted to expand on the efforts that took place during the Super Bowl festivities, where the homeless were taken from the streets, fed, and allowed to watch the Super Bowl. He wanted to provide a year-long service for the homeless, so he created this clinic and called it Super All Year. When I heard about this, I thought, 'Beaumont can help in more ways than just nursing.' I knew our nurses would participate because they're all happy to do that kind of work, but then I thought that Beaumont could do even more. We made a plan to do their lab work. Within a week, we were doing their radiology.

"We're also working with the Detroit Rescue Mission and have somewhat adopted that clinic. Nurses and doctors volunteer, we give them all our old mattresses, and much more.

"We opened another community center called Safety City. It's a program designed for kids to teach kids about trauma and how to be safe, and we do other programs there too."

"I particularly like the support given to nurses at Beaumont, and the more active collaboration between nurses and physicians. I like the culture of safety and quality, and the determination to be number one in those areas."

DEAN CAPUTO, R.N.

Registered Nurse
Administrative Manager, 5 North
Beaumont, Royal Oak

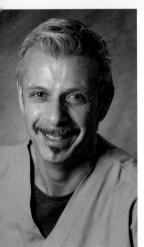

"I am a guy. Do I multi-task?

"That's the kind of question that pops into the minds of most women when they meet a male nurse. Patients will say, 'Oh, you're a male nurse?' No, I'm a nurse.

"The word 'nurse' has come through history with a female connotation. As soon as a male goes into nursing, you're automatically gay, automatically feminine, or 'not a man.' That was definitely the stereotype, but it's starting to change. Male nurses have no problem with female patients. Body parts are body parts; once you've seen one, you've seen them all. It's never been a discussion for me, unless the patient is very old or just has her own problems with male nurses, but it doesn't come up that often. It's hardly even considered. We're very discrete and stress privacy. I've had no complaints.

"There are cultures that don't allow a man to touch a woman, and we just get female nurses for that patient. Some men don't want female nurses bathing them. We try to be in tune to that and just swap the assignment. I try never to put two male nurses on an assignment, but always a male and a female."

"I've been a nurse for 25 years. Back then, I didn't know what to do with my life. I was raised in Michigan, but not interested in the auto industry, and was working as a coordinator in the ER at St. John's Hospital, and watching what nurses were doing. I saw that I could make money in the field. Yes, I care for people, but I also wanted to make a decent living. I went into nursing school and I've never regretted it. Working in a predominantly women's field can be difficult because of the labeling. Male nurses have to set a certain ground rule. We're not just here to help lift patients.

"I've been here at Beaumont for over 20 years, and worked my way up to being a manager in a unit. In 5 North, we care for surgical, cardio-vascular, thoracic, trauma, and vascular patients. When I'm

hiring, I try to change the mix by hiring more men. The dynamics have changed, and it's so nice when there's more of a mix. Women watch how they're acting, and it can be surprising how compassionate and caring the men can be. I have 140 staff, and when I started 90% of them were women. I think it's about 70% now. If I could be 50/50, that would be great, because it's more like real life. A healthy mix cuts down on the things that happen when there are all women or all men in a given situation.

"Fathering has changed over the years. My father worked all the time and wasn't visible in the house that much, but I've been very involved in my family. I worked nights, so I could do all the things I wanted to do with my kids. My son swears to this day that my being available during the day was the great thing; of course he didn't realize how many hours I was working at night. I love that I had the flexibility to do that.

"I always considered the financial aspect. People like to think that nursing is a 'calling,' and there's a degree of that, of course—we like to take care of people, we're social types, nurses are co-dependent, and cold fish don't go into nursing. But I also had a family to raise and a life to live, and I looked at the income. Everybody looks at that when choosing a field of work, but for some reason people don't think that nurses do.

"Since I've changed the mix some, the patients love it. Female patients respond very well to the young male nurses coming into the field. Sometimes it's like the nurses are their sons, or they just like the attention, and there's nothing wrong with that. Many older women absolutely insist on having a male doctor, even a male OB/GYN, but they don't want a male nurse helping them take a bath. They've had the images stuck in their heads for decades, and it's in the culture. We don't try to change them. We're here for their comfort."

THE MIDDLE-MEN AND -WOMEN

"Nursing is really the glue that holds everything together, but the respect goes to the doctor. However, doctors are beginning to respect nurses. It's a growing factor. Younger doctors today are learning how much nurses really do and that medical treatment should be more of a collaborative effort than just, 'I said so.'

"The old joke about doctors' thinking they're gods and everybody else is here to assist them comes from the fact that we ask doctors to do godlike things and they have to have superhuman self-confidence. But they also have to treat the people with respect who have their ears and eyes out for your patients 24 hours a day, 7 days a week, when you can't be there. We're the ones who make sure you're called if something changes.

"Beaumont is really trying to change that focus and make us more of a team. Our philosophy has changed and we're much more cohesive.

"I have a long history of working in the ICU. Being a guy, I never had a problem speaking up. The older nurses were trained to say, 'Yes, doctor,' 'Yes, doctor.' I couldn't do that. I challenged. When I was first starting out, there weren't many male nurses, and I was very loud-mouthed. I'd stick up for my patients and also for what I believed. I used to get frustrated because the residents would come through and when they didn't know anything, they were our best friends. We'd teach them, assist them, show them how to do things, and the next year when they come through, they treated us like garbage because they thought they knew everything and didn't need our help anymore. Well, we let them know this wasn't going to work anymore. If we're going to help them, when they come back they need to have respect for us."

ALL DAY, ALL NIGHT, ALL THE TIME

"One of the difficulties of nursing as a career is that it is a 24/7 job. Somebody has to be here all the time—nights, Saturdays, Sunday, Christmas, Easter, Hannukah—and we all have to do it. We give up our family time, our personal time, and a regular sleep schedule. Now that I'm a manager, I really try to be sensitive and fair. The hours are part of the job, but I want to be sensitive about what my staff is giving up. We may find that our kids are proud of us and get a good work ethic from seeing us go to work while other people are having time off. I love working nights because I feel so autonomous.

"Things are getting much better. Nurses today do technical things at such a high level that doctors have no choice but to accept us in medical partnership. Now that we're moving to a more wired technology with Electronic Medical Records and super-elite computer capabilities and medical equipment, some of the older nurses are just retiring, while for the younger nurses and doctors, it's a whiz. And they're teaching the doctors. It's a hard transition, especially for the older doctors, some of whom have never worked with a keyboard at all, but I really have to give these guys credit for trying something that's so new to them. Nurses are helping them. Nurses are becoming the hingepin around which everything else revolves."

"People don't really relate to what nurses do until they're patients in hospitals. We don't just pass bedpans. We're the eyes and ears of the doctor, and we are your advocates. We watch those subtle clues that are going on during the night when nobody's there, then act to keep you safe and healthy. It's a wonderful profession. I encourage more men to go into it. We're a big part of the reason people leave the hospital and go home and get back into society."

5.4% of the 2.1 million registered nurses in the United States are male. Men make up 13% of all new nursing students. Here a male nurse administers to a patient.

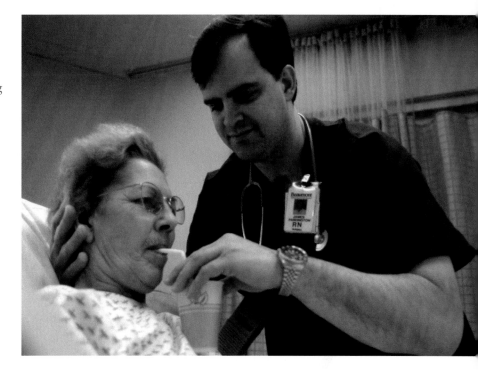

7

THE GROWTH OF ACADEMICS: THE MADER ERA

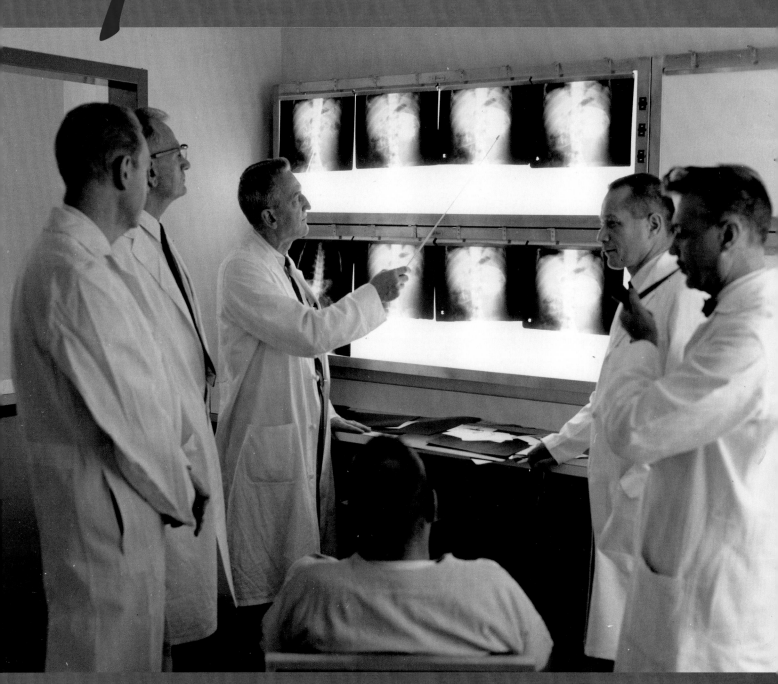

What Kind of Hospital is This?

William Beaumont Hospital was conceived as a community hospital of 238 beds, with primarily local doctors, mostly private practitioners. Underlying that goal, however, was a bigger plan gelling in the minds of the founders. That bigger idea was displayed, literally, by the foundation of the building. Though the original hospital was a five-floor structure, a thick-enough foundation was laid to support ten floors. They knew. Even before it was built, before it even had its ultimate name, Beaumont Hospital was ordained to grow.

The hospital was crowded with patients even in its first three years, and expansions took place in the late 1950's and '60's to accommodate a burgeoning local population—more stories, more offices, a bigger emergency room. Those changes reflected more people, more health problems, more accidents, but not until Dr. Ivan Mader became the Corporate Medical Director in 1970 did the hospital grow not only in size, but in the types of medicine that could be practiced there. Dr. Mader had his own ideas for the growth of the hospital, and facilitated the birth of myriad new departments. Beaumont was taking long strides toward becoming a medical center for the modern era.

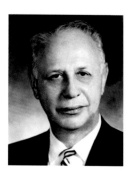

Harold W. Longyear
Chief of Staff
1965–1970

TOM THOMPSON
ON THE EARLY LEADERS

"**D**r. Ivan Mader and Dr. Yoshikazu Morita had been full-time faculty members at Wayne State Medical School. When Beaumont decided to upgrade its teaching programs in 1969-70, the Board of Directors decided to hire senior faculty from a recognized medical school. There was a third doctor, Dr. McCaughey, and these made up the three prominent Wayne Medical School faculty who decided to leave there completely and come to Beaumont. Dr. Mader became Chief of Staff, Dr. McCaughey was a GI specialist and Director of Medical Education, and Dr. Morita, a nephrologist. They were all board-certified internists. With their arrival, Beaumont moved quickly toward a sudden surge of growth in new departments."

EVEN EARLIER
"Prior to Dr. Mader, Dr. Harold Longyear had been a part-time Chief of Staff. This was before the top physician administrator was called 'Chief Medical Officer.' Before Dr. Longyear, Admiral Scarney was part-time Chief of Staff. There were a couple before that. They were very part-time administrators, and essentially full-time practitioners. When Dr. Mader came, he came in as a full-time medical administrator. He started to aggressively hire full-time chiefs—not just as medical educators, but full-time chiefs of departments. That was in the 70's. He held the position for twelve years, growing the hospital department by department."

We have examples like Dr. O'Neill in cardiology, who was on the rise. He wasn't a superstar yet, but he was on the way there. He developed Beaumont's cardiology, and it grew and prospered. The other cardiologists could have said, 'Well, he's taking away from us,' but they didn't. They also grew and prospered. He brought in so many new programs that it helped the other doctors in the department.

IVAN MADER, M.D.

Vice-President of Education, Beaumont,
Royal Oak, 1962–1969
Corporate Medical Director, 1970–1982

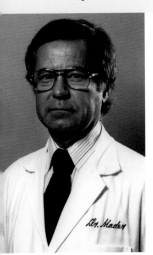

"In 1962, I sensed that Beaumont was

on the brink of something big and had terrific potential. I was the Director of Medical Education then. The hospital had been open about eight years and had only two approved residencies–medicine and OB-GYN. Surgery was on probation and approved for only three years instead of the normal four. The irony is that Beaumont was not recognized then as a good place to get training or to work as a physician.

"By 1966, we had thirteen interns. From a portion of the fees from reading electrocardiograms, I had established a cardiology fund to support fellowships, equipment, research, and cardiac nurses. There were no accredited cardiology specialists at all. A couple of general internists were self-styled cardiologists, but I wanted the Board-certified cardiologists to read all the EKGs. That action was controversial. The internists insisted, 'We can read EKGs; we always have.'

"It was always a chore to convince people that if a new service prospered, with new personnel and new departments, then all of us would prosper together. The prospect of change is always threatening, and it's no different in the field of medicine."

"I was named Corporate Medical Director in 1970. We established a retinal surgery program with laser capability and reactivated the Beaumont Research Institute. The Institute had been organized in 1966, but had been inactive. We also established the Neuro-Education Center in pediatrics. The same year, Beaumont hosted a radio-pharmaceutical workshop which attracted nationwide participation. The governing Board then made a controversial decision that Board certification in a specialty

would be mandatory for a staff appointment. The medical staff did the vetting and the Board held the power of final approval–a situation that often led to complaining and controversy.

"I thought we needed a dialysis program, but this led to more controversy. Some argued, 'We don't need renal dialysis at Beaumont. We've gotten along without it for years. Why should we need it now?' Nevertheless Dr. Yoshikazu Morita and I were convinced there was a need in the community and we pushed ahead.

"The original KOLFF Kidney Dialysis Machine was large and cumbersome. Today, the dialysis units are much more compact. What a job it was to get that original machine ready to use! Cellophane tubing was used for the conduit of the blood, and there were frequent leaks. The dialysis program at Beaumont has flourished, and today it is an exemplary part of the hospital's program, especially considering that there were once people who thought it wasn't needed.

"We began offering a series of seminars at Beaumont about electronics in cardiology, drawing a nation-wide audience. By that time, I had brought some Board-certified cardiologists from Wayne State University despite great resistance. In 1972, we developed the Audiology Service and did the first kidney transplant. We established a neonatology unit, were approved for an orthopaedic surgery residency, and established a small-animal laboratory at the Research Institute. In 1973, we instituted full-time, salaried physicians in the Emergency Center. Prior to that, emergency duty was assigned by rotation or on a voluntary basis, which was not conducive to consistently good care.

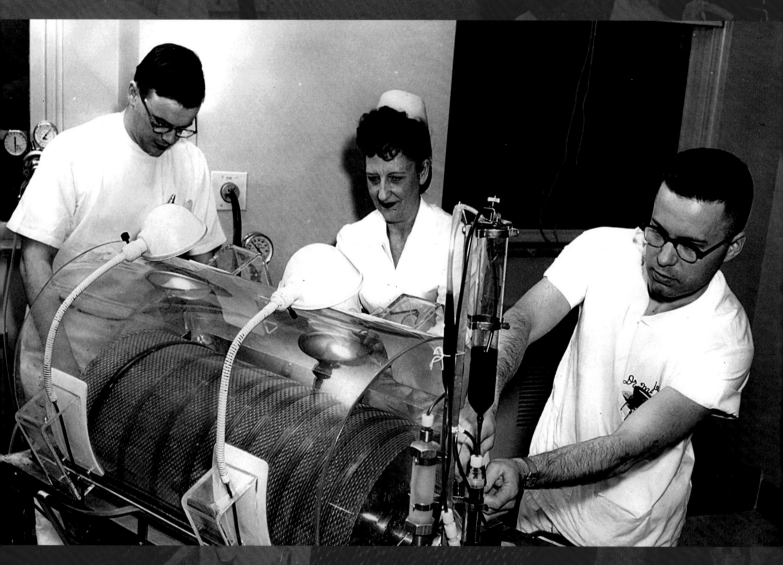

One of the early artificial kidney
machines. Dr. Mader is on far right.

Handwritten: *Memo to myself*
Mader

SUBJECT: DEPARTMENT HEAD MEETING

A Department Head Meeting was held on December 11, 1972, at the Troy Hilton. In attendance were Drs. Grekin, Byberg, Arcari, Ingold, Welsh, Morita, Kurnetz, Margulis and Mader.

University affiliation was discussed and it was generally agreed that, while we should continue to explore all avenues with respect to Wayne State University, Michigan State University and the University of Michigan, that there seemed little ~~likelihood~~ likelihood of anything concrete developing with those institutions in the foreseeable future. It was concluded to continue to talk with the Oakland Medical Education Association, keeping in mind always the interests of William Beaumont Hospital as first and primary. It was also agreed to begin exploratory talks with Dr. Dawson and Oakland University to see whether or not any possibility of medical school development could occur at Oakland University, either as a freestanding instutition or possibly along the "Berkley" plan wherein the University would provide the pre-clinical or basic science years and a large independent hospital the clinical or ward training.

Dr. Mader provided this memo to document that the idea of Beaumont as part of a medical school started as early as 1972.

"Also in 1973, we started a Pediatric Intensive Care Unit, and a plastic surgery residency was approved. There was a major expansion of the cardiovascular laboratory. In 1974, we received approval for a nuclear medicine residency program and established both an otolaryngology and urology laboratory. We had an international symposium of hip pathology, and were approved for a therapeutic radiology residency.

"By 1975, we had 12 approved residency programs--medicine, surgery, OB-GYN, pediatrics, urology, orthopaedics, plastic surgery, diagnostic radiology, nuclear medicine, therapeutic radiology, clinical pathology, and anatomic pathology. For some time I had been urging the Chief of Urology to apply for a residency program. He was nationally known in the field, but resisted going for a residency program because he thought Beaumont was not yet worthy. So I invited the Professor of Urology from Wayne State to give a talk at Beaumont and that proved to be the right motivation. Within a month, we had a residency in urology.

A GLIMMER IN DR. MADER'S EYE

"On September 11, 1972, I made a memo to myself. I'd been talking to Dr. Dawson at Oakland University about whether there was any possibility of a medical school at Oakland University. This was the very first time anyone thought about Beaumont's having a medical school affiliation, and I think it is the first time anyone considered it at Oakland University."

AND THE DECADE IS ONLY HALF OVER

"Around 1975, we did the first open-heart surgery at Beaumont. We were also approved for colon-rectal surgery and ophthalmology residencies. Again, when I recruited a colon-rectal specialist for the staff, the general surgeons were up in arms. They had always done that type of surgery and they resented my bringing in specialists. But we were on a track to improve and expand our medical capabilities, and specialists were essential for that.

"We were also building the hospital in Troy, which would open in 1977. In 1978, the family practice residency was approved. The 1970s had been a decade of expansion and innovation for William Beaumont Hospital, and by the end of the decade, it was Beaumont *Hospitals*, plural.

"In 1981, the Ferndale Clinic was opened as a means for Beaumont to reach out to the community. In 1982, Beaumont was approved for a residency in physical medicine and rehabilitation. In 1983, we applied for an Emergency Medicine residency and it was subsequently approved. We had research grants at that time of $300,000, up from zero.

"Then, on a Monday morning in 1983, I was summarily fired—just after being reappointed as Medical Director by the Board. It came as a complete surprise, since I had just been reappointed.

"Why was I fired? I was told that they didn't think that I had the vision or the drive for the position. Considering the bountiful growth of the hospital through the 1970s, there were obviously other politics involved. Any time one is building a large institution, or transforming a small one into a larger one, there will be concerns, complaints, and controversies. Some peope wanted to remain mavericks within the system, and I insisted that they abide by the corporations rules and by-laws, including new rules, and rules that were evolving.

"Then there was the whole new hospital in Troy. Many of those self-styled 'mavericks' went to Troy to supposedly, 'do it again.' By that time, however, Beaumont had a certain reputation, certain standards and rules, and the hospital in Troy had to comply if it was going to be a Beaumont Hospital. It fell to me to rein them in and assure Troy's success.

"I've thought about this a lot over the years, particularly the last two or three years since I have retired. When I began at Beaumont, John Poole was Chairman of the Board and his vision was that the hospital should grow to be a major medical center. He told me, 'Ivan, tell me what you need and I'll get the money for it.'

"We worked well together, but I also rubbed a few people the wrong way. That's the way things go sometimes. But I'll compare what happened in the years of my tenure at Beaumont against anyone else's accomplishments.

AND THE REST IS HISTORY

"I didn't leave Beaumont, but stayed and practiced internal medicine until I retired in 2007. Internal medicine is a wonderful field because one sees everything in one form or another. The Internist is the doctor who decides whether the patient is sick. Then you proceed one way or another; send the patient this way or that, for certain treatment, or perhaps to a specialist, whatever is needed. Sometimes a specialist's vision is too narrow. We certainly need specialists, but many patients can end up with too many specialists and no doctor. An Internist gets to know a patient over time and should have a broad knowledge of medicine to serve that patient's needs.

"I was in the right place at the right time. I believed that if pediatrics flourished, if cardiology flourished, if urology flourished, then Beaumont Hospital and I would flourish as well. During my tenure as Corporate Medical Director, Beaumont grew from a community hospital into a major two-hospital teaching and research institution that is now university affiliated. I am very proud of what I accomplished at Beaumont. I also must acknowledge and give credit to the superb medical administrative team that offered support and encouragement during those years of growth."

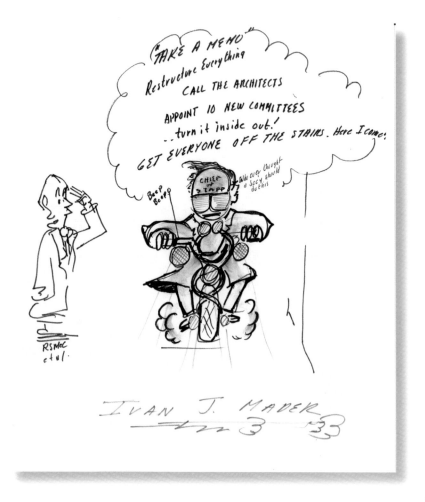

YOSHIKAZU MORITA, M.D.

Former Chair, Department of Internal Medicine
Beaumont, Royal Oak

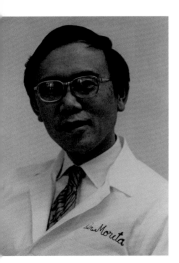

From Dr. Carl Lauter

"When I came to Beaumont, we didn't

have a huge cancer operation at that time the way they did at Wayne State Medical School. Bone marrow transplant is one of the rare things we don't do at Beaumont. One of my teachers at Wayne State was Dr. Yoshikazu Morita. Dr. Morita was the head of the Nephrology Division, the kidney division, a leader in that field, certainly in Michigan. He was one of the first people to do dialysis and was involved in some of the early transplant programs in the Detroit area.

"Dr. Morita is a very important person in the history of Beaumont. He was one of my role models. He was a brilliant clinician and teacher, tough as nails, totally demanding of hard work, and he would embarrass the heck out of you if you did bad work, but you could learn very much from him and if you emulated him, you would be a good doctor. Sometime later, he came to Beaumont and was appointed Chief of the Medical Department.

"Unfortunately, Dr. Morita had an unexpected death. Dr. Gerald Weintraub was Vice-Chief of the department. When he was going through Dr. Morita's papers, he found a note under 'Work in Progress' that said 'Recruit Lauter.' Dr. Weintraub moved up to Chief of Medicine, so now the Vice-Chief position was open, and that job appealed to me.

"Dr. Morita was very important to Beaumont. Until Morita took the job, Beaumont was still a local hospital with doctors who were locally known. When Morita came aboard, suddenly Beaumont had a major figure at the head of the Medical Department, a person with a national and international reputation, who was a known leader in his field, regarded and respected by people in the kidney field all over the world. He was a huge step forward. Suddenly they had a face on the Department of Medicine who was a major personage. He was one of the people brought in from the outside to take over a department and bring it into the 21st Century."

GERALD WEINTRAUB, M.D., WHO SUCCEEDED DR. MORITA AS CHAIR OF INTERNAL MEDICINE, ON PRIVATE AND SALARIED DOCTORS

"One feature about Beaumont that everyone should appreciate is that we built a cadre of full-time doctors, employed by the hospital, and private-practice doctors who are self-employed. Beaumont was out front with the blended model. There has always been tension in the medical profession between salaried doctors and private practitioners. Beaumont manages to blend them. Not always harmoniously, and there is some competition, but we have doctors here who would otherwise be full-time at the University of Michigan, Wayne State, or Henry Ford, because they don't want to be in private practice. They want to practice medicine, have a good income, but don't want to run an office, send out bills, or be employers. We recognize that.

"I was involved in recruiting some full-time doctors. It's difficult, because we want to be fair to the private practitioners and not alienate them. Some of the palace coups we've had over the years have had to do with the private practitioners feeling they weren't getting a fair shake. They're small businessmen, have offices, pay rent or own a building, have to get bills out, deal with insurance companies, while employed doctors don't have to deal with all that.

"Tension has always been there, but we work it out. Beaumont really is an outstanding hospital."

CARL LAUTER, M.D.

Professor of Internal Medicine, Oakland University
William Beaumont School of Medicine.
Director, Division of Allergy and Clinical Immunology.
Department of Medicine, Beaumont, Royal Oak

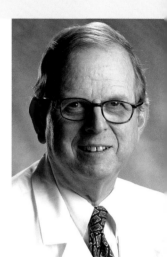

"I've been at Beaumont since July of

1980. I came from Wayne State Medical School, where I was on the teaching faculty. I'm an internist, and my field is adult patients' infectious disease, which is a specialty of internal medicine.

"The Assistant Chief of the Medical Department and the Assistant Program Director at that time, Dr. Gerald Weintraub, recruited me to Beaumont. I came here with the idea that I would learn the job, and eventually take over his job of running the Medical Department, which I did in 1982, when he was promoted to Associate Medical Director. I became the Program Director of the Internal Medicine Residency and the Chief of the Department of Medical Services, which includes internal medicine, internal medicine specialties, and related fields such as dermatology, neurology, psychiatry, and physical medicine and rehabilitation.

"Over the years, the job became more onerous, with more paperwork. I was canceling patient appointments, canceling assignments, canceling teaching jobs, just so I could be in more meetings. Finally my bosses told me I would have to give up teaching and patients and become a full-time administrator in order to do the job right. I thought about it for several weeks, then resigned.

"That was 1992, and I was 52. I gave them a year's notice, and they kept me on as a teacher/administrator and gave me a job as head of the Adult Allergy Division. It was a position I've held ever since, one of relatively little administrative duty, so I was able to do my other duties as well."

"Beaumont wanted infectious disease specialists, and I was originally trained in infectious disease. There was only one other salaried full-time doctor in the Infectious Disease (ID) Division, Dr. James Colville, who was one of the first people to have a university-style appointment in Beaumont hospital, other than people who might be department heads. Even the Corporate Medical Director, now called the Chief Medical Officer, was not full-time. The director then was Ivan Mader, the head doctor of everything at Beaumont, but he continued to have a private practice and outside consultation jobs with health insurance companies, and that was considered okay. Today it would not be considered okay, but it's an evolving system. Today it would be a conflict of interest to have outside positions and also working for a hospital that pays you a nice salary and expects you to be here working full-time. Dr. Colville was a model.

"Dr. Colville and I had to arrange how we would work together on infectious disease, since we were now two salaried doctors at Beaumont Hospital, I with administrative duties in the Department of Medicine and he with administrative duties in the Department of Pathology and Microbiology.

"In the early 1980's Dr. Colville asked to be relieved of the Infectious Disease duties for personal reasons, so I took over the duties of the Chief of the Medical Department and the program director of the residency, and for a couple of years I was also running the ID division."

IN THE BEGINNING

"I went to Wayne State as an undergrad, brown-bagging it and taking the bus within the City of Detroit. I was accepted to other medical schools, but turned them down because we couldn't afford for me to live outside the home. My father had died, leaving my mother a widow with three children. With loans

"I really fell in love with infectious disease." — Dr. Lauter

and scholarships, I got through Wayne State Medical School in 1965, did my internship at Henry Ford Hospital, a year of residency at Detroit Receiving Hospital, and then 'volunteered' in the U.S. Air Force. If you didn't volunteer, you got drafted, and there was a physician draft, so I volunteered. I spent two years doing internal medicine work for the Air Force in Illinois. It was actually an excellent experience.

"I really fell in love with infectious disease."

"Infectious disease was attractive to me because I love microbiology and infectious disease as applied microbiology. I loved studying about germs and the immune system. In the Air Force, we dealt with young people and the most common illnesses were infections. I really fell in love with infectious disease.

"I joined the faculty of Wayne State from 1973 to 1979 as an infectious disease specialist assigned to the Cancer Department, so I spent my time primarily being the head infectious disease consultant and coordinator with the Oncology Department. I became more heavily involved with cancer-related infectious diseases. It became a sub-specialty of mine in the field of infectious disease, dealing with what we call immuno-compromised post-infections.

"When I did my training in allergy and immunology, that was partly because I wanted to be a better infectious disease doctor, not necessarily an allergist or immunologist. It tracks back to the work I did with cancer patients. I also deal with people who are born with immune deficiencies. Most of my teaching is not in the classroom, but in small group sessions or at the bedside."

BEAUMONT AS A COMMUNITY RESOURCE

"I run a clinic for immunodeficiency in adults. There aren't many immunologists for adults. Most of the immunodeficiency that isn't caused by medicine is taken care of by pediatricians because its congenital. The Wayne State Allergy and Immunology Program has a huge pediatric immunology clinic, but almost no adult patients. Several years ago, the program director there arranged for their trainees in the Wayne Program to spend Thursday mornings with me in my clinic, so we at Beaumont are a resource for the community. We're involved in teaching throughout the Metropolitan Detroit area.

"Over the years, the Infectious Disease Division, started by Dr. Colville, joined by myself, has grown to its present strength of five full-time salaried academic professor-type individuals who teach, do research and see patients in consultation. It's a feather in our cap that Henry Ford Hospital and other hospitals are recruiting our people to head their departments.

"So our division currently headed by Jeffrey Band, M.D. is a resource for the whole community. We're very proud of that."

ROBERT LUCAS, M.D.
Chief of Surgery and Medical Director, 1972–2000
Beaumont, Royal Oak

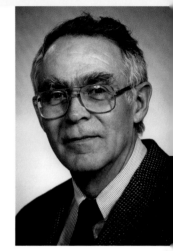

"I was recruited here by Ivan Mader,

the Medical Director at that time, and Fred Arcari, who was Chief of Surgical Services. The residency program was relatively new then, and had some problems. I had trained at Wayne State and was in practice at Grace Hospital, and I was asked to come here to run the residency program. This was the early 1970's. I ran it for ten years, and I think we made it a first-class residency program.

"In the early '80's, there was a change in administration, and the new Chief Medical Officer, Julius Rutzky, asked me to take on more responsibility by being an Associate Director and take on the emergency room, surgical pathology, and radiology. That was an interesting four years, but all things change, and eventually I went back into private practice. I retired in 2000. I'm almost 80 years old."

WHAT IS GENERAL SURGERY?

"General surgery covers breast surgery, endocrine surgery, especially thyroid, all abdominal surgery—stomach, gall bladder, pancreas, colon—and things like hernia repairs, and for a short period I did some vascular surgery before it became a sub-specialty of its own.

"These things that were part of 'general surgery' started to bloom in to sub-specialties in the '70's. There were things that had always been natural specialties, like orthopaedics, neurosurgery, urology, ear-nose-throat, ophthalmology have been around a long time because they all have reasons why they've become their own specialties. Things like endocrine surgery, bariatric surgery, vascular surgery, and colo-rectal surgery are all outgrowths of general surgery. They developed because doctors felt more comfortable doing one thing well, if they could make a living, and of course they want to be recognized as specialists so they could have residents and train fellows and so on.

"Also, things change. Vascular surgery, for instance—when I was first in practice, probably half my practice was vascular surgery. We did our own radiology, our own arteriograms and so on, then radiology departments got more sophisticated they began to do most of the radiologic procedures. In the last twenty years, endovascular surgery has become a major part of that. Vascular surgery is all done as open surgical procedures—aneurysms, corotid arteries, arteries and veins—but when a fellow from Argentina developed a way of putting in an endo-stent to treat aortic aneurysms, and that slowly revolutionized the field of vascular surgery. Surgeons had to be adept at doing arteriograms and working with X-ray equipment to insert these things. That was the first big thing in separating vascular surgery from general surgery.

"Then came endovascular dilation for people who have artery stenosis, which opens the artery with a balloon, just as with the coronary arteries. Soon came stents for vascular dilations and eventually vascular surgery branched into its own whole new area and became a specialty.

"In 1970 John Poole brought in Ivan Mader

and the group he brought with him, brought in the teaching program, and improved the quality of the institution. When I arrived, my goal was to build a surgical residency program so that the emergency room could call at any time and someone would be available, and that all the departments would have high-quality surgeons. I helped hire Dr. Diokno. He really did a magnificent job building the urology department, and I'm proud of that."

BRAVE NEW WORLD OF LITTLE HOLES

"Surgery has changed tremendously. Laparoscopic surgery has been a big revolution. Gall bladder surgery is minimally invasive where we used to make a big incision. General surgeons were actually a little late getting into that area. Gynecologists were way ahead of us.

"Laparoscopic surgery involves two, three, or four little holes, depending upon the procedure. Then the abdomen is inflated and a camera goes in, then other things to do the surgery. It involves almost no pain and the patient can be out of the hospital the next day. Just at the end of my career I did laparoscopic gall bladder work. Even kidneys can be removed laparoscopically. This is a beautiful, major improvement and has replaced many very big operations."

TRAUMA SURGERY

"Beaumont came at an opportune time, to an ideal location. When I was going through surgical residency and was first in practice, Beaumont was a basic community hospital. When they started expanding the institution, they began a residency program, and gradually grew into much more because of people with great vision. The advantage

of having a good residency program is that there was always a senior resident in the hospital, day or night, who was a fifth year resident. We would alternate on-call in the surgery department and other departments as well. For the general surgeon, there are emergencies other than trauma, like appendicitis, perforated ulcer, GI bleeding, and other surgical emergencies.

"Our trauma team is run by general surgeons who are trained in trauma and critical care. Head trauma goes to neurosurgeons and orthopaedics get bone injuries. Beaumont has a great trauma service, a marvelous program, and highly trained trauma surgeons.

"The first person to see a trauma victim was the resident, then the senior resident if it was serious, then they would call a surgeon and have the patient in the operating room by the time the surgeon arrived. At the present time, there's a trauma service covered by about six people who also cover emergency surgery. The senior resident will be down in the ER, and immediately the on-call surgeon is called and must be here within twenty minutes. It has worked out very well."

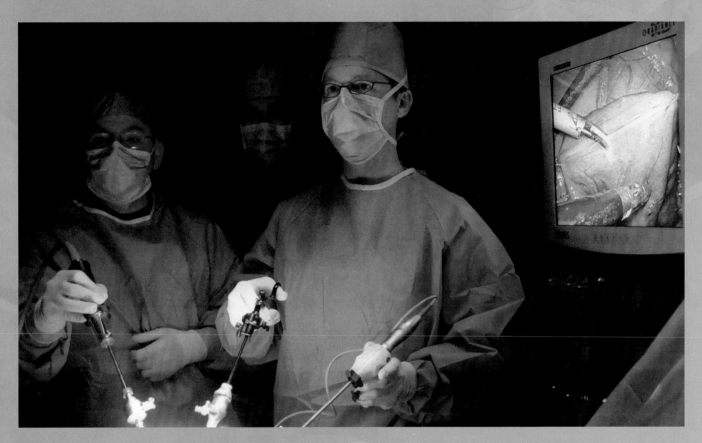

Beaumont surgeons, led in this picture by Kevin Krause, M.D.,
leading bariatric surgeon at Royal Oak, performing laparoscopic
surgery. The camera inside the abdomen allows the surgeon to see
and operate by looking at the TV monitor while manipulating the
instruments that are inserted in the abdomen through little holes.

A. NEIL JOHNSON, M.D.

Senior Vice President and Associate Chief Medical
   Officer for Clinical Operations, 2009–2010
Beaumont Hospitals

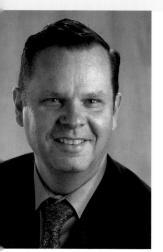

"I'm A. Neil Johnson, and I

never tell anyone what the "A" is. I keep that a secret. Nobody can ever guess. I came to Beaumont on January 2, 1975. I was always in a big hurry, so I got out of medical school at Wayne State University in three and a half years. The academic people at Wayne didn't want me to come here. They thought I was going to a country club and I'd be ruined. I liked the environment at Beaumont. It was a pleasant place to practice, with nice facilities, but still academic. I viewed it as a hybrid even then.

"Internal medicine cuts across all the major systems of the body, mostly in adults. Whether it's pulmonary, infectious disease, heart disease, the internal medicine doctor has broad knowledge to navigate the human body, develop a relationship with the patient, focus on common medical problems like blood pressure, diabetes, heart failure, lung disease, asthma, COPD—the lion's share of problems. Family medicine gets broader than general internal medicine, covering all age groups. The training is similar, but it encompasses children's medicine as well. Some family doctors even do obstetrics.

"Believe it or not, we didn't have enough specialists in the '70's. In those days, the general internist was king. All patients were admitted to the general internist. Even cardiologists didn't admit a patient. A mild myocardial infarction heart attack was admitted to the general internist, and a cardiologist was consulted, because back in the '70's they couldn't do angioplasty. They could only tell us to adjust this or that medicine. They were truly consultants.

"But that changed. The world of medicine changed at the hospitals in 1983 when Diagnosis Related Groups were put into place. There are over five hundred of them. It's a designation by CMS for Medicare/Medicaid reimbursement. If you have this DRG, the hospital would be paid X amount, and they bundled payment for in-patient care and diagnosis. Before that, it was on a cost basis. The

hospitals made lots of money. A general internist would put a brand new diabetic in the hospital, just to put him on insulin and adjust his sugars. A patient with a bad peptic ulcer would be admitted to the hospital for a week just for bed rest and a bland diet, just to take him out of the stress of the world.

"A general internists lifestyle before 1983 was highly collegial, with good communication, very involved in the hospital. He would come in the morning, have twelve or fifteen patients to see, see all his colleagues, he would know all the nurses by first names, he would go to lunch with other doctors, discuss cases, then go to his office in the afternoon.

"Well, after DRG's, those things went away. The world of the hospital dramatically changed. The internist no longer had twelve patients in the hospital, but only one or two. Patients were treated outside of the hospital, or had very limited hospital stays. Advancements in technology meant that all myocardial infarctions went straight to the cardiologist. Specialists and sub-specialists began to burgeon in a variety of medical fields. The general internist became a kind of triage doctor. As my former mentor said, 'You're expected to be expert in everything, but you're really not expert in anything.' The internist became more of an office doctor.

"We began to lose our interaction with colleagues, the hospital was calling while we were trying to see people, and it was just inefficient for thirteen doctors to go back and forth to see one or two patients. The internist found it hard to keep up with new clinical protocols. When we spent half the day in the hospital, keeping up to date was no problem, but that was no longer the pattern. It was getting uncomfortable. Our patients had the idea we were just not showing up to take care of them.

"By 1993, we were increasingly frustrated. We got an idea that was fairly innovative and creative, and new in the country. Myself and another doctor left our office and came to the hospital, to take care of hospital patients only. That's what became known as a 'hospitalist' doctor. Because we were a large group, the financial viability of the hospitalists was covered by the rest of the group. We were still members of Troy Internal Medicine Group, and on the front door of Troy Internal Medicine were the words 'Hospital Consultants' and the names of myself and the other hospitalist from our group.

"We explained all this to our patients, and it worked very well. We freely shared information, which is still a challenge in today's world and also the reason that information technology (IT) is so important. Having electronic medical records and informational flow across the country is critical today.

"In those days, though, we had a personal tie. Patients could call us, knew us well, could fax records to us, and we could pick up a person's care fairly easily. That's something I work on in my new role—transitional care. There are still all kinds of problems with transitional care. Grandma can do well in the hospital, but when she gets sent home, she doesn't know how to read the medication list, doesn't take her medications, and comes back four days later in heart failure. So within our group, we had this excellent communication which allowed us to be very successful.

"It was still important for the hospital to serve the community and patients who came in and didn't have a doctor, so Beaumont started hiring doctors, who then got patients from those coming through the ER who didn't have doctors. There was a growing number of hospitalists, both employed and private. The concept became popular and even surgeons would ask us for consultations. The other doctor who had done this with me in 1993 began teaching a rotation of internal medicine resident doctors on the pre-operative validation of patients. For instance, what were the key things to look for regarding the different types of surgery before going in? And there were peculiarities, like drugs, that needed to be considered."

"So it's 1993 and now I'm a hospitalist, I'm in the hospital all the time and see opportunities, watch operations, and there's always a way to improve things. There was inefficiency. I graduated from Wayne in '75, and back then we had to be very independent thinkers. Even though a radiologist would look at an X-ray, we would look at it ourselves. Check everything. Take nothing verbally. The patient's life was on the line. If we got wrong information and assumed it

was correct, there could be a gross error. We were really taught to be a little paranoid and confirm everything ourselves, but that kind of mentality is not necessarily good for teaching teamwork.

"What medicine had to learn, primarily doctors, was how to be members of teams. That was, and still is, a huge transition for doctors and medical schools. I'm hoping our new medical school is going to train doctors to be parts of teams, and how to function well that way.

"I became Chairman of the Utilization Management Committee, which looks at operations, length of stay, what's the best practice, how to promote quality, reduce costs, and looking at transitions from the hospital in case a patient is going to a nursing home or home care. I did that for seven years, till 2004.

"Later I was named Vice-President of Ancillary Services. The other VP was Leslie Rocher, Vice-President of Clinical Services. I had anesthesiology, pathology, radiology, physical medicine, rehabilitation, and he had medicine, surgery, pediatrics, and OB/GYN. He is now the Medical Director of the Royal Oak hospital.

"What medicine had to learn, primarily doctors, was how to be members of teams. I'm hoping our new medical school is going to train doctors to be parts of teams, and how to function well that way."

"I was head of the Ultimate Site Secure Division, the ambulatory division of Beaumont's home health and Beaumont's nursing homes. I had the whole out-patient spectrum. In October of 2009, I became Associate Chief Medical Officer of Clinical Operations. I'm combining all my past experiences in some way. I look at the continuum of care, from the doctor's office to the hospital, home care, and nursing home. Are we preventing illnesses? What are primary care doctors doing? Are they using the best protocols in their offices? Are we maintaining the highest quality of care on the outside? How well do we prevent re-admissions? Do the patients get mammograms, PAP smears, colonoscopies? Are cancers diagnosed early, saving lives and cost? Are the most effective drugs used? Are we getting the best high quality service in a way that is cost-effective? That's the goal."

JOHN MUSICH, M.D.

Chair, Department of Obstetrics and Gynecology,
Beaumont, Royal Oak, 1983–2006
Vice-President and Director for Medical Education,
Beaumont Hospitals, 2006–2010

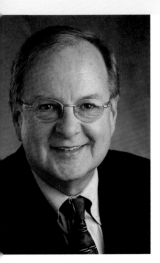

"I was introduced to Beaumont

Hospital when I was still a resident at the University of Michigan from 1972 to 1976. One of my professors became my 'professional father'—Dr. Jan Behrman. Dr. Behrman was an internationally renowned specialist in infertility. He left the U of M in 1977 to chair Beaumont's Obstetrics/Gynecology Department and to run its residency program.

"I did a lot of work with Dr. Behrman when I was a resident. In 1976, I went into the Air Force for two years, and during that time I was undecided about whether I wanted to go into general OB/GYN practice or do a fellowship in reproductive endocrinology, which was Dr. Behrman's field. Well, he made short work of that decision.

"Dr. Behrman was one of the first surgeons to do laparoscopy to the United States. When he came back from a trip to England, he smuggled the first laparoscope into the country with the equipment tucked in his pant leg. Obviously, security wasn't what it is today, but he smuggled it in and started doing laparoscopy in 1971."

FROM BEAUMONT TO CHICAGO AND BACK

"I came to Beaumont for the first time in 1978 to do a two-year fellowship in reproductive endocrinology and fertility. After that, I looked at other places, a possible position at the Cleveland Clinic, and at Henry Ford Hospital, but stayed at Beaumont for a year. In '81, I joined the faculty at University of Illinois in Chicago. While I was there, Dr. Behrman approached me about coming back to Beaumont. I came back to the department on May 1, 1983.

"At the time, there were serious considerations given to starting an in-vitro fertilization program at Beaumont. I was getting settled in, preparing to get started with that, when Dr. Behrman walked into my office on June 1st and said, 'John, on July 1, you're it.'

"'I'm what 'it'?'

"He said, 'You're taking over as Chair of the OB/GYN Department and Residency Director on July 1.'

"All of a sudden, on July 1, 1983, the job was mine. Jan was going to devote his full attention to the IFV program. So the administrative and program duties were suddenly mine.

"I was glad to return to Beaumont. While here as a fellow, I was blown away by the tremendous obstetric and gynecological patient volume in the department, much more than I was exposed to as a resident at the University of Michigan. I was eager to remodel the core clinical services, develop sub-specialty services and, as a consequence, reconfigure and greatly strengthen the residency program both clinically and academically around a 'hybrid' teaching physician core of both private physicians and newly recruited full-time faculty physicians.

"I never could have come to Beaumont at a better time. About a year before I came, our Board of Directors had recommitted themselves to the notion of becoming an academic medical center of pre-eminence in the United States. It was a very dramatic goal.

"In the mid-'80's, I was able to recruit some very dynamic faculty physicians, develop the department, expand the size of the residency, and get consistent five-year maximum accreditations from the Accreditation Council for Graduate Medical Education. That's the body in Chicago that is responsible for granting accreditation to teaching hospitals and to residency and fellowship programs.

"We were able to grow into one of the most successful in-vitro fertilization programs in the country. We developed a cancer unit and a premier high-risk obstetrical unit. We developed a fetal

> "So often, what you end up doing in medicine is very dependent upon the specialty of the person who has influence on you."

imaging unit that, as far as I'm concerned, is second to none in terms of what they can do, and is the most academic division within the department.

"We were able to change the culture of the residency program and recruit a higher caliber of residents. The program became much more academic and disciplined. One of the highest compliments I was ever paid came from the then-Chairman of the program at Ohio State, Steven Gabbe. He described Beaumont's program as 'a powerhouse in non-university OB/GYN programs.' Steve always went out of his way to tell Ohio State students who wanted to go into OB/GYN to 'do yourself a favor and take a look at the program up at Beaumont.'

"It's a great accolade for this program to be recognized as one of the three or four premier non-university residencies in obstetrics and gynecology in this country."

"There was no way I could ever have scripted a more gratifying professional life than I have had. It's due to the opportunities Beaumont has given me. By being able to participate here as a Chair and Residency Director, I was able to catapult from the local activities and responsibilities to become very involved nationally. For nine years I was on the Council for Resident Education in Obstetrics and Gynecology, called CREOG. It's a kind of super-sub-committee of the American College of OB/GYN. I was its education program director for three years, responsible for two national-scope meetings every year, and for the last three years I was the Chairman. To date, I'm the only non-university residency director who has ever been a CREOG Chair.

"I've always been a joiner, always doing things outside of my local scope. I've been able to do these things, and many more, because Beaumont gave me the springboard, enabling me to be in a position

of contributing and learning on the outside, then bringing ideas back, which in turn allowed us to make improvements and do things more on the cutting edge. I'm extremely proud of where we are with graduate medical education. I have no problem recommending Beaumont as a great place to work or practice."

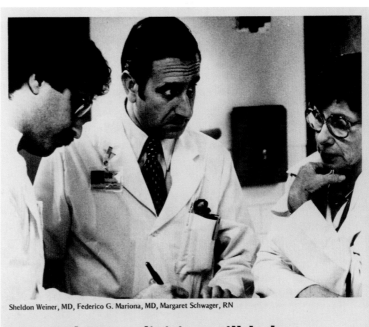

Sheldon Weiner, MD, Federico G. Mariona, MD, Margaret Schwager, RN

New Ob/Gyn division will help women with problem pregnancies

The new chief of Beaumont-Royal Oak's Division of Maternal and Fetal Medicine had barely established himself in his 6-Central office in mid-December.

organized. The more general things are already here," he said. "The center represents a team effort to provide quality obstetrical care."

The center will include a perinatal labora-

NANCY BRUSKE

Former Administrative Director for Continuing
Medical Education (CME)

"I've been employed at Beaumont

Hospital for many years. When I started in the Medical Education Department, two or three residency training programs were approved. The department's function was to recruit medical students for our training programs, assist the department chiefs in preparing a curriculum for the interns and residents, maintain the on-call schedules and conference schedules, and serve as a 'home base' for all house officers, regardless of specialty. At that time, immediately following graduation from medical school, physicians were required to serve a year in what was called a 'rotating internship.' During that year, the intern rotated through several specialties in preparation for making a career choice.

"The Director of Medical Education was Dr. Ivan Mader. I feel that the reason the medical education program is as strong as it is today is due to his solid leadership in the infancy of Beaumont's medical education program. He was brought to Beaumont from Wayne State University, and determined that internship was the cornerstone on which to build a strong educational program for physicians. He established parameters against which potential interns would be judged. For many years, this small hospital was unable to attract medical students to our internship program because the applicants didn't meet his high standards. With

diligent recruiting and a reputation for excellence, Beaumont began to attract desirable candidates for the internship program and many of these physicians continued in our residency programs. The number of residencies gradually increased and, with the platform of the high quality internship, the number and caliber of residents increased incrementally to our current 19 residency and 18 fellowship training programs."

A BEAUTIFUL PLACE

"The day I walked into Beaumont, it was beautiful. It was a small community hospital determined to have a friendly atmosphere and provide comfortable surroundings. It resembled a hotel more than a hospital. The hospital has endured major changes and growth, but it has never lost its loveliness and welcoming atmosphere.

"The Board of Directors has always been extremely progressive and, at Dr. Mader's urging, embraced medical education as part of Beaumont's mission. With the building blocks of a beautiful structure, continuous renovation and updating with the latest technology and a superb medical staff, Beaumont Hospital has grown into a powerful force in the medical arena, into an institution that has a national impact.

"Although the hospital has always offered continuing medical education to its Medical Staff, the Continuing Medical Education program (CME), as it is structured today, emerged when the State of Michigan began requiring practicing physicians to submit documentation of their participation in CME activities in order to renew their licenses. The hospital was originally approved by the State of Michigan through the Michigan State Medical Society to provide continuing

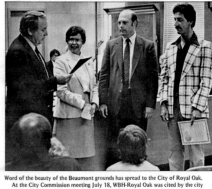

William Beaumont
Hospital System
Royal Oak, Michigan 48072

July 29, 1983

Beauty of hospital campus wins award from City of Royal Oak

Word of the beauty of the Beaumont grounds has spread to the City of Royal Oak. At the City Commission meeting July 18, WBH-Royal Oak was cited by the city Beautification Council for its efforts to protect and enhance the environment and

Cytotech grad wins OHEP award

Joann Kush, a 1982 graduate of Beaumont's School of Cytotechnology and of Oakland University, has won a research award from the Oakland Health

educational programs and grant CME credits to physicians who attend. Doctors are required to have 150 continuing medical education credits for each license renewal cycle.

"In 1994, one of my responsibilities was to help achieve national accreditation for the hospital's CME program. This accreditation allows the hospital to accredit conferences and seminars for CME credit. The credits granted can be used by physicians for re-licensure and specialty Board certification throughout the United States. If an institution is accredited by a state medical society, those credits can only be used within that state and the immediate surrounding states. With the usual foresight, Beaumont sought to offer conferences and seminars from which CME credit could be attained by physicians throughout the country. This status is granted by the Accreditation Council for Continuing Medical Education (ACCME). This organization functions in conjunction with the American Medical Association and several national specialty organizations and boards.

"Beaumont is accredited to provide continuing medical education for physicians. Currently offers approximately ninety regularly scheduled conferences, some monthly, some weekly and some daily, and approximately thirty medical education seminars, ranging from half a day to a week annually. My role, along with the rest of the CME Department, is to assure that the hospital abides by the ACCME's accreditation standards and guidelines."

"SMALL" CONTRIBUTIONS

"My contribution to Beaumont's success has been relatively small, but all employees contribute in ways most of the public don't even realize simply by our attitude. I always felt this was one of my contributions to the residency and CME programs as well as to patients—that I always try to be helpful to people, because that's my role. I always try to remember and remind others that, as employees, we are here to serve the physicians and our patients. They are our customers—the physicians are the ones who bring patients. Patients are the ones who ultimately support our salaries. Without both of them, we wouldn't have our jobs nor would we have a hospital."

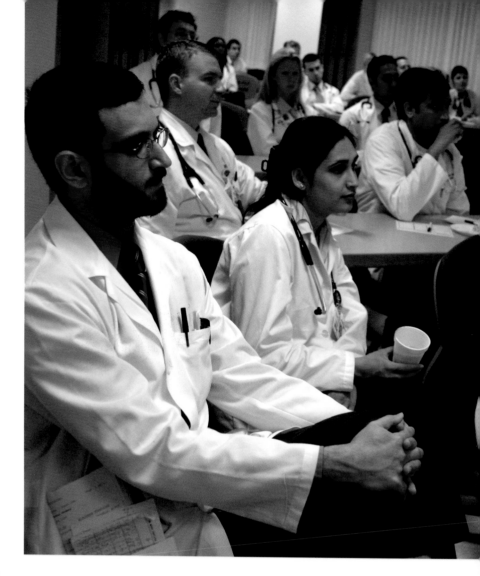

JAMES GRANT, M.D. ON THE NEWEST RESIDENCY PROGRAM AT BEAUMONT

"Beaumont has the largest complement of graduate medical education (GME) programs of any non-University based institution in the country. But despite our size, we were still lacking programs in some key areas, anesthesiology and pain medicine being a prime example. Recognizing the need to have an anesthesiology program, and despite being well over the 'cap' for residency spots, approval was given to begin the formation of a solid GME program. The development of a residency in anesthesiology would be the first new program for Beaumont since the physical medicine and rehabilitation program was launched in the mid 1980's. After much work, numerous and lengthy meetings, and an extensive site review, the Beaumont residency was approved by the ACGME in May 2009. Roy Soto, M.D. was appointed Program Director. The first class of six post graduate trainees entered in July 2010. This addition really begins to make complete the post-graduate offerings of Beaumont."

BEAUMONT HOSPITAL IN TROY 8

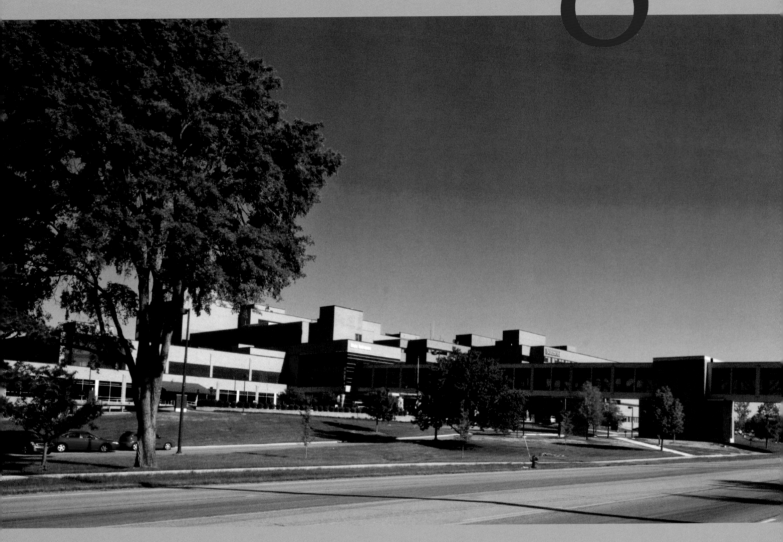

DR. REID ON BEAUMONT, TROY

"The Troy hospital started out just like Royal Oak, and it's growing faster than Royal Oak grew in the initial phases. It's going to be a huge facility. And it's growing with quality, not just expanding."

A Place Called "Troy"

Troy, Michigan, once only part of the Detroit doughnut of suburbs populated by employees and suppliers of the American automotive industry, has now gained acclaim for another reason; a reason that has made Troy a new destination city and a place of healing.

That reason is a hospital built in a confluence of undeveloped fields, spanning a highway that marks the boundaries of two townships: the modern hospital called Beaumont, Troy.

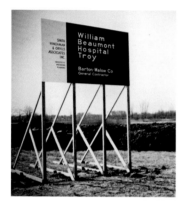
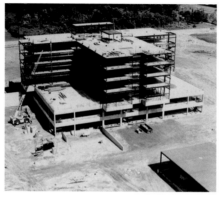

Beaumont, Troy was built on a 48-acre site on Dequindre, south of M-59. The six–story original hospital was equipped with medical-surgical, pediatric, intensive-cardiac care and emergency services, serving the people in Troy, Sterling Heights, Utica, Avon and Shelby townships, Rochester and northwestern Warren.

Silence, serene and tranquil, drenched in peace
Butterflies flirting with flowers and the leaves
Rippling waters of the lake – the cool breeze
Caressing the crops, the dwellings and the trees . . .
The winds blowing, whistling and whispering . . .
Beaumont is coming, Beaumont is coming . . .

In the farms? In the wetlands? Quite baffling.
Certainly, the City of Troy needs such a blessing.
The trucks unloading, the direct roads unending,
the architects planning, the corporate financing . . .
The electrical heating and the hammers pounding,
the concrete pouring, the steel re-enforcing . . .

And, lo and behold, out of the clear blue sky
arose the beautiful, majestic Beaumont nearby.
Slim and slight, petite and bright and shy,
gaining confidence and the momentum by and by.
Ambulances with sirens and RN's par excellence,
Surgeons with prudence, volunteers omnipresent,
Computers with intelligence, administrators' diligence,
Acting in concert with rhythm and cadence . . .

Now enters our patient, with hope and insight,
Confident of personal care by day and by night,
Relaxed, reassured, in love at first sight,
Says au revoir, spreading the word with delight.

And so the dream goes on, from hospital
to office building a patient-care model
Dialysis and telemetry with CCU colossal,
ER and OR, imaging and radiation triumphanl.
Pride and passion, dedication and affection,
A gentle touch, a kind word, a timely action,
Lots of laughs, a few tears, but a connection . . .
A healing hand and a heart of compassion.

by Prem Khilanani, M.D.

Troy Hospital Admits 5,000 in First Year

Since it opened on May 1, 1977, Beaumont-Troy has served the citizens of Troy, Sterling Heights, Utica, Avon and Shelby townships, Rochester and northwestern Warren in greater numbers than expected.

Almost 5,000 patients have been admitted to the 200-bed facility since that date. Planning for the hospital began in 1973, and construction began in 1974. Now it is functioning smoothly as a major part of the William Beaumont Hospital System.

The Emergency Center has treated a total of 15,816 patients, with specialists in emergency procedures dealing with everything from sore throats to the most severe trauma cases.

"Pediatric Services, a service unique to the area, was added only months before the hospital's completion," says hospital Director Kenneth J. Matzick. "It has exceeded the most optimistic expectations, with regular office medical services provided for 9,189 young people since its inception."

Part of Beaumont-Troy's success can be attributed to its carefully planned system of shared services with its parent hospital in Royal Oak. Participating in the Shared Services program are dietary, data processing, linen service, accounting and other departments.

Bulk purchasing and storage in Royal Oak add to the savings.

"Duplication of many expensive facilities and operations has been eliminated," continues Mr. Matzick, "resulting in very tangible savings.

"Less tangible, but just as real and invaluable to the hospital are the dedication, enthusiasm and just plain hard work of our employees, volunteers and medical staff members.

"With a difficult first year behind us, we are better-prepared and ready to accept the challenges of the future, confident that the people of the Beaumont System can meet them."

The Founding of Beaumont, Troy

by Prem Khilanani, M.D.

Professor of Interal Medicine, Oakland University
William Beaumont School of Medicine
Chief, Division of Hematology and Oncology, Beaumont, Troy

It was a picture-perfect view—nature in its full panorama, unraveling the mystery and glory of life. The birds were gossiping uninhibited, the butterflies carrying tales from flower to flower, the deer feasting without fear and the rabbits running around aimlessly. The sky was blue, the rays of the sun filtered through the clouds and bounced off a lake, and the swamps were a reminder of creation unaltered. The flowers provided color and fragrance, and the leaves in the landscape formed the background. In the distance were the tall elm, ash and maple trees, covered on the ground by evergreens. The hawks were circling the skies and provided local security. Everything stood still, and there was silence, and nothing changed.

This was the northeastern corner of the city of Troy, Michigan.

The next moment, as if by a miraculous stroke, the scene changed dramatically. Here now stood Beaumont Hospital, Troy. This was an entirely different landscape. It was a landscape of human beings with various ailments, others extending themselves in the arts of caring, sharing, relieving pain and suffering, of communicating and connecting, human beings with excellence, commitment and dedication. This was God's little nursery for humans in need of care.

For the staff, the Beaumont hospital in Troy created a miracle. They were the pioneers. They had left their safe and secure environments and set out for uncharted territory. They made it happen, for they were a determined, dedicated, tenacious, principled and devoted group. They did not work as departments, but as a family. Everyone knew each other and everyone pitched in to help set up, pack and unpack and transfer, fighting hard to get the resources and make the hospital happen, and make it grow.

At first there were more employees than patients. Those lucky patients were smothered with care and showered with respect. Patients were valued and everyone went out of his way to please a patient.

In the late 1960's, there was a growth spurt in the city of Troy and a realization that a state-of-the-art hospital was needed. Dr. Norton Cooksey was appointed by the city of Troy to explore this option. At his cottage up north, he had a brainstorming session that resulted in a report presented to the city.

The Hospital Council identified six essential criteria which would have to be fulfilled before a new hospital could be constructed: First, the new hospital should substantially replace any existing inadequate facilities on a roughly equivalent basis, since no one knew what the need would be for hospital beds in the next five years in that area. Second, it should have an extremely close operating relationship with a large hospital organization, to enhance quality of care, achieve economic efficiency, and provide medical expertise. Third, a broad ambulatory care program should be an essential ingredient from the outset. Fourth, an effectively functioning mechanism would have to exist to ensure that the residents of Troy had direct and continuing input into the formulation of the new hospital. Fifth, qualified physicians currently practicing in and around Troy should be guaranteed access to the hospital. Sixth, the project must be financially feasible, from the viewpoint of the institution itself, and also from the viewpoint of the seven-county community.

The city of Troy then requested bids and proposals for the construction of the hospital. The main four applicants were Troy Tri-Hospital Corporation-- consisting of Ardmore Hospital and Warren Memorial Hospital—Henry Ford Hospital, William Beaumont Hospital, and Madison Community Hospital. There were a series of votes for the selection of a single provider, and finally the winner was William Beaumont Hospital Corporation.

The Beaumont Hospital Corporation met the challenge and fulfilled the six criteria identified by the hospital council. They entered into agreement with the Tri-Hospital Corporation to take over and

Beaumont, Troy opened its doors to the community in May, 1977 with 278 physicians in 35 specialties. Our 200 bed hospital admitted 2,508 patients, performed 2,030 surgeries and treated 9,942 patients in our emergency center.

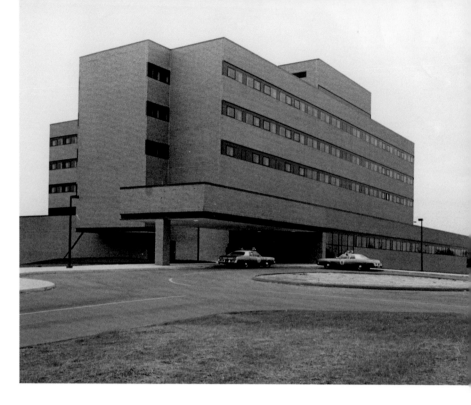

manage Ardmore and Warren Memorial Hospitals and eventually absorb them, providing justification for approximately 100 replacement beds in the new hospital. Initially, only the medical, surgical and pediatric beds with basic ancillary services were provided at Troy. The obstetrical and psychiatric patients were admitted to Beaumont, Royal Oak. Patients requiring cardiac catheterization, open heart surgery, neurosurgery, neonatal intensive care, pediatric intensive care, cobalt therapy, kidney dialysis and transplantation, certain laboratory and diagnostic radiology services, nuclear medicine, and physical medicine and rehabilitation were also provided at the Royal Oak facility.

Eventually, complete facilities to handle all types of routine emergency and walk-in patients would be established, as well as facilities for laboratory and radiology services, and other diagnostic procedures. The city was assured that local representatives would be made members of the Beaumont Board. A Credentials and Qualifications Committee would certify to the Board the specific areas of competence of applicants seeking appointment to the staff. This would ensure that qualified physicians practicing in and around the Troy hospital would be guaranteed the opportunity to have access to the hospital.

And finally, a financially feasible, viable and independent institution was promised by the Beaumont Hospital Corporation. At present, the hospital has a surgical, medical, cardiac, and pediatric intensive care units, an ER, a radiation department, open-heart surgery, oncology, hospice, a cancer center, PET scanner, brachytherapy and stereotactic radiosurgery, and the da Vinci surgical robot.

So this is how a wonderful hospital was made in the place of swamps and butterflies.

FEDERICO ARCARI, M.D. ON BEAUMONT, TROY

" The hospital that is probably the hospital of the moment is Beaumont, Troy. It's younger, it was able to grow with not only medical science but the science of other than pure medicine—radiology and all the extras. It's the hospital that has grown up in the period of time when we started to limit the number of days people stayed in the hospital. That hospital developed just at the beginning of that episode in the history of medicine. As a result, it's probably one of the most modern hospitals built for the time—that is, one-day surgeries, short-stay surgery—the idea is to get patients up on their feet and avoid pneumonia and staph infections, boredom, stress on the family—all those things."

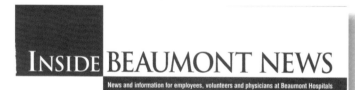

News and information for employees, volunteers and physicians at Beaumont Hospitals

July 26, 2010

First robotic surgery performed at Beaumont Hospital, Troy

Beaumont Hospital, Troy now has the *da Vinci Si®* Surgical System, the newly refined, most-up-to-date robotic surgery system. On July 19, Kenneth Kernen, M.D., director of Urology, and Jason Hafron, M.D., urologist, performed a laparoscopic robotic prostatectomy, the hospital's first minimally invasive surgery using the da Vinci system.

"The robot is an enhancement to our already successful multidisciplinary prostate cancer program," says Dr. Kernen. "It combines the knowledge and skills of the surgeon with precise manipulation of surgical instruments. It has transformed surgery for prostate cancer because of the technical and clinical advantages in terms of visual magnification and refinement in an area that can be difficult to operate on using traditional techniques."

By enhancing precision, robotic surgery can improve surgical outcomes by reducing trauma to the body, blood loss, the need for transfusions and post-operative pain and discomfort. Robotic surgery can also result in a shorter hospital stay and a faster recovery and return to normal daily activities when compared with traditional open surgery.

All three Beaumont hospitals offer various types of robotic surgeries with da Vinci systems. Beaumont, Troy will initially perform robotic urologic surgeries, later expanding to thoracic, gynecologic and colorectal surgeries.

"The high-definition, 3-D vision provides superior clinical capability, while the new technology will allow us to perform single-incision urologic surgery," says Dr. Hafron.

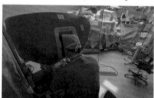

Kenneth Kernen, M.D., performs Troy's first robotic surgery, a prostatectomy, using the da Vinci system.

the 3-D image with hands and wrists naturally positioned relative to his eyes. The system translates the surgeon's hand, wrist and finger movements into precise, real-time movements of surgical instruments inside the patient.

"We are very excited to have robotic technology at Beaumont, Troy," says Roger Howard, M.D., senior vice president and medical director. "Our patients will benefit from having highly trained physicians with access to advanced surgical equipment to provide them a safer and potentially quicker recovery time."

Surgeons operate the robot while seated comfortably at

KEN MATZICK ON BEAUMONT, TROY

"The sentinel event that started me on the path to CEO at Beaumont was the opportunity to plan, design, and operate the Troy hospital in the early 1970's. I was in my early 30's and that project gave me experience that served me well over time. I then had the opportunity to run the Royal Oak hospital for a number of years, then became Chief Operating Officer, and then CEO.

"When Beaumont decided to build a second hospital in Troy, there were already numerous hospitals in southeast Michigan, but there wasn't a hospital in that area. Beaumont Royal Oak was a 700-bed hospital and jammed to the gills. We had to close our OB-GYN department to new doctors because we had run out of OB capacity. We were restricted in several departments, with a large number of doctors. Residents who graduated from our programs were frustrated because they wanted to be on staff and we couldn't accommodate them. It was a good problem, but a problem nonetheless in terms of adding capacity.

"There was a volunteer planning group in the Detroit area called the Greater Detroit Area Hospital Council, and they were very politically connected to the State licensure folks and convinced them to endorse a new hospital in southeast Michigan. We had done our demographic studies and knew that the four communities of Rochester Hills, Troy, Sterling Heights, and Shelby Township were the fastest growing communities in the area. Interestingly, our hospital is located at the intersection of those four communities.

"We worked with the State and got the support of the local planning councils, with the agreement that we would acquire and close two relatively small hospitals that were on provisional licenses with the State: Memorial Hospital in Warren and Ardmore Hospital in Ferndale. We had to acquire them, then also operate them through the time it took to build Beaumont, Troy. We took on their Board members, their doctors, their employees, and created a subsidiary company to merge with them. As we built Troy, we gradually closed those hospitals down.

"This took a number of years, which helped us develop what we called 'Beaumont Shared Services'–dietary services, centralized business office services, warehousing, purchasing—and an infrastructure to serve both hospitals, Royal Oak and Troy, for these services. This worked out well because we didn't have to build duplicate facilities that otherwise we would have to staff if we were starting a hospital from scratch. It also allowed us to spin off Beaumont Shared Services Company, which was a purchasing, supply and logistics company that at one time operated in three states, had five warehouses that served several non-Beaumont hospitals and health facilities around the area.

That's how we ended up in Troy. It was the right place to be relative to population growth, there was an expressway there—M-59, which was called 'The Golden Corridor' because it was and still is developing rapidly. We picked a good spot, and growth just took off and has not stopped to this day."

Ken Matzick, newly appointed Beaumont, Troy hospital director, (center) is shown the architectural model of the new facility.

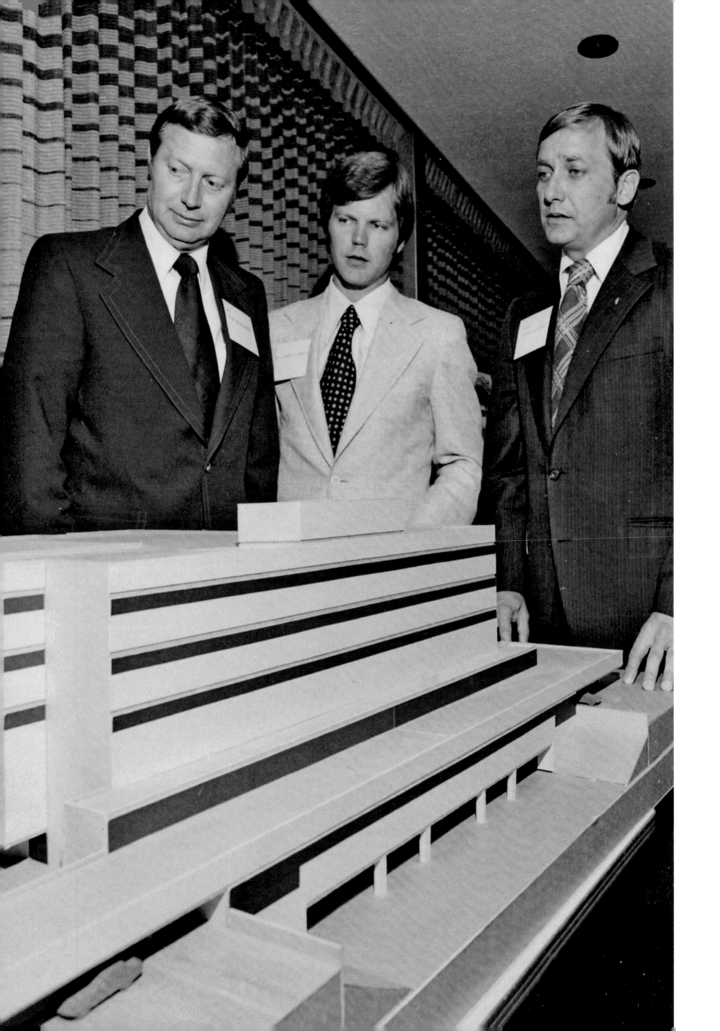

THOMAS M. BRISSE

Senior Vice President, President
Beaumont Hospital, Troy

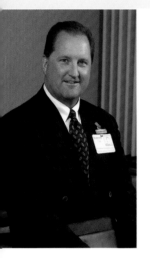

Thomas M. Brisse is senior vice president and hospital director of Beaumont Hospital in Troy, Michigan. Prior to his January 2007 appointment, Brisse had served as vice president of operations since 1996 at Beaumont, Troy. He has more than 20 years of experience in health care, 19 of which have been at Beaumont.

Currently, he has administrative responsibility for 394 beds, $430 million annual revenue, 2,500 FTE's, 26,500 admissions, 3,400 births, 70,300 emergency visits, 19,000 surgeries and 1,100 physician member medical staff.

Brisse began at Beaumont in 1987 as a management engineering coordinator. In 1992, he became the administrative associate of the Beaumont Reference Laboratory. Beginning in 1996, Brisse held key hospital operations positions at Beaumont, Troy: assistant director, associate director and senior associate director, before being named vice president of operations.

He earned his Bachelor of Arts and Master of Health Services Administration degrees from the University of Michigan.

Brisse is a member of the American College of Healthcare Executives and the American Hospital Association. He is also past operations chairman of the Joint Venture Hospital Laboratories and past publicity chairman of the Michigan Health Management Systems Society.

"Beaumont, Troy continues to grow and thrive. I expect to see the Troy campus add more tertiary services, and grow to a 450-500 bed hospital within the next five years. Despite the economic downturn over the last two years, the decision to invest in a major expansion at Troy has proven to be a very sound decision as the surrounding communities continue to grow, the population continues to age, and Beaumont, Troy continues to be recognized as the preferred hospital in the local market.

GENE MICHALSKI, CEO OF BEAUMONT HOSPITALS, ON TROY

"When Ken Matzick asked me to return to Beaumont, Troy after a five-year term at St. Frances of Evanston in Illinois, I said I'd come back, but not to just manage things. I wanted to grow the hospital. I didn't want to come back as the CEO of Troy, but Ken said it wasn't the Troy I had left. There was a nursing home partnership to manage, and a home health agency, and I would be in charge of ambulatory services, which needed a lot of work. I told Ken I would come back if he would give me the freedom to grow the hospital.

"Five years almost to the day, I returned to the Troy hospital. I had gone away to work as CEO in an integrated health system, and come back just as Beaumont was blossoming into an integratd health system. What's really interesting, and I never thought it would make a difference, is that my Catholic experience in Chicago would be helpful in some way. Well, Beaumont was just about to absorb Bon Secours Hospital in Grosse Pointe, Michigan. This time I was on the acquiring side. And guess what—Bon Secours had a hospital, a home health company, a nursing home—it was a mini-St. Frances of Evanston.

"Evanston is a very nice older suburb on the shore of Lake Michigan, north of Chicago. Grosse Pointe is an affluent community on the shore of Lake St. Clair, in a suburb of Detroit. Very similar demographics, and similar hospitals in how they were managed. For me, history was repeating itself.

"The Troy hospital at that time was 189 beds. It's now 454. It'll top 500 shortly. We've increased by more than 2 ½ times. We launched the hospital's first joint-venture ambulatory care center, out at North Macomb, included a joint-venture surgery center, and syndicated a joint-venture medical building. Doctors could now own a piece of the medical building. That was a first. And now we have five nursing homes.

"I expanded the Troy hospital from a basic community hospital to an emerging tertiary care facility with open heart surgery, radiation therapy, MRI's, CT scanners, and now we have robotic surgery."

KEN MYERS
ON TROY

" In 1973, the planning agencies concluded there was a need for a 200-bed hospital in Troy. There were six others in the bidding to build the Troy hospital. The bidding process was very competitive. One of the proposals was submitted by two small 50-bed hospitals, Ardmore and Warren Memorial. We decided to combine our proposal with theirs. Ardmore and Warren Memorial would cease to exist, would come under the Beaumont umbrella, and we would then build the Troy hospital. To make a long story short, our Boards all agreed to do that, and that won the approval of the planning agencies. That's how we received the opportunity to build Beaumont, Troy.

"Of course, when hospitals merged or are absorbed, you're dealing with medical staffs and hospital employees who are suddenly going to be working for another entity. They were eager to join because we assured them of membership on the Troy staff, with privileges to be determined. Those privileges would be based on Beaumont's standards.

"Mergers are often difficult, but actually very few physicians or employees ended up leaving. The merger worked very well, and we were able to bring almost everybody up to Beaumont standards at Troy.

"We opened the Troy hospital in March of 1977 as an extension of Beaumont, Royal Oak with very few problems. We accomplished our concept of a satellite hospital with shared services. The planning agencies saw that we weren't going to duplicate services. Even the laundry was done in Royal Oak, as was food preparation. It's only thirteen miles and worked well, saving quite a bit of money. We opened up with high-quality patient care, and costs were about 10% lower than if Troy had been a free-standing hospital.

"Troy has grown to such an extent that it's no longer a small hospital, but is now a hospital on the cutting edge of medical technology and patient care."

DAVID FORST, M.D.

Professor of Internal Medicine, Oakland University
William Beaumont School of Medicine
Corporate Vice Chief, Heart and Vascular Services
President, Medical Staff, Beaumont, Troy, 2006–2010

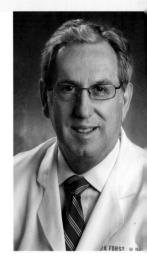

"In 1980, I completed a cardiology fellowship and came to Beaumont, Troy with the hopes of building a cardiovascular program that was renowned for providing outstanding medical care at a very affordable cost. Resources were limited. PA referred to a loudspeaker system, there were no computers or cell phones and many services were yet to be established. A cardiologist had to be at the bedside, day or night, whenever the need arose. In order to succeed, doctors, nurses, administrators and support staff had to work together. This spirit of collaboration and collegiality enabled us to grow into a full service hospital that continues to receive national recognition. This includes our heart surgery program, opened in 2003.

During my years at Beaumont, I have served as Chief of Cardiology and President of the Medical Staff at Troy. Presently, I am Vice Chief of the Beaumont Heart and Vascular Service. It has been a privilege to work with outstanding people, writing clinical guidelines, developing new programs, establishing high performance standards, engaging in research, teaching residents and helping launch our medical school. Best of all, every day we get to work in a beautiful facility with state of the art equipment and dedicated colleagues.

Many challenges remain. Never has there been a greater need for high value, innovative healthcare. Our team-based pursuit of excellence bodes well for the future. Not only have we built a hospital equipped with top technology and a first class staff, we have established an enduring culture of multi-disciplinary accountability and compassion. In addition, sharing knowledge with our colleagues at the Grosse Pointe and Royal Oak campuses has enhanced our ability to achieve the clinical outcomes that our community deserves. The last 30 years have been great, the next 30 years will be even better. At Beaumont, Troy, impossible is only an opinion.

RICHARD HERBERT, D.O.

Chief of Intensive Care, 1977–2007

Senior Vice-President and Medical Director, Beaumont,
  Troy, 1993–2006

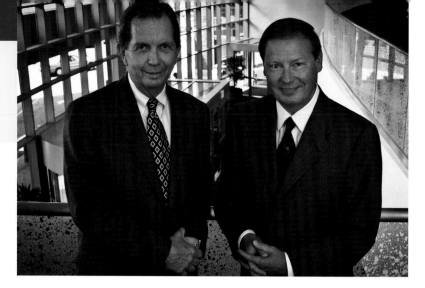

Dr. Herbert with Gene
Michalski, CEO

"I'm the kind of doctor you don't want

to have. You'll likely see me when you are in the Intensive Care Unit. I take care of you after you've been through the Emergency Room and and have had emergency surgery. We manage all the ventilators, take care of serious post-operative patients—open heart surgery, brain surgery, pneumonia, collapsed lungs, lung cancer, emphysema, asthma . . .

"Beaumont is unique in that the hospital has been focused on private practice and has always been on the cutting edge of medicine, which is the way most doctors like it. Doctors are largely independent sorts; they like to work *with* people, but don't like to work *for* people.

"I'm the former Medical Director of Beaumont, Troy, and I started there the day it opened in 1977, in charge of the Intensive Care Department, until I retired from my administrative practice in 2007. In real life, I'm a Pulmonary and Critical Care physician, and the managing partner of an 18-doctor, 6 physician-assistant group. In reality I had two jobs—Medical Director at Troy, and my practice.

"When the Troy hospital opened, Macomb County was mostly strawberry and mushroom farms and cornfields, farms that now have historical markers on them if they're still standing. We started before the building was even finished. It was going to be a 200-bed hospital, growing in increments, so we started with thirty beds in 1977, and all the beds were full. Everybody wanted to come to the shiny new Beaumont Hospital.

"We had doctors from two smaller hospitals with which Beaumont agreed to take some of their staff, and it was a callenge to put the Beaumont brand on the new facility with doctors from such varied

backgrounds. The doctors from Royal Oak were used to having house staff, residents, interns, students, who provided additional patient care. At Troy, there was no house staff. There were attending physicians and nurses. The nurses really bore the brunt of the responsibilities for medical care. If not for the strong nursing staff at Troy, the hospital wouldn't have been nearly as successful. As a result, we had a very close bond between the medical staff and the nursing staff, with a very collegial relationship and mutual respect. At the time it was unique.

"There were some high-quality physicians coming from other hospitals, some of whom were mature, but by no means over the hill, and we were able to steal some of them because they saw the opportunity now becoming available in the suburbs. We had some excellent specialists and sub-specialists as our medical leadership with regard to medical and surgical expertise. Good orthopedists, good surgeons, internists and plastic surgeons, good thoracic surgeons—it was an opportune time in the 1970's when the handwriting was on the wall about what was going to happen to Detroit. It was only ten years after the riots of 1967, and the migration to the suburbs was becoming apparent. The outer communities were growing, especially with the auto companies' being located out in Sterling Heights along Mound Road, and GM and Chrysler in Warren."

SUB-SPECIALISTS

"Troy was set apart from other hospitals by its solid representation of sub-specialists, whereas at other hospitals there were general internists and general surgeons who cared for many 'general' problems.

Troy was much more specialized. Colo-rectal surgery was well-defined, and even in the mid-1970's we had people who just did gastro-intestinal surgery. The whole concept of a sub-specialty was relatively new in the field of medicine. But if you were a child at Troy, you had your appendix taken out by a pediatric surgeon, even if it was a routine appendectomy.

"We had gastrointestinal surgeons, thoracic surgeons who did only thoracic surgery, thoracic surgeons who only did thoracic surgery. We also had nuclear medicine physicians who were really nuclear medicine physicians, not radiologists who also did nuclear medicine. We had good radiologists, and also radiologists who were trained mostly at Beaumont in interventional work—some who just did vascular, or neuro, or mammography. It put us well ahead of other area hospitals."

A PLACE FOR PIONEERS

"The presence of Gerald Wilson, an innovator in the area of breast surgery, had a big impact. He was a vascular surgeon who decided he was going to do breast surgery. It's a unique field—more emotional, takes finesse, takes a certain kind of personality . . . the doctor can be a genius, but if a patient has cancer and the doctor has no sensitivity, genius doesn't matter. The patient won't have confidence in him. Dr. Wilson was a master. He had such a huge following that there weren't enough hours in the day for him. He was truly a grandfatherly/father-scholar all wrapped up in an extremely competent surgeon. A great mix. He developed breast surgery into a sub-specialty. While he probably wasn't the first, he was certainly a pioneer.

"Troy was, and is, a place for pioneers. While I was the Medical Director, we started the open-heart program at Troy, and I'm very proud of that because we really had to push for it. It turned out to be one of the most successful programs in the state with regard to volume—heart surgery is high-volume—and results. We had the second-best outcome statistics in the state for bypass surgery.

"A community hospital program is different from a teaching hospital's. A teaching hospital has a number of residents and nurse clinicians, physicians' assistants and many layers of support.

"When the hospital started, we had gynecology, but no obstetrics. Then, the patients would go elsewhere for deliveries. As this suburbia grew into a bedroom community, there was more demand for obstetrics and the Beaumont Board of Directors let us open obstetrics services. That was about 1993.

"Then the question became what to do with the babies. We didn't have a special unit for babies born a little jaundiced or a little small, and were faced with the dilemma. Should we transfer the baby to Royal Oak, and leave the mother at Troy? Making a new unit was a hard sell to the Board of Directors and administrators, who didn't approve of duplicating facilities when we already had capacity for OB at Royal Oak. The alternative was a hard sell to the mothers—'You know that baby you just had? You won't be able to see him for a while.'

"Parents didn't like that. Ultimately, we got a neonatalogist from Royal Oak to come out and staff the nursery, and we developed a special-care nursery which was a huge success. We had very good outcomes, and patients and doctors loved it.

"Now it's evolved into a neonatal intensive care unit and takes care of all kinds of babies. It's a matter of growth, evolution, maturation. We had a blueprint, but we didn't have a plan; the department grew up in its own time, and we made it work as we went along."

AT THE END OF THE DAY IN ICU

"In the Intensive Care Unit, more people survive than don't. It will never happen as fast as you want it to. But your loved one is here. In all likelihood, he'll get better. We often don't know how long it will take. We'll update the family every day. There are times when you have to dig in for the long haul.

"I learned a long time ago to never ask the family, 'Do you want us to turn off the ventilator?' They're not qualified to answer. There's a difference between prolonging life and prolonging death. We should provide the individual some dignity. We have to act as the advocate for the patient. If he or she could speak, what would he say? If we're at the point where the only thing we can offer is futile care, a good physician will make the decision and the family can ratify it.

"I retired from Beaumont Medical Administration, but I still run our private practice. I've seen thousands of people live and way too many people die. Life is a series of passages. Every day of patient care has been pure pleasure for me."

ROGER HOWARD, M.D.

Vice-President and Medical Director
Beaumont, Troy, 2007–2010

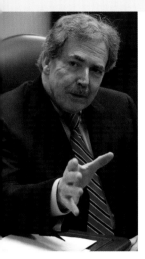

"I started out at Michigan State University

with a major in forestry. It was the late 1960's, and I'd been swept up by the social climate of the times. I was really interested in natural sciences, natural resources, sociology, psychology, Russian language and literature, German theatre—anything I could put my hands on that appealed to me.

"In my senior year, just to make money, I became an admitting clerk on the midnight shift at one of the Lansing hospitals, and then an orderly, back when we still had orderlies. Orderlies were primarily males who did male-type things. We put urinary catheters in male patients, gave males their bed baths, carried things, set up things. I was the single midnight orderly in a ten-bed intensive care unit. The people who seemed the most satisfied were the physicians.

"I went back to Michigan State and asked what I needed to go medical school. They looked at my transcript and said, 'Man, you have done nothing to qualify yourself for medical school!' So I stayed on an extra year and immersed myself in organic chemistry, physics, and all the things necessary.

"I took my first surgical rotation at Receiving Hospital in the middle of Detroit. It was an incredible experience with all the trauma and gunshot wounds, and the Chief Surgical Resident got me interested in surgery. Then I heard about this Beaumont Hospital out in Royal Oak.

"Beaumont was a small community hospital, but it was very busy. I spent a month here and discovered they were doing actual elective surgery, not just trauma, and volume-wise they were doing much more of it. Maybe this was where I'd like to train. They encouraged me to come. My advisor at Wayne was a surgeon and when he found out, he just went nuts. He thought I was throwing my life away to go to this little community hospital out in the middle of nowhere!"

"I did five years of surgical residency here, then joined the practice of one of the young surgeons on the staff, Dr. John Murphy, who was in a very busy four-man private practice. In 1977, he said, 'I've been going out to this Troy hospital quite a bit. I'm going to try to make a mark out there.'

"John became one of the founding fathers of the Troy hospital. In 1988, John and I heard about laparoscopic cholecystectomy. At first, I thought it was the dumbest idea. I told him, 'John, we have the perfect operation for removing the gall bladder. Why do we want to screw around with it?' But we decided to take a look. We each went at separate times to the University of Chicago for training on fairly large pigs, and when we came back we set up a little pilot study with ten patients. We did the first laparoscopic removal of the gall bladder at Beaumont.

"We weren't formally supported or teaching anyone—we just wanted to try it. We came together cautiously and carefully, and took it upon ourselves to make this advancement."

SYSTEMS THINKING

"In 1999, I found myself drawn more into the administrative world. They had a new Department of Care Management and needed a physician-director, so I went into administration. I began to learn the things you don't learn in medical school: systems thinking. I went to one of the local MBA programs, which was one of the most eye-opening experience in my life. I learned how differently we clinicians think as opposed to managers, how differently we lead and focus, how autonomy is a great asset that sometimes gets in the way of making a system function. Every day I remember thinking, 'Boy, I wish I'd known this twenty years ago. I would've run my

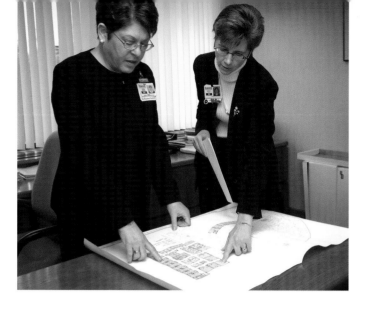

Heidi Shepard, RN, MSA and Nancy Susick, MSN, RN, NE-BC, Vice President and Chief Operating Officer, Chief Nursing Officer for Beaumont Troy, discussing a new project at Beaumont, Troy.

professional life and my business differently.

"I drifted away from my surgical practice and become more involved in medical administration. I would stick my nose into anything at Troy. I was appointed Associate Medical Director and aggressively pursued improvements.

"For instance, the average length of stay for patients was very long. There were misalignments where the physicians were paid by the day, whereas the hospital received one single fee no matter how long the patient stayed. This had been an adversarial relationship because the hospital always wanted to know why a doctor wasn't getting his patient on his way.

"I said, 'You know, this isn't working. Let's look at our system and rearrange things so physicians can't fail. Is our physical therapy being taken to the patient on time? Is it being done in the morning so we can get it out of the way? Are we responding with testing? If a doctor orders a cardiac test, is it done that afternoon or are we waiting two days? Before we even talk about physician behavior, let's fix every delay and problem in our model and bring everything to the table.'

"I had never thought like that before. We cut our length of stay from 5.8 days to 3.9 days. Not only were we more profitable, but we were freeing those beds, so our admissions rose. We looked at getting people admitted from the ER to the floor. If the floor is not efficient and functioning, the people get backed up in the ER, the ER gets jammed up and takes forever, and sometimes it even has to close. If you have an ER that's closing while you still have empty beds upstairs, there's a problem that needs fixing.

"So we redesigned the communications, policies and procedures. The floor nurses said they were getting five or six patients at once, because doctors would often wait till the ends of their shifts to route their patients upstairs. We got the docs together and devised what we called 'admission by appointment.' We guaranteed that we would send no more than two patients at a time to any unit, but that we would do it in half-hour increments, spreading the admissions throughout the doctor's shift.

"Dr. Richard Herbert retired at the end of 2006. I assumed the position of Medical Director. At the same time, Tom Brisse became Troy's new Hospital Director.

"This had been the furthest thing from my mind, but here I was."

TALK TO ME, BABY

"One of my first advancements was within the OB department, and I'm very proud of it. The department had grown to delivering 3500 babies a year, and it seemed almost irresponsible not to have a neonatal intensive care unit. Normal delivery of a baby is at forty weeks, and the OB staff wanted to care for patients who might deliver as early as twenty-eight weeks, but Troy only had a standard nursery. Any premature babies were shipped to Royal Oak. And that can be a risky venture.

"So, one of my first jobs was to call the Chief of Pediatrics at Royal Oak. I told him, 'We really want this neonatal activity at Troy. Let's see what we can do together.'

"We got a great neonatologist, the second-in-command at Royal Oak—David DeWitte—who arranged for all the neonatologists to rotate through both hospitals. Dave took the quality of care and the

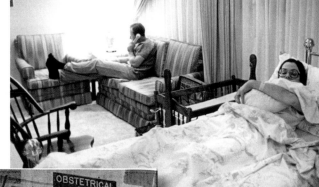

A family relaxes in the new obstetrical birthing room at Beaumont, Troy that were completed in 1992.

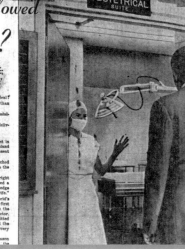

Should Dads Be Allowed In the Delivery Room?

MOST HOSPITALS SEEM TO AGREE HE'S A BAD RISK THERE; HERE'S A MAN WHO VIEWS IT AS A 'TERRIBLE EXPERIENCE'

By Frances Givens

MUCH like scattered, hesitant soldiers grouping before a barricade that is to be taken, young fathers these days are gathering strength to storm that heretofore holy of holies—the delivery room where babies miraculously come to life.

Slowly over the long years they have come closer to baby—through hospital and Red Cross schools for expectant fathers—and now they insist on witnessing the dark mysteries—and the ordeals—of the delivery room.

This is something new and startling in obstetrics. In the past fathers have been the complacent "dogs" around hospitals, being shunted and kicked around by doctors, nurses and anesthetists, coweringly grateful for any little crumb of information given them.

The worried father, pacing the floor and gnawing his fingernails, being pushed aside and walked upon by everybody, is a stock joke.

Not anymore—perhaps.

Father wants his information first-hand and will get it—perhaps.

Anyway the obstetrical revolution is on. Whether or not it will die aborning is still a question.

Doctors, generally, certainly don't want the delivery room littered with unpredictable husbands.

Do wives want their husbands to share their ordeal? Would most husbands rather pace the floor than watch at close range the agonies of delivery?

Whatever, whichever—just who is behind this miniature revolution, only time will tell.

Most hospitals agree the requests to enter the delivery room are increasing rapidly.

Thomas W. O'Connell, a lawyer, broke into print in newspapers across the nation when he sued Highland Hospital in Rochester, N. Y., to permit him to be present in the delivery room when his third child was born.

His daughter Jean arrived before the case reached the courts but O'Connell says he intends to continue the suit in behalf of other fathers. His arguments:

A father has "the inherent natural and moral right to be a witness to any treatment or service rendered a member of his family. To know of his own knowledge the specific services or treatments rendered to his wife."

Movie Star Gina Lollobrigida, one of the world's most beautiful women, who gave birth to a son, her first child, in late July, refused to permit her husband in the delivery room during the birth although he is a doctor.

It seems the husband, Dr. Milko Skofic, was admitted to the delivery room in the beginning but put out at the request of the mother-to-be before the actual delivery began.

Most hospitals seem to agree the primary reason father isn't allowed in the...

level of neonatal medicine at Troy way up. We now have a 13-bed neonatal ICU. I just appointed him Chief of Pediatrics at Troy. We're delivering women way down to twenty-eight weeks now, and just delivered the first set of triplets in the history of the hospital.

"We have an open-heart program which we fought for about four years ago. Again, there was resistance. It's a problem that Beaumont is competing with itself and has to think more like an integrated system in which no branch of Beaumont is minimized. Looking at just the numbers, we do about 300 cases of open-heart surgery a year at Troy, with primarily one open-heart surgeon, Dr. Eric Hanson, who is helped by his partners on staff at Royal Oak, and we have outstanding outcomes— rates of mortality and complications that are lower than many places."

THE FUTURE

"We want to build up our trauma program at Troy, and do it in a 'system' fashion so we can all benefit. We just tripled our ER size and finished a 120,000 square-foot ambulatory care center for much of our outpatient work, across the street and connected by an enclosed bridge that spans Dequindre Road, which is a city boundary and also a county boundary, so two cities and two counties are connected by the Beaumont Bridge.

"What will Beaumont, Troy look like in three or five years? What kinds of services do we want to provide? We likely won't ever be a Royal Oak, a formal academic medical center, but we'll take part in the new medical school in some fashion. Then again, if optimum care, high quality, safe practices and constant learning continue at Troy, then I guess we are an academic center. There will be a great opportunity for medical students to use the Troy facility, which some do today.

"As we get bigger, many of our employees fear losing our sense of family, but as Tom Brisse always says, culture is built one person at a time. I just hope that I, as one person, have been part of maintaining and building that culture."

PAUL MISCH, M.D.

Professor and Chair, Department of Family Medicine,
Oakland University William Beaumont School of Medicine
and Beaumont Hospitals

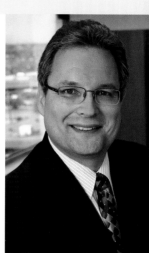

"I thought I had my plans in place, but

then an accident and a major injury changed the course of my life.

"I came to Beaumont in 1981 as a medical student and went to the Troy hospital for the Wayne State University Family Medicine Program. I was energized that it was a new program, and Troy was new, and I was impressed by the faculty. When I graduated, they encouraged me to stay on as faculty.

"My plan was to go into private practice with four colleagues who had gone through residency with me. We couldn't all do that at the same time, so two went into practice and I stayed on at Beaumont to teach for a year. As the end of the year approached, on a freezing rainy day I went to my residency director and gave my notice. I went outside after giving my notice, slipped and fell on the ice, right on my keister.

"Severe back pain began to occur, and got worse as the week progressed. I had a herniated thoracic disk in the middle of my back, pressing on my spinal cord. It's an unusual injury and I could end up paralyzed. I hadn't been smart enough to line up medical or disability insurance before giving notice, and here I had a potentially life-long situation in which I might be paralyzed. I called Beaumont and sheepishly asked whether I could retract my resignation.

"They allowed me to stay on, keep my benefits and have my surgery, which was very successful and restored the use of my legs. I felt a great indebtedness to Beaumont that they allowed me to stay and maintain my insurance. I told my partners that I was going to commit to staying at Beaumont, and that's how I became an employed physician for Beaumont.

"That was a great decision for me. I have a passion for teaching, and after a couple of years they asked if I'd like to be Residency Director."

MEDICAL EDUCATION

"Family medicine is the only residency at Troy. At the time, Royal Oak was being developed as a sub-speciality hospital with the idea of competing with the Mayo Clinic, the Cleveland Clinic, the University of Michigan—that type of institution— and was well on its way to becoming an academic powerhouse. I was impressed that our 'founding fathers' decided on family medicine for the Troy residency. They could've put any kind of training program out there. Troy was more community and primary care oriented.

"Family practice residents work in pediatrics, internal medicine, OB and surgery, and actually do better in community hospital settings than in university-based settings. Universities are designed to teach very much about very little. That's why we have researchers who are not just internists, but who are gastroenterologists; they're not just gastroenterologists, but they focus only on the liver, and not just the liver, but just hepatitis C. And they get grants on a particular virus that causes hep-C. The focus of universities is really on sub-sub-sub-specialization. Primary care takes the opposite approach. We don't just focus on the disease, but on the entire individual—how the disease affects you not only physically, but emotionally; how it affects your family who are trying to support you. We need to know how to treat that disease, but to help prevent it in the future if you have a family history of the disease.

"Beaumont did a course called 'Introduction to the Patient,' for first and second year medical students. They learned basic physical exam skills, how to do the basic history on patients, and worked on case scenarios. We developed a third-year clerkship for Wayne State medical students in which they could learn all about family medicine and work side by side with us in the office and the hospital. For fourth-year students, we offered electives and sub-internships.

"I strongly felt that I didn't want to be a Residency Director who was just inbred from the program. I should bring something new. One way to do that is to be in private practice and bring those skills back, but I didn't have that option. I asked to take a year's sabbatical to go to Duke University to learn administrative skills and some teaching skills, so I could come back to Troy and improve the program. At the time, Duke had the most renowned faculty development program, designed for primary care physicians to improve their leadership skills, administrative skills, teaching and research skills. Duke had the highest status of any program in family medicine. They had the ability to make participants feel as if there was no higher profession than being a teacher in primary care, and that primary care was an important and inspiring specialty.

That's what I've always been proud of at Beaumont—this setting of integrity. They back up their administrators, so we have confidence to act.

"I came to know my stuff as well as anyone at Duke, and won the Teacher of the Year Award while teaching there. I had a core set of skills and the confidence to come back to Troy and be a leader in medical education.

"Between keeping me when I needed surgery and letting me take the Duke fellowship, Beaumont earned my deep commitment. That's what I've always been proud of at Beaumont—this setting of integrity. They back up their administrators, so we have confidence to act.

"We focus on the patient, so you don't feel you're lost in the system. The majority of patients have the common diseases, not the sub-specialty diseases, so it was brilliant to put family medicine in a community-hospital setting. The residency program flourished at Troy, and the whole hospital embraced it. At the residency graduation, everyone turns out—the surgeons, the internists, the pediatricians and obstetricians—everyone comes and there's ownership of that residency. Those young doctors feel embraced and supported, and many of them stay

at Troy or affiliated with Troy.

"The hospital leadership might identify a location where we need some primary care docs, and encourage young doctors to establish practices in these areas that we expect to be successful. They send patients in to Troy from these areas, and that helps the Troy hospital be a strong hospital. We have the same relationship with the family medicine program at Beaumont, Grosse Pointe."

AND HERE COMES THE GOVERNMENT

"In October of 2009, Dr. Diokno asked me to oversee not just family medicine, but primary care within the whole Beaumont system. Primary care encompasses internal medicine, family medicine, pediatrics, and obstetrics. There are some unique difficulties, because medicine is transforming. With all these governmental pressures and decreasing reimbursements, for the first time we have doctors who can't make it. They're not able to get loans to support their practices. So doctors are hurting and struggling, particularly in primary care, because they tend to be the lowest income earners in the spectrum of doctors. They see patients, then drive to the hospital to see one or two other patients, then back to the office—they can't do all that driving and all that paperwork without much reimbursement. They've had to start depending upon hospitalists, doctors who work in hospitals, to take care of their hospitalized patients.

"In the past, hospitals never cared about what was going on outside of the hospital, but that's no longer the case. We have to arrange for smooth hand-offs of patients and information, for safety and quality.

"And now this year, the government came out with a new set of requirements which require the primary care doctor to track the patient throughout the system. It's called 'Patient-Centered Medical Home.' Now doctors have to change how we practice medicine. Until now, we'd set up an office and patients would call for appointments, and the doctor would treat whatever the ailment or condition was. Now we're supposed to take care of patients we may never have even seen. Let's say a person works at General Motors and GM says he has to sign up for a health care plan, and that plan requires picking a primary care doctor from a list. The idea is that the doctor will eventually pick up that patient. But many patients never go in. These are phantom patients, but the doctor is suddenly responsible to know all these patients, know their conditions, and if the patients don't come in, the doctor is supposed to get them in, identify their problems, get them to specialists and keep them out of the emergency rooms. If a phantom patient in my patient pool, someone I've never seen, someone who has never called me, ends up in the ER, that becomes my problem.

"The doctor has to make sure that someone who has never established care with him comes in every four months if he needs a blood sugar check for diabetes or some other problem. If the docs don't do that or can't keep up, we get penalized in terms of how much the insurance companies reimburse us. That means weekend and evening hours. These new laws take the responsibility of personal health away from the patient and put it on doctors. It's a dramatic increase in work load.

"This will probably have the result of driving many doctors out of private practice. The government thinks everything can be institutionalized.

"Part of my role for primary care is to figure out ways to help doctors who have been saddled with these requirements."

AMBULATORY SERVICES

"Since taking this job, I've learned about how much of the hospital isn't in the hospital. We have out-patient surgical centers, sleep labs, dialysis units, physical therapy, home health care, all scattered throughout southeast Michigan. We have hyperbaric chambers used for diabetes or wound care, occupational rehab facilities, cardiovascular rehab, all on off-campus sites, probably 70 different locations. My role is to look at those areas from a medical perspective and push for high and higher quality. Our ambulatory division has the highest patient satisfaction scores, in the top percentile in the country."

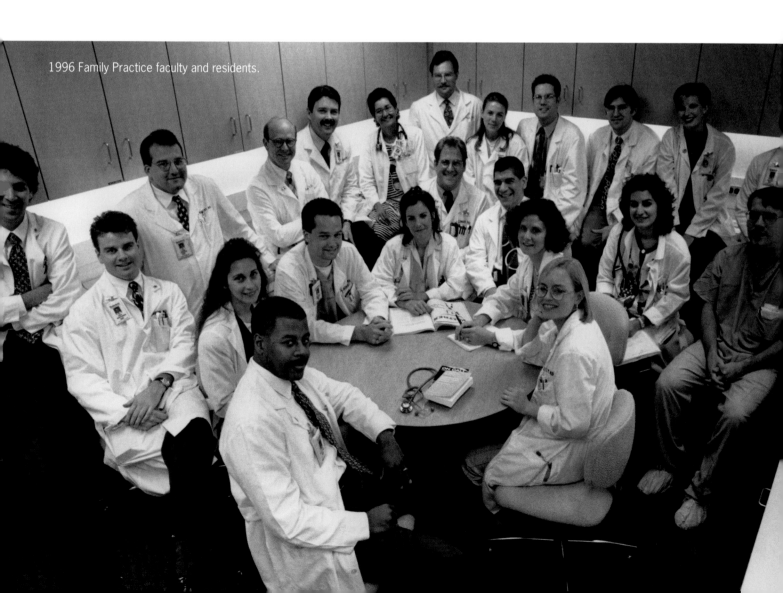

1996 Family Practice faculty and residents.

THEODORE TANGALOS, M.D.

Assistant Professor of Family Medicine, Oakland University William
Beaumont School of Medicine
Attending Staff, Family Practice, Beaumont, Troy

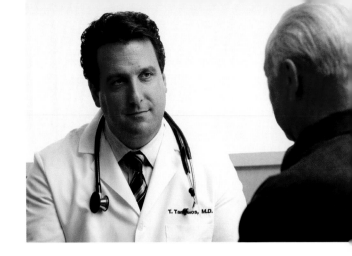

"I grew up in Shelby Township.

I'm pretty much a local yokel, grew up in our family's Greek Restaurant, where I worked to pay the bills during med school. We were very family-oriented, very ethnically connected.

"I was accepted as a family practice resident at Beaumont and graduated in June of 1998. I planned to open an office with my partner, Dr. Steven Kotsonis, my best friend from college and medical school. We went to the hospital to buy used equipment. We knew we wanted to be on staff at Beaumont.

"They said, 'Well, you were a resident here, and we'd love to have you in the Outreach Program so you can be employed for two or three years, establish yourselves as Beaumont physicians and not have to be on staff at multiple hospitals. We'll also send you referrals to people who are looking for Beaumont physicians.'

"That built a very strong loyalty between us and Beaumont. By the third year, Kotsonis and I were independent physicians on staff at Beaumont, Troy. Because of our loyalty and because we were busy, we didn't pursue other hospital systems. If specialists are well trained, and make patients comfortable, they make our practice look better and us as physicians look better.

"We have 10 physicians, 70 employees, and also run an urgent care center in the Beaumont building on Hall Road. It's open 10 PM to 10 AM, 365 days a year, and has helped decompress the Emergency Room by absorbing the colds, coughs, small cuts, bruises, and sprains. The ER wants people to come in for heart problems, strokes or something more intense, but if the hospital's full with colds and coughs, they have to shut down their E. R. It's been

a good marriage. We send acute problems to the hospital, and serve as a beacon in Macomb County for people who are looking for doctors.

"We have loyalty to Beaumont because they treated us well when we were first starting to flap our wings. We now have ten physicians in three different locations and ours is one of the busier practices for the hospital. We're still exclusively connected to Beaumont rather than branching out to other hospital networks.

"In the current economic climate, with fears about where health care is going, many doctors want the comfort and cover of being employed by hospitals, have a lot of back-up, work regular hours, don't want to worry about paying bills or running a business. For me, that didn't work. I grew up in a family business. I wanted to be in private practice. It's a very individual choice. The more entrepreneurial physician may join us as a partner in our practice, while someone with other interests might choose the employed model. And you'll find these all at Beaumont.

"At our practice, we take care of people from birth to the grave. We're all Board-certified in family practice. We see newborns at the hospital, and our oldest patient is 105. She just stopped driving about a year ago."

THE PUSH FOR QUALITY

"People will always look for quality health care. Medical professionals who do a good job, stay above board and have high levels of quality will still be sought out and I hope be compensated for what they do. If the free market is allowed to compete, the best products will come out eventually. There are always humps and bumps, but there's fraud and abuse in the government too. I'm Greek, so I saw how medicine changed drastically in Greece from the mid-70's, when they became very socialist there, to how it's practiced now. It's really a shame. In Greece, you have to have your significant other or a family member stay with you and do your nursing care, bring towels in, and change sheets. Unfortunately there are very unethical practices, like making sure you tip your doctor to so he treats you or puts you in line. There's a lot of corruption in that regard, which ethically I think is very bad.

"The thing I like the most about Beaumont is the very high level of quality required of physicians whom they take on staff, from primary care all the way up to the pediatric cardio-vascular surgeon, and it's still in a community setting. We function as a teaching hospital, and now we're connecting with Oakland University for a med school, yet we still have that community feeling that it's not an overbearing 2000-bed system in the middle of a large city where they don't know your name and you're just a number.

"Then, from a doctor's standpoint, Beaumont is still a beacon where a person with an entrepreneurial spirit can survive, strive, and become very successful, as opposed to many other hospital systems where they're really trying to become more of an ownership model, telling doctors what their requirements are, where and how much they should work, what structures and requirements they have, and this is all the benefit and fruits they can get out of their labor. Beaumont still strives to keep that entrepreneurial flame alive, to allow young, innovative physicians to try things outside of the box to better help their patients and the hospital system."

YOUNG ENTREPRENEURS

"Dr. Robert Reid signed our first lease, which allowed us to start our practice. Tom Thompson is the godfather of our practice, because he blessed us to be in the Outreach Program. Dr. Richard Herbert is the person who put it together for us. Kotsonis and I were just looking to hang a shingle and buy some equipment, and Dr. Herbert was the one who put us together with the Outreach Program. If it weren't for Dr. Herbert, this ten-physician-strong practice would never have been here. So forward thinkers like Dr. Herbert, Dr. Reid and Mr. Thompson allowed this program to go forward. The fruits paid off very well, and we are a busy and large practice. I hope that offsets the fear of investing in young physicians as health care costs are compressed in the future. The young entrepreneurs will drive good things for medical care if they're given the kind of support Beaumont has given us."

9 GIANT LEAPS: THE RUTZKY ERA

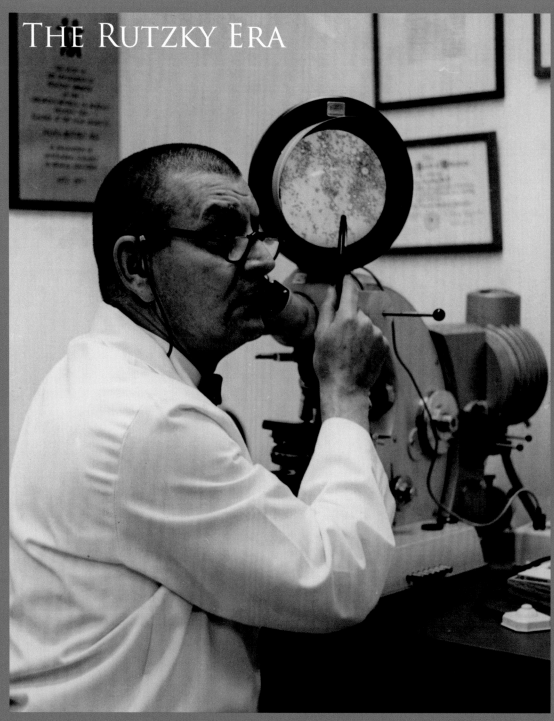

THE STAFFING SURGE OF THE 1980'S

The next giant leaps would occur under Dr. Julius Rutzky, and that was to bring in multiple doctors from all over the country and the world, to seek out the highest-quality physicians, many with national or global reputations, and recruit them to Beaumont as full-time employees of the hospital. The Board of Directors and the directors of the hospital determined that Beaumont should become a truly great independent academic medical center.

According to Dr. Musich, "You're not going to do that on the backs of a staff of private practitioners. You have to have a cadre of full-time, salaried physicians. When I came to Beaumont in '83 as Department Chair, my position was a fifty-percent salaried position. There were no full-time positions. When I left the Department Chair position in 2004, after 21 years, there were 21 full-time salaried physicians. The hospital had committed the resources and to build a department that would provide maximum clinical care, opportunities and quality for patients and also serve as a foundation for what would become recognized in the mid- to late-'90's as one of four or five best non-university training programs in the country in my field of Obstetrics and Gynecology."

THOMAS THOMPSON ON THE STAFFING SURGE OF THE 1980'S

"In 1982, Dr. Mader was followed in the Chief Medical Officer (CMO) position by a full-time clinical pathologist, the Chief of Clinical Pathology, Dr. Julius Rutzky, a pediatric oncologist. Dr. Rutzky believed he had a mandate from the Board of Directors, from the Chairman, Mr. Garrett Mouw, to develop Beaumont into a world-class medical center. In his mind the basis for that would be prominent, well-recognized, distinguished chiefs of departments. He set about finding those people.

"His process to find them was to contact three or four very prominent people in a particular field, say oncology, and ask, 'Who are the best oncologists in the United States?' So he would get these very prominent people in the country, and retain them to be his advisors in his search for whatever the field was. From them he would get a list of five or ten well-recognized doctors. He would then pick out names that he recognized, or that were repeated on the lists, and narrow it down. He found Dr. Martinez, Dr. Diokno, Dr. Comstock, Dr. Lorenz, Dr. Maisels, and many others, many of whom are still here today.

"It was a good cause and a good thing to do. Dr. Rutzky was absolutely convinced he was doing the right thing by recruiting stars. There was never a doubt in his mind. The only problem is that bringing in these big names in various fields began to antagonize or threaten others on the medical staff. Some were fearful of how competitive superstars would be. The local doctors were understandably concerned that the big names in their fields would attract patients away from them.

"Many of the private staff felt threatened and lobbied at a very high level. They started calling their patients who were members of the Board. Finally, somebody got tired of getting calls at home and told Ken Myers, the CEO, to do something about it. That led to the departure of Dr. Rutzky and the addition of Dr. Federico Arcari.

"Dr. Arcari was primarily a private physician. He may have done some part-time teaching, but he was primarily a private pediatric surgeon, which was what the private staff wanted: a Chief Medical Officer who knew what it was like to be in private practice. So we entered another new era.

"Dr. Arcari, in spite of the fact that he was born in Scotland and his mother lived there her entire life, his father was Italian and Dr. Arcari clearly had the Mediterranean temperament. However, there was no doubt in anyone's mind that if there were some right thing to be done, and he was convinced that it was right, that was going to be done. If that doesn't happen, if a person in command can't make hard decisions, no matter how likeable the person is, if he's not capable of doing unpopular things, it's not good.

"Dr. Arcari recruited Dr. William O'Neill from Ann Arbor, because the former co-Chiefs of Cardiology had reached the point in their own careers and in the development of the department that it was time to find new leadership in cardiology. Dr. Gordon died a few years back, and Dr. Gerald Timmis is still reading EKGs to this day.

"So we had this period of prosperity and peace when Dr. Arcari was here, and a period of harmony when Dr. Reid was here. Then came Dr. Ron Irwin, who was very young at the time and couldn't wait for things to happen. He was an oncologic orthopaedic surgeon. He was probably the youngest Chief Medical Officer in Beaumont's history, and was anxious for things to happen quickly, probably too quickly for a big hospital's quasi-bureaucracy can make things happen, so he stayed a relatively short time as CMO. He was good-looking and a good speaker, patients liked him, and he went back into private practice as an oncologic orthopaedic surgeon with a partner. He was recruited by the McLaren system, and currently practices at Mt. Clemens Regional Medical Center.

"Following him, then CEO Ken Matzick picked a salaried physician who had been an academic success at Ann Arbor, and was recruited to come here by Dr. Rutzky and Dr. Robert Lucas, Chief of Surgery, and had been very successful as a professor. The offers that we made, as we always did then, outbid medical schools, and we got the prize. That was Dr. Diokno. He has a great temperament, personality, and gets along with everybody. He was an outstanding professor, a *real* researcher as opposed to people who do it as a hobby; he brought in National Institute of Health grants. NIH grants are very hard to come by, but they also bring with them an extra amount in a formula the government uses, which pays an extra 50%. If you're an NIH researcher and bring in NIH grants, you're very valuable. We have very few people like Dr. Martinez and his group, Dr. Diokno and the Department of Urology, who do an outstanding job of getting grants from outside Beaumont."

"Sometimes, to be in command you have to be bold and brash. If you're not putting people off, you're probably not being effective. You have to do things that won't be popular. It's rare to find someone who can be in command and also be someone everybody likes. We're especially fortunate to have Dr. Diokno as our CMO now. He's one of those rare finds with that just-right personality to lead Beaumont into the future."

Some of the physician leaders that Dr. Rutzky recruited included (clockwise from top left): Drs. Christine Comstock, Robert Lorenz, Jeffrey Maisels, Charles Main, Ronald Krome, Ananias Diokno, and Alvaro Martinez.

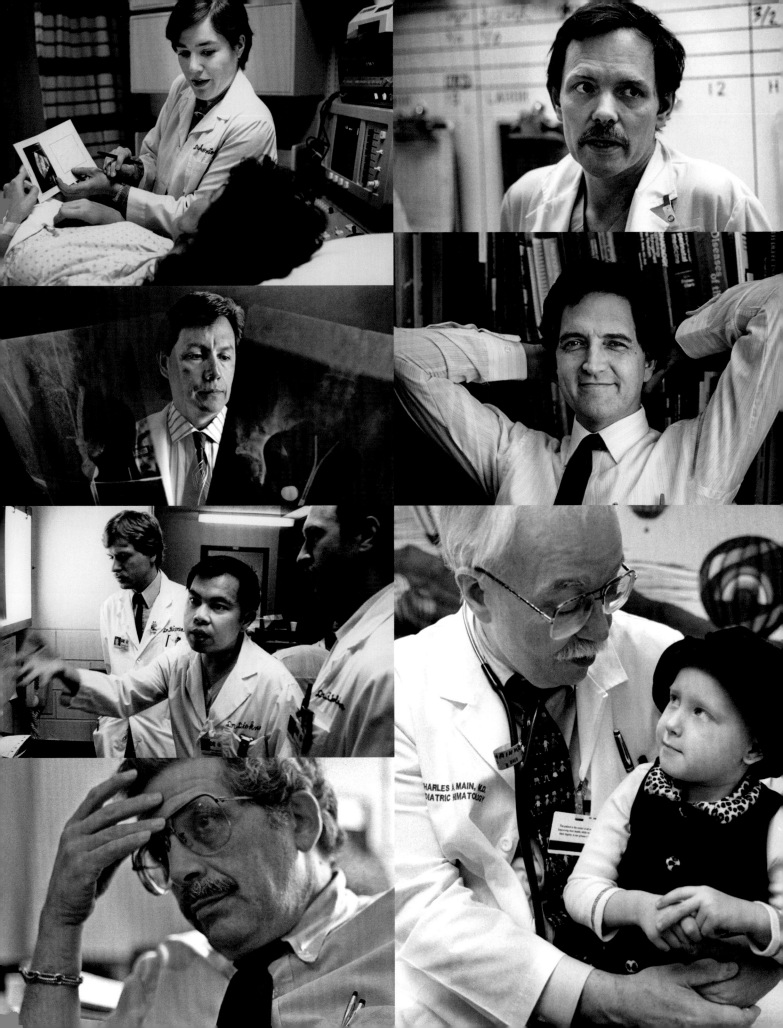

CHARLES MAIN, M.D.

Associate Professor of Pediatrics, Oakland University William
   Beaumont School of Medicine
Chief, Division of Pediatric Hematology and Oncology, 2004–2010
Beaumont, Royal Oak

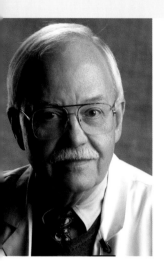

"We take care of patients with hemophilia,

sickle cell, anemia, blood disease and cancer. I'm not in private practice; I'm a hospital employee here at Beaumont.

"I grew up in Detroit, went to Cooley High School, went to Wayne State University for one day, quit, and went into the Army. My father was a truck driver in Detroit and my mother worked at a Cunningham's drug store. We lived in a very small house. I didn't even have a bedroom. I slept on the couch or on the porch. I had to get out of there. The next day, instead of going back to Wayne, I just kept going all the way downtown and signed up for the Army and went away. When I got back, I was a very different person. I'm not sure I would even have succeeded if I had stayed in college. But after two years in the Army, I was different.

"I met my mentor while in medical school at Wayne. His name was Julius Rutzky. Dr. Rutzky was everything I thought a physician should be . . . hard-working, dedicated to his patients, and he was voted by our class to be the outstanding teacher. I went directly into pediatrics and was looking for a practice to join, when he asked, 'Would you like to go into pediatric hematology and oncology with me?'

"It's funny, because the first day I spent on pediatrics in medical school, I came home and told my wife, 'I can't wait to get out of there. It smells, everybody's crying, they can't answer a question—it's very frustrating. I can't wait till this month is over!'

"Well, by the end of the month, I loved it. The children were so forgiving, and if you do the right thing with them, for the most part they get better. After a year of my internship with senior citizens, I realized you can do all the right things and still many seniors don't get better, so pediatrics was the field for me."

"RUTZKY'S PEOPLE"

"Dr. Rutzky came from Brooklyn, and he was a tough, tough guy. I had seen him at a meeting in which he voted one way and everyone else voted the other way, and he wouldn't let the meeting disband until he had everybody convinced to vote his way.

"In 1968, I was in a fellowship for pediatric hematology and oncology when Dr. Rutzky came to me and said, 'On Labor Day, I'm going to Beaumont. Do you want to go with me?'

"I said, 'If I don't go with you, I don't have a job!'

"So on that 3-day weekend, we moved our stuff to Beaumont. There must've been twenty or thirty people who came with us—nurses, lab techs, desk clerks from pediatrics. For a long time we were known as 'Rutzky's people.'

"For me to have a boss like him in the young part of my life was perfect."

CHILDREN: NOT JUST LITTLE ADULTS

"Children aren't just little adults when it comes to pediatric oncology. For one thing, they can tolerate, pound for pound, more chemotherapy than an adult. They tolerate medicine better, they have younger kidneys, younger liver—we can take away quite a bit of the liver from a child, and it will regenerate. Several times I've had oncologists for adults come to me and ask, 'What protocol do you use for X?' and when I tell them, they ask, 'How can you get away with giving doses like that? If I gave a dose like that, my patient would be in the hospital for three weeks!'

"Kids just recover that much faster than adults. The tipping point must be somewhere in the 20's, because we don't see it.

"People also ask why the results are so much better in treating children with cancer than treating

JOHN MUSICH, M.D. ON DR. JULIUS RUTZKY

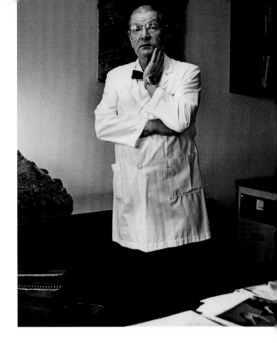

"Julius Rutzky was a visionary. He was a hematologist/oncologist from New York who came to this area initially at St. Joseph's in Pontiac. He was a dynamic individual and truly knew what greatness was. He reached out to recruit the best people in the country. I wasn't recruited by Rutzky, but he kept me on in obstetrics and gynecology as the chair.

"The Urology Department was probably ready to tar and feather Julius Rutzky because he brought full-time physicians to a department that had been purely private practice and a very powerful unit. But Rutzky stood by his guns. He knew it was going to be great under Ananias Diokno's leadership.

"Rutzky brought in Dr. Alvaro Martinez, a world-renowned radiation oncologist, Stanford-trained, who came from the Mayo Clinic. About two years after that, he brought in Dr. Jeffrey Maisels, a newborn intensive care specialist from Penn State. It was an incredible and vibrant time to be at Beaumont."

---

adults with cancer. Well, for one thing, kids have mothers. A mother is going to make sure her child gets to his appointments and takes his medicine, and the compliance with pediatric oncology is almost 100%. It's very rare to have a no-show at an appointment. The mothers will drag them in if necessary."

AN UNFORGETTABLE CASE

"All the cases stick with you. You think they won't, but they do. Thirteen years ago, I had my gall bladder out. I was on the oncology floor because there was a bed crunch. While there, I saw someone I knew walking toward me with her son—on the *oncology* floor. I really hoped I was not about to have this young man as a patient. But here he was, he did have cancer, and we did end up taking care of him.

"A couple of weeks ago he came in and wanted to have his picture taken with me. I asked why.

"'You probably don't remember,' he said, 'but before you started chemotherapy on me, you recommended that I store sperm and freeze it. I didn't want to. I was 18 or 19 and just wanted to get the treatment over with and get on with my life.'

"I had told him, 'The day will come when you'll be happy you took this advice. You have to do it before we start chemotherapy.'

"So here he was, thirteen years later, married to a wonderful woman, and they wanted to have a family. And they had healthy frozen sperm. Now they have a healthy, beautiful baby boy. The dad wanted a photo of me holding the baby, and when we took the picture, he said to his little son, 'Smile for Dr. Main, because if not for him, you wouldn't be here.'

CHILDREN WITH LEUKEMIA

"With children who have leukemia, the cure rate used to be about 2%. Not long before that, it was zero. That 2% went to 4%, then 6%, to a point now where it's somewhere between 85% and 90%. If a child comes in with leukemia, he has an 85 or 90% chance of being cured, whereas with leukemia forty years ago, he had a 98% chance of dying.

"You're still giving poisons to children. We're looking for ways to get to 100% without putting the kids through the distress we have to put them through now."

"I enjoy being at Beaumont today as much as I did when I first came here in 1968. It was a lot smaller then . . . there were baseball diamonds and tennis courts out there, and we had hospital picnics out on the grounds. Certainly the people I've worked with in pediatrics have constantly pleased me with their availability and conscientiousness, and what good physicians and nurses they are."

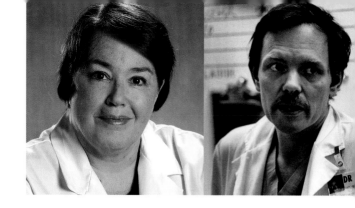

CHRISTINE COMSTOCK, M.D.

Professor of Obstetrics and Gynecology, Oakland University
William Beaumont School of Medicine
Director of Fetal Imaging, Beaumont, Royal Oak, 1984–2010

ROBERT LORENZ, M.D.

Professor of Obstetrics and Gynecology, Oakland University
William Beaumont School of Medicine
Director, Maternal Fetal Medicine, 1984–2010

Dr. Comstock: "We met as medical students. Somebody had stolen my car from the streets of Chicago that day, and I needed a ride home, and this young man gave me a ride. He proposed when I was an intern at Children's Hospital, and here we are thirty-nine years later with two children.

Dr. Lorenz: "I'm trained in OB/GYN with a subspecialty in maternal/fetal medicine, which is high-risk pregnancy. I did all that training at the University of Michigan and I was looking for a job. She was only part way through her residency when I got a call from the chairman at Hershey, and she yells into the phone, 'Where's Hershey?'

"It's in central Pennsylvania, Penn State University. We were there for five years, had our first son, and by then a friend of mine, Dr. John Musich, had moved to Beaumont and asked me to take a look at a job.

"That was twenty-five years ago. We moved back, and we actually live two blocks from the house I grew up in. The first night, I was up all night delivering a baby, and when I drove home I actually drove back to the old house."

Dr. Comstock: "We came here in 1984, part of an influx of people hired by Dr. Julius Rutzky. He had a vision of Beaumont as an academic institution and was trying to replace part-time chairs with academic chairmen and acquire sub-specialists Beaumont did not yet have."

IN THE WOMB

Dr. Lorenz: "We work in the Department of Obstetrics and Gynecology. I'm the head of the new Division of Maternal/Fetal Medicine. We do high-risk consultations and care for patients and do procedures to help the regular OB/GYNs when they have particular problems during those pregnancies.

A big part of obstetrics and gynecology now is imaging, and Chris does fetal imaging and obstetrical ultrasound.

Dr. Comstock: "Our work stops at delivery. In the delivery room, we turn everything over to the pediatric team.

Dr. Lorenz: "Many patients have potential problems with the unborn baby. In the past, the doctor would send the patients for an ultrasound, then perhaps for an amniocentesis to check the amniotic fluid to check the chromosomes; if there's a problem, the patient goes to the pediatrician to talk about what that means for the baby. It's like a cocktail party game; for a family that's under stress and worried, even the simplest diagnosis compounds the worry.

"I decided that the better mousetrap was to quickly get all the doctors together in one room, go over the information, bring the family in to meet everybody, lay out a plan, answer all their questions, produce a document that gets distributed to every member of the team, and that document sits in labor and delivery. When they come in, everybody knows what's going on and care can be coordinated.

"The internet has changed everything. We try to have the meeting quickly after the diagnosis, but within three hours the patients have been on the internet and they'll have the good and bad right in their hands. It's good in that patients are empowered to participate in their health care. The challenge is to help them understand what's valid and what isn't, because anybody can post anything."

Dr. Comstock: "If they leave Fetal Imaging with a diagnosis, we give them a list of reputable websites that pertain to their problem, so they're not just going on anecdotes. Also, hospitals give a lot of teaching now to parents."

PREGNANCY AND DIABETES

Dr. Lorenz: "A common high-risk problem is diabetes, acquired during pregnancy or before. We're a referral center for diabetes. We have a multidisciplinary approach. We have a social worker, a nutritionist, a nurse-educator, a medical endocrinologist, and the high-risk obstetrician, and we work with the obstetrician who's going to do the delivery. There's a direct relationship between how high the blood sugar is and the risk of miscarriage, stillbirths, birth defects, and trouble with delivery. We get as close as we can to normal and improve outcomes.

"Seventy years ago, diabetics couldn't have babies. The blood sugar's being so high would have killed the pregnancy. We've evolved. At first it was a couple of shots of beef-pork insulin a day, and the patient measured her urine dipstick for glucose levels. Today women have monitors and measure their blood sugar eight times a day. Many have a computer pump device; the pump considers what the blood sugar is, how many carbohydrates the woman is going to have with a meal, and she programs it to give the proper amount of insulin over time. It leaks in a little bit of insulin continuously for each meal, just like a normal body does.

"Newborns of diabetics have problems that can be controlled or reduced by controlling the mother's blood sugar. Jaundice, breathing problems, low blood sugar, and trouble feeding are common. We have these women calling or faxing three times a week with their blood sugars. We read the numbers and make adjustments, because over the course of a pregnancy insulin requirements go up at least 100% because of the physiology of pregnancy.

"The relationship of blood sugar to birth defects and miscarriage actually relates to the blood sugar at the time of conception. We try to identify diabetic women who want to have babies, and bring them into this program before conception. At any given time I'll have a dozen or more women who are planning to become pregnant, and we're doing all their diabetes care to normalize the blood sugar to reduce the risk of complications.

Dr. Comstock: "Before the strict control of blood glucose, there were many more deformed babies. They can have short legs, heart defects, brain defects—we hardly see those anymore because of the strict control of diabetes."

Dr. Lorenz: "In about 1981, a New England Journal

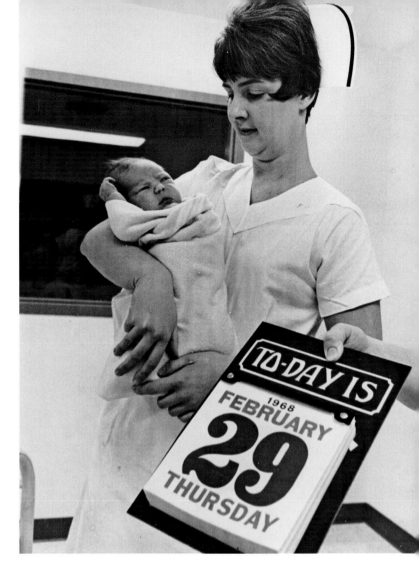

Beaumont's first leap year baby.

article showed that diabetics that had the worst blood sugars at the first OB visit had a 21% rate of birth defects. Now, that's huge. The general population is 3%. Diabetics who had the best blood sugars had a rate of birth defects of 4-5%. So right there, we can reduce the rate of birth defects by a large factor just by controlling blood sugar. This is what we ought to be doing with everybody."

MORE COMPLICATIONS

Dr. Lorenz: "Kidney transplants, heart disease, cancer patients—those are typical medical problems we see in obstetrics. Other types of problems are the lady with triplets, the lady with twins, the lady with a birth defect, and the lady who delivered her last child at five months of pregnancy. For some conditions we sample the baby's blood while he or she is inside; put a needle in under ultrasound, find the umbilical cord, draw blood, and do a test on it. Sometimes if the baby has a low blood count, we can even give the baby a blood transfusion at the same time. The technology related to obstetrics has advanced tremendously."

THE SECOND PATIENT

Dr. Comstock: "One of my colleagues is a pioneer in 3-D and 4-D ultrasound imaging. Fetal imaging is really for diagnosis, but it does expand the bond between parents and the unborn. Of course the family wants to see the baby. It's hard for them to understand that we're also doing a medical test and the objects are very, very small. We're trying to look at the heart, which is the size of a thumbnail, and we're trying to look for one-millimeter defects.

"Fetal imaging has changed obstetrics because throughout most of history we had no way of looking at our second patient, which is the baby. Today we can follow growth, look for defects, look for flow of blood in the cord to the placenta or in the brain, or tell when the baby is anemic. If the baby might be anemic, we look at the middle cerebral artery's blood velocity. If it's high, the baby is preserving blood for his or her brain, shunting blood from the body to the brain. It might be due to a virus or RH disease, where the mother has antibodies to the baby's blood. We have a much-expanded role in treating the baby before he's born."

GLOBAL CONTRIBUTIONS

Dr. Lorenz: "Chris' division is internationally known for their contributions in research about the fetal brain, the fetal heart, and they've established screening methods that have changed the way we approach a number of different fetal conditions. They're really made a major contribution far beyond Michigan."

Dr. Comstock: "Radiology was doing the OB ultrasound when I came here. I had to get equipment, and hire people, but I was lucky because it was at a time, 1984, when there was a huge growth in ultrasound. About five years after I got here, I hired Wesley Lee from Baylor University, and he is internationally known. He has figured out how to use the 3-D and 4-D technology in diagnosis and provides seminars nationally and internationally.

"We're used to looking at the surface-type 3-D,

in which we can see the baby's face, but the more helpful one is where we can dissect all the tissues away and look for the structures under the face. Does the baby have a cleft lip or palate? Along with other people, Dr. Lee has developed a technology to see the fetal heart pumping, the direction of blood flow, and all the vessels that go in and out, and the image can then be turned around for another view. They're trying to improve the diagnosis of, for instance, abnormal drainage of the veins that go into the heart, because that can cause a baby to die right at birth."

Dr. Lorenz: "If we find a heart defect, we gather the pediatric cardiologist, the neonatal doctors, the ultrasound people, the genetics people, the obstetrician, and ourselves, and try to determine what exactly is the structural problem. With some heart defects, the baby's heart isn't going to work right for the first couple days and will require cardiac surgery. Others will be a problem within the first year. Long before the end of the pregnancy, we make a decision and pick a site of delivery in a place where cardiac surgery can be done on newborns."

Dr. Comstock: "When we do screenings, we're sorting that out. Does this heart look normal? Is there a diaphragmatic hernia? There's a very long checklist of what might be discovered. We use checklists so we don't miss anything. We also designed our computer program so that if we miss something, it tells us."

CORPUS COLLOSUM, AND OTHER BRAINY THINGS

Dr. Comstock: "Corpus collosum is a bundle of fibers that connects the right and left brain. I was the first person to find it in the fetus and describe it. Since then, there's been a huge amount of literature about it. If a baby has it, he can have one of 180 syndromes, most of which are bad. So it helps in counseling patients.

"Another contribution was a paper out of our unit written by Dr. Richard Bronsteen which has changed how people deal with choroid plexus cysts, little cysts found in the brain that are more frequent when a person has three copies of the eighteenth chromosome, which is bad. When that work first came out, everyone who had a choroid plexus cyst got an amniocentesis to check for extra 18th chromosomes, but someone in our unit published a paper saying that if the hands and heart are normal in the presence of these cysts, amniocentesis wasn't necessary. We extend our examination to look for the hands, and get a complete view of the heart. That has become a world-wide standard now and has cut down dramatically on the number of amniocenteses."

"The most important contribution I made was back when I was here by myself. I noticed a few hearts that were pointed to the left shoulder or over to the right. Normally the heart is pointed at forty-five degrees. I figured out what the normal axis was by looking at 200 normal babies. Then I looked at everyone who had an axis to the left and to the right, and found that babies with an axis to the left often have abnormal great vessels—the aorta, pulmonary artery—so it's a good, simple screening tool. If we see an axis to the left, we have to extend to an echocardiogram to make sure the heart vessels are normal."

Dr. Lorenz: "I do ultrasound only under certain circumstances, just to figure out something, brief and targeted, but this axis check is so simple that I know if the axis is wrong, I have to get somebody to look at it. It's a neat way to sort patients and not miss something more serious."

THE "FASTER" TRIAL

Dr. Lorenz: "The FASTER trial really revolutionized screening."

Dr. Comstock: "It stands for 'First and Second Trimester Evaluation of Risk.' It was a National Institutes of Health multi-center trial. Beaumont was one of two places that were not university hospitals. We were the only hospital in the Mid-West in that trial. Beaumont contributed a large number of patients to that trial. There were 33,000 patients, and Beaumont was 6th out of 20 in the number contributed. That trial changed screening for chromosomes. It's a blood and ultrasound test, applying to all women of all ages. No longer is it the rule that women over 35 are offered amniocentesis to check for Down's Syndrome. Most of the women who have babies with Down's Syndrome are less than 35 years old. The test developed from this trial showed that we can pick up abnormal chromosomes

in about 90 to 95% of women, so amniocentesis is no longer the first choice for diagnosis.

Dr. Lorenz: It's a better mousetrap that results in at least as high detection rate for Down's with a lot fewer amniocenteses, which is an invasive procedure with some risks. With this, we only need to do five amniocenteses to discover when Down's syndrome exists. Before that, it was hundreds. This markedly reduced the number of interventional procedures."

Dr. Comstock: "The reason we were chosen was that the lead investigator knew we had a very organized unit and did a large number of cases. She later modeled her unit at Tufts University after ours, because she was so impressed."

Dr. Lorenz: "With the support of Beaumont, I've been involved in the American College of OB/GYN for some time, I'm currently on the executive board, and district chair for the Mid-West region. It's given me a chance to contribute nationally to practice guidelines, work on legislation for women's health care, which wouldn't have happened if I didn't have the support of the institution. I've volunteered twice on the Navy's hospital ship *Comfort*. The ship went to Indonesia for the relief effort after the 2004 tsunami. It was a remarkable experience to see what those people had to face and be able to help. Many hospitals would say, 'No, you can't leave for a month.' Beaumont was very supportive and other doctors moved in to cover my responsibilities while I was gone.

Dr. Comstock: Beaumont has given me what I needed, when I needed it. I never asked for more than I needed, but they've never denied me anything. It's been a good place to work."

A nurse checking the vitals of a premature baby inside the incubator.

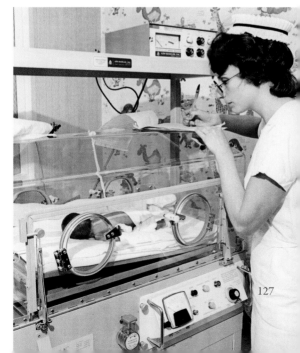

JEFFREY MAISELS, M.D.

Professor and Chair of Pediatrics, Oakland University
William Beaumont School of Medicine and
Beaumont Hospitals

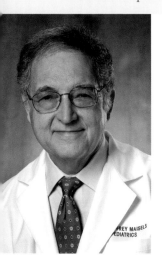

"I'm a neonatologist. I take care of sick babies.

Neonatology is a field that has changed dramatically over the last four or five decades and the outcomes for sick newborns and, particularly, for tiny premature infants are entirely different today from what they were when I started in this field more than forty years ago.

"I was born in Johannesburg, South Africa. I finished my medical school training at the University of the Witwatersrand, Johannesburg, in 1961, and came to the U. S. in 1966. I wanted to leave South Africa because I didn't want to bring up my children in the apartheid system which existed then. The chair of pediatrics at Harvard, Charles Janeway, arranged for me to get a job at the Northshore Children's Hospital in Salem, Massachusetts, where the witches come from. I spent a year there and then six months as the Chief Resident of the Medical Outpatient Department at the Boston Children's Hospital before starting a fellowship in neonatology at the Laboratory for Neonatal Research, Boston Lying–In Hospital and Harvard Medical School. These were the peak years of the Vietnam war and the U.S. Army needed doctors, so before I could finish my fellowship, I was drafted into the Army Medical Corps.

"During my fellowship, I had developed a special technique for measuring carbon monoxide production in newborn infants. This is measure of the rate of hemoglobin catabolism (breakdown). It is also a measurement of the rate of bilirubin production so it can tell us why a baby is jaundiced. Fortunately for me, the fellow who ran the hematology research lab at the Walter Reed Army Institute of Research in Washington, D.C., wanted a person who could do these measurements in adults. So I was assigned to Walter Reed instead of

wherever they would've sent me including Vietnam. In order to go there, I had to agree to serve for three years instead of two which is the regular time in the draft. Needless to say, I was happy to do that.

"I spent three years at Walter Reed, where I did some research both in adults and in babies. Then I got a job as the Chief of Neonatology at the new Pennsylvania State University College of Medicine in Hershey, Pennsylvania, where they make chocolates, and I stayed there for 15 years.

"When I started there, I was the fourth person in the pediatric department. By the time I left, we had developed a regional neonatal intensive care program with babies transported by ambulance, helicopter and fixed wing transport from sixty hospitals in twenty-four counties. We took care of many Amish babies. They delivered their babies at home, but if there was a problem they would come to us.

"Then, I came to Beaumont. Dr. Robert Lorenz had completed his training in Hershey and was the head of fetal and maternal medicine here at Beaumont. His wife, Christine Comstock, is the head of fetal imaging. They were visiting Hershey and told me that Beaumont was looking for a new Chairman of Pediatrics. So I gave Bob my resume, and a couple of weeks later I got a call from Dr. Julius Rutsky, who was then the Chief Medical Officer. I came here in August of 1986 and I've been here ever since."

"I've been involved nationally in my role as the head of the Subcommittee on Hyperbilirubinemia of the American Academy of Pediatrics. This committee develops guidelines to help pediatricians take care of jaundiced babies. We make bilirubin all the time, but our livers get rid of it. In babies, the liver is not yet mature. In addition, they produce more bilirubin than we do and that is why almost all babies develop some degree of jaundice. Most of the time this does not cause a problem, but if the bilirubin level gets very high, it can cause brain damage. So that is why we monitor the bilirubin levels in all babies and we treat them with a special kind of light if the bilirubin levels get too high. This light treatment, called phototherapy, is very effective in lowering the bilirubin levels.

"I've done a lot of research on how to use these phototherapy devices most effectively, and I have continued to measure the rate of bilirubin production in babies using the carbon-monoxide technique although it has now been automated and is a much simpler technique than the one I originally developed. I have also done research on methods for measuring the baby's bilirubin level in the skin. This provides instantaneous information and avoids the need for a blood sample.

"I'm now the head of Beaumont Children's Hospital, which officially opened in 2009. We can take care of all sorts of children's ailments and injuries, and make life much better for Beaumont's young patients."

Jeffrey Maisels, M.D., Pediatrics, was the recipient of the 2007 APGAR award from The American Academy of Pediatrics for having a continuing influence on the well being of newborn infants. Dr. Maisels was the first physician to describe the use of a rebreathing technique to measure carbon monoxide production in newborns.

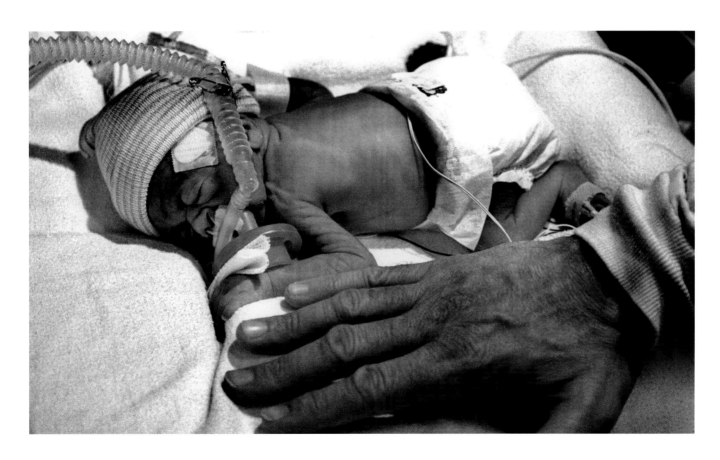

ANANIAS DIOKNO, M.D.

Chair, Department of Urology, Beaumont, Royal Oak, 1984–2007
Executive Vice-President and Chief Medical Officer,
  Beaumont Hospitals

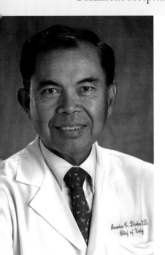

"After twenty-three years as Chairman

of Urology at Beaumont, I had built a department that was one of the top fifty in the country, according to the *U.S. News and World Report* ranking. One of my former students and residents, Jay Hollander, joined me a year into my chairmanship as the Director of Education and later as Program Director of our Residency program. Evan Kass, a former resident at the University of Michigan, joined me as well, as Chief of the Division of Pediatric Urology. These two, in addition to Jose Gonzalez, who was already an attending at Beaumont when I came here, were instrumental in the success attained by the Urology Department.

"I was able to increase the length of the residency from five to six years, and the number of attending urologists from eight to thirty-eight. All these urologists, in one way or another, contributed also to the success of the department. These urologists represented every possible sub-specialties in urology, including cancer care, bladder dysfunction and incontinence, pediatric urology, stone diseases, infertility, prostate diseases, erectile dysfunction, robotic surgeries, and many others.

"Our research programs were very active. The department was continuously funded by the National Institute of Health (NIH) since 1984. It was during this period that I received the coveted NIH MERIT Award. We have established very robust clinical trials that made it possible for many patients to receive drugs and devices that were not available elsewhere because they were still under trials.

"We had successful philanthropic fund raising, thanks to the help of Jose Gonzalez in introducing Mr. Peter Ministrelli to our department. Peter and Florine Ministrelli were so generous that they started funding our International Fellowship program. We had Fellows from Argentina to Zambia, from China

to Russia, many who are now practicing or leaders in their countries. Mr. Ministrelli was so impressed with our progress that he donated multi-millions of dollars in funds in perpetuity to support the department's research and education. This is now known as MPURE—the Ministrelli Program for Urologic Research and Education.

"Part of the funding was also to establish the Peter and Florine Ministrelli Distinguished Chair in Urology. I had the honor of being the first 'occupant' of the Chair.

"One long-term plan of my chairmanship was to develop a succession plan. I had groomed a successor, Kenneth Peters, who succeeded me on July 1, 2007. I had accomplished everything in my vision for the department, and by 2006 I was on maintenance mode. I was ready to retire.

"In June of 2006, my secretary got a call from Ken Matzick, the new CEO of Beaumont Hospitals, who asked to see me right away. I thought maybe he had some prostatitis or BPH or something. When he came into my office, I was sitting behind my desk and he was like my guest. He told me confidentially that he was considering picking his own Chief Medical Officer. He was a new CEO and of course wanted to model the hospital system after his own ideas.

"There were quite a few of the vice-presidents who would qualify for that, who were popular and good leaders, someone who was already on his or her way to a higher position.

"Mr. Matzick said he was also looking for someone who had been successful as a department leader and in developing a residency program, who was respected in the United States as a teacher and program leader—someone who would be good at bringing in funds and philanthropy, a researcher himself, and a very respected clinician nationally.

"'I have consulted the Chairman of the Board,' he told me, 'and we're unanimous in our choice for this person. And that is you.'

"I sat back in my chair, shocked. I have never been in medical administration leadership except for being Chairman of Urology. I never aspired to be a CMO and I was ready to retire in a year. At that time I was already 64 years old, but he told me that they would suspend the rule about retiring at 65 for me.

"I started calling people. My wife, my partners, and my confidants. I emailed my four children. Even before this, people had told me that I had a lot of respect and influence at the administrative level. They said that when I spoke, people listened. Really, I just say what I think is right, fair, or best for a patient, but I had apparently made an impression.

"At this level of my career, this may be a good ending for me. Never in my wildest dreams had I imagined being the Chief Medical Officer at Beaumont. And here I am."

Besides Dr. Diokno's active practice as seen in this picture, he had a robust international fellowship program, thanks to the generosity of the late Robert Flint and later by Peter and Florence Ministrelli. He trained over 40 fellows from 4 continents, from Argentina to Zambia.

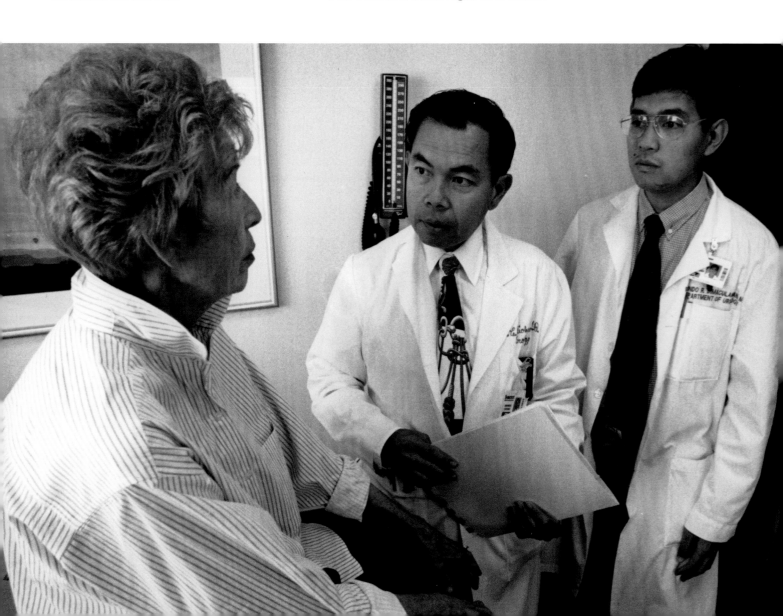

10

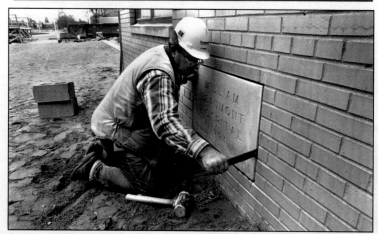

Pipeline

For employees, medical staff and volunteers at Beaumont, Royal Oak   October 25, 1993

Good for another 40 (or more) years

Charles Suder, of Jones and Simpson Mason Contracting, cements in place the hospital's 1953 cornerstone.

The cornerstone wa... the north side of the S... Wing Oct. 12. According... Design/Build, it had be... location just west of th...

The wall in which the cornerstone had been installed was demolished as part of the Critical Care Tower construction. The cornerstone then was...

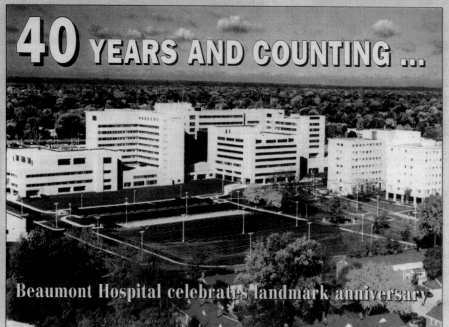

40 YEARS AND COUNTING ...

Beaumont Hospital celebrates landmark anniversary

DUANE MEZWA, M.D.

Professor and Chair of Radiology, Oakland University
William Beaumont School of Medicine and
Beaumont Hospitals

"I started at Beaumont in 1979,

when there were 16 radiologists. I was the sixteenth. At our maximum we were 82, between Royal Oak and Troy. I think we have about 75 right now, including several who are part time.

"Radiology uses multiple means to look at the human body and determine why someone may be ill. We may use magnetic resonance imaging—MRI. We use sound waves with ultrasound. A CT-scan, or CAT scan, is 'computed tomography'; CT uses energy waves to make a two-dimensional X-ray image. PET scan is 'positive emission tomography.' Its a type of nuclear medicine. In nuclear medicine, we actually use radiation that is being emitted.

"There is a variety of techniques we use under the term 'radiology.' CT is very good at showing large tumors, but sometimes tumors can look like normal anatomy. We can now use nuclear medicine to pick up areas of unusual metabolic activity—in other words, if there's a tumor that is rapidly using glucose, a PET scan will identify those areas that are turning over quickly. There might be a normal-looking lymph node that lights up on PET, then we can fuse the CT image on top of the PET and find that it's an abnormal lymph node with abnormal activity.

"Nuclear medicine is good for function, and CT is good for looking at gross anatomy. Putting the two together is called 'fusion imaging' and that's what we're doing with our PET/CTs and SPECT/CT—marrying a CT with images of different slices through an organ.

Dr. Mezwa reviewing
intestinal images

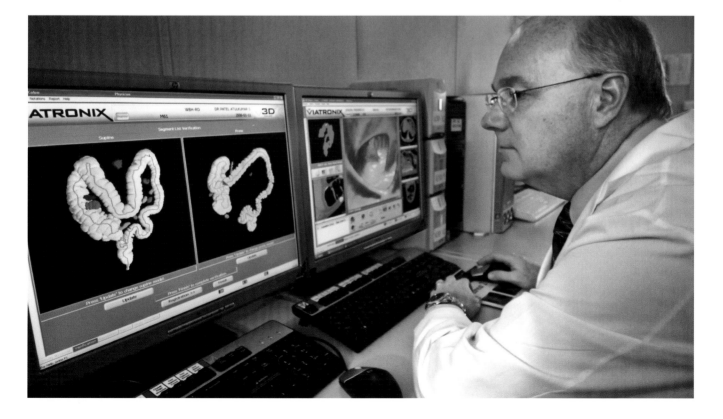

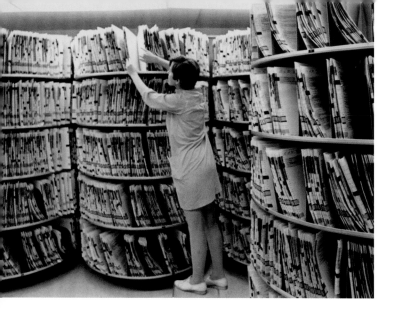

X-ray images are now digitally stored and electronically viewed eliminating huge storage space and personnel time to store and locate films.

"Nuclear medicine involves injecting radioactive materials into a patient, and as the body emits radiation we measure how much radiation is emanating. Using radiation that is tagged to certain particles causes those particles to go to different parts of the body. We use sulfur colloid if we want to look at the liver, because it goes only to liver tissue. A tumor will appear as a big empty spot.

"If we can tag using monoclonal antibodies, antibodies attracted to a tumor, and tag the radiopharmaceutical right onto it; it will be able to deliver radiation right to the tumor."

"In the old days, radiologists were actually Board-certified in everything. They did diagnoses and therapy, but that broke off years ago. We have physicians who specialize in nuclear medicine, radiologists who do diagnosis, and radiation oncologists who do therapy.

"We use ultrasound and MRI to help guide us during biopsies. So not only are we diagnosing, but today radiology is far more involved with treatment as well. For example, in our angio-interventional area, I have radiologists who will ablate liver tumors. In other words, they use radio frequency and high heat or cold to take a liver tumor and freeze it or burn it so the patient doesn't need surgery, or they'll get the tumor down to a point at which it's easier for a surgeon to extract whatever is left. If we're not able to ablate, we put a catheter in and deliver chemotherapy right to the tumor. There are fewer side effects for the whole body if we hit that tumor directly. We have another technique with which we combine nuclear medicine with radioactive seeds, and put them directly into the center of the tumor.

"Women with uterine fibroid tumors used to face surgery to remove them. They're benign, not malignant, but cause a lot of pain. Today, for women who would otherwise be getting hysterectomies, we can embolize those tumors—cut off the blood supply. That will either make surgery much easier or even eliminate the need for surgery.

"We're on the forefront of a study with our breast surgeons to look at small breast tumors, involving putting a needle in the right place and eliminating that tumor. The patient walks out with a bandaid and goes back to work the next day, instead of having surgery.

"We weren't doing these things ten years ago. Today our radiologists are able to use their skills to do these procedures. These are all new techniques."

"Today, we look at organs. In the future, we want to get down to the cells. We're hoping to be able to deliver therapies at an even smaller level—at the cellular level—and be able to detect tumors before we can even see them, by utilizing nuclear medicine techniques and tagging pharmaceuticals to a radio nucleotide that goes directly to the tumor and doesn't go anywhere else."

X-RAY TECHNOLOGIST OR RADIOLOGIST?

"A radiologist is not the same as an X-ray technologist, which is a common mistake in perception. The X-ray technologist is the person who actually takes the X-ray. They know how to get in there and scan. That's not the expertise of a radiologist. I could not take an X-ray. We're taught to read them, and that takes a long time, and the learning process is never done. We have to re-certify every ten years, go back and take the test to prove that we've kept up on our skills. I'm involved with the American Board of Radiologists, so I sit on the Board that gives that exam. There are fifteen of us around the country who are on the Board and help develop the exams for our residents. We want to make sure that when someone goes to an office that says 'Certified by the American Board of Radiology,' that means something. Patients need to check that.

"In Michigan, there's no requirement for technologists to be certified. Anybody can turn a

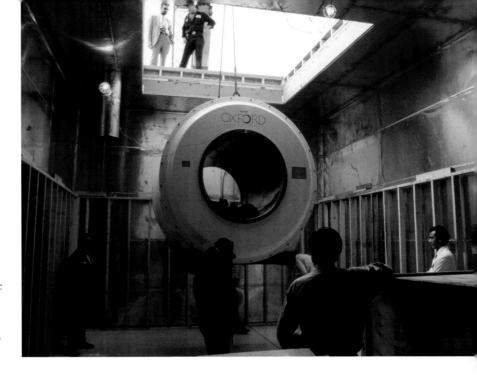

machine on and take an X-ray. Our students go to school for two years just to learn how to take X-rays.

"In our department, we've taken the approach that we are highly specialized. We're also 24/7 in the ER. We have nine radiologists who do nothing but emergency radiology. We have neuroradioloists and body imaging radiologists who are experts in CT and MRI. We have four pediatric radiologists, three full-time and one part-time who also does some musculoskeletal imaging. Children are special, not just little adults. They have their own diseases that we don't see in adults. We want to make sure we keep those films in the hands of experts.

"There are many good general radiologists out there, but we want people to know that if they come to Beaumont, they're going to get that higher level of expertise."

"When I first started in 1983, you couldn't get a CT-scan after 5 o'clock. They turned the machine off. And at that time, CT was just a scan of the head. Now it's for the whole body. It used to take twenty or thirty minutes to generate a study. Today, with our Flash CT, the patients are done in less that two seconds for the entire body. You fly through the machine with far less radiation. The equipment is getting very sophisticated, and the beautiful thing is that we have no idea what the next black box will be. We don't know what will be the next great diagnostic tool."

THE PHYSICIAN'S PHYSICIAN

"Radiology is highly intellectual and you're never done learning. You read every day of your life and the stimulation never stops. You're a consultant to doctors. You are the physician's physician. Often you may not get the thanks and respect from patients, because they don't know you're doing a great job. Every now and then you might get a thank-you note from a patient for finding a cancer that nobody else saw while you were looking at a mammogram for tiny grains of white dots that tell you it's an early cancer. And we're getting better and better at finding these things early.

"We need to get out there and tell the world that we are the faces of radiology. We're their doctors' consultants, the imaging experts who will help

determine what's wrong, because the doctors sent you to us."

"We get people who are engineers, physicists, people who like math and science, who want to continue learning. The best and the brightest are going into radiology. Beaumont's residency is one of the best in the country."

RADIOLOGY IN THE NEW MEDICAL SCHOOL

"The next big thing for us is the medical school. I am the Chair of Radiology for the medical school. We'll have a large role in teaching anatomy, and radiology with our MRIs and CTs, and correlating with gross anatomy. Our radiologists will be involved with many of the committees throughout the school. We're going to have a new rotation in the fourth year that is going to be like no other rotation anywhere in the country. We're going to concentrate on teaching how to decide which method of imaging should be used in various cases, and what is appropriate, whether lab tests change anything for the radiologist to consider, and what's the best bang for the buck."

Installation of the magnet for an MRI machine being lowered into place.

LESLIE ROCHER, M.D.

Professor of Internal Medicine, Oakland University
William Beaumont School of Medicine
Senior Vice-President and Physician-in-Chief
Beaumont, Royal Oak

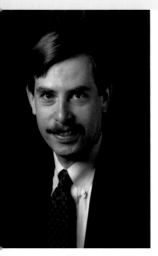

"I became Chair of the Department of

Internal Medicine at Beaumont, Royal Oak, in 1992, three years after initially coming to the hospital to serve as the section head in nephrology and director of transplant programs. By that time, the Department of Internal Medicine had grown to local prominence over the years under the leadership of Drs. Morita, Weintraub and Lauter. The department had grown substantially and developed several training programs, including an internal medicine residency and fellowships in multiple disciplines. Many of the best doctors in our community had relocated their practices to be affiliated with the department.

Partly as an outcome of this dramatic growth, by that time it became difficult to find doctors to accept new patients being admitted to the hospital through the emergency room. It was not uncommon to have ten to fifteen admissions, even back then, in the late evening and early morning hours, presenting without a Beaumont primary care doctor. The initial strategy had been to mandate an on-call program for all general internists to accept such patients. Given the size of the staff, this meant call every six to eight weeks. This didn't work too well. Even by that time, the pressures of a large outpatient practice coupled with inpatient work was stressing the medical staff. Doctors would come in early in the morning, make rounds, go back to the office and see outpatients, and frequently need to come back in the evening. If they had call and admitted several patients through the night, they were too physically exhausted to care for their outpatients the next day.

We came up with a new idea. We offered to eliminate the call requirement, and in its stead, hired a doctor to accept all of the unassigned new admissions from the emergency room. I was concerned this might not be popular, as the vast majority of the medical staff was in private practice, and new doctors often built their practices from

such emergency room referrals. Nonetheless, this idea was greeted with open arms, and our hospitalist program was inaugurated in this fashion in 1992. It soon became evident that this program was destined to grow. It was very difficult for internists to care for their acutely ill patients when they were simultaneously in their outpatient offices, often at substantial distance from the hospital. These hospital-based doctors now not only cared for the unassigned patients admitted at night, but could also provide care to inpatients at any time of the day, as their practice was based exclusively in the hospital.

Over time, as outpatient practices have grown, the majority of our medical staff have divided themselves into outpatient-based internists or inpatient-based internists, these being designated as hospitalists. While this has produced some challenges in continuity of care for patients, in the aggregate, it has permitted our patients to receive better inpatient care, and allow doctors a much better control of their schedules and personal lives. This is a trend that has been seen at virtually every American hospital, but I think our program must have been among the first to initiate such a service.

Through the 1990's and into the first decade of the 21st century, the department of medicine continued to prosper, the admissions in 1992 were 39,000 per year, in 2000 they were 53,000 per year, and in 2010 they were 56,000 per year. The academic stature of the program has also grown on the basis of its outstanding postgraduate training programs in internal medicine, geriatrics, gastroenterology, infectious diseases, hematology and oncology, and cardiology. Over this time period, hundreds of peer-reviewed publications, book chapters and other educational materials were published by the members of the Department of Internal Medicine and its related specialties.

DR. ROCHER ON TRANSPLANTS

"Beaumont has a long history of providing care to patients with end-stage renal disease. Renal transplants were first performed here in 1972. The program was one of our first models of effective multidisciplinary care of patients. When I arrived, the transplant team was reorganized with a small core of doctors and nurses focusing on the care of these patients. With this commitment, the program grew rapidly and became one of the larger programs in Michigan. The surgeons Mark Frikker, Robert Threlkeld and Steven Cohn, along with urologists Jay Hollander and Bill Spencer, grew the transplant program to over sixty kidneys a year, a big number then. The outcomes also improved steadily. Success rates with living donors were on the order of 95% at one year and for deceased donor kidneys on the order of 90%. Our outcomes were as good as the best transplant centers in America Our program was the first in Michigan to make routine use of pediatric en bloc (both kidneys in one unit) kidneys; they functioned quite well. This approach shortened the waiting time for some of our patients. Our program also began a collaboration with the University of Pittsburgh to access immunosuppressants that were not yet FDA approved. Several patients with refractory rejection were initially sent to the University of Pittsburgh for initiation of the investigational drug FK506 and were then followed up at Beaumont. This program made the difference for a dozen or so patients. Since then, this drug, known as tacrolimus, is widely used in transplants.

In the late 1980's and early 1990's, we also started a heart transplant program with Dr. Jeffrey Altshuler serving as the surgical director. About fifteen people received hearts, many of whom survive to this day. The program was ultimately closed by us due to a relatively small volume of hearts available in Michigan.

A new chapter in Beaumont's transplant history began in 2008, when Dr. Alan Koffron came to serve as the new director. Under his leadership, the obligatory certificate of need was obtained, and the first liver transplants were performed at Beaumont in 2010."

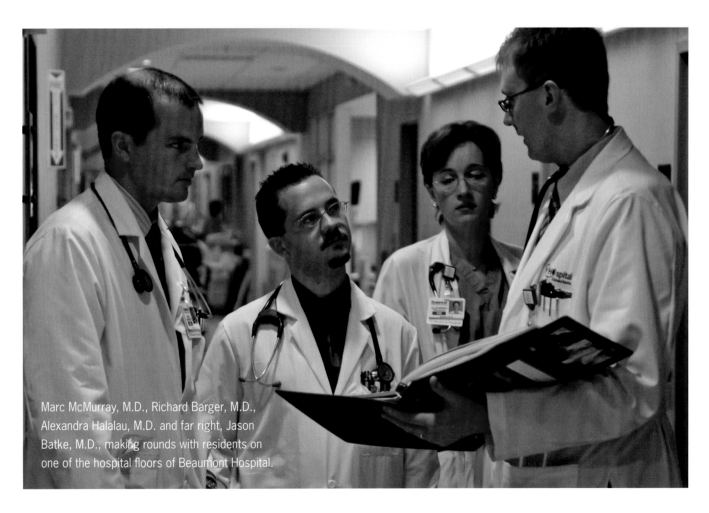

Marc McMurray, M.D., Richard Barger, M.D., Alexandra Halalau, M.D. and far right, Jason Batke, M.D., making rounds with residents on one of the hospital floors of Beaumont Hospital.

MICHAEL MADDENS, M.D.

Professor and Chair of Medicine, Oakland University William
Beaumont School of Medicine and Beaumont Hospitals

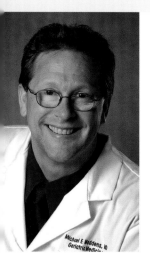

"My involvement in the hospital started

in 1988, when Mr. Garrett Mouw, one of the Board members, convinced the Board to make geriatrics one of its areas of special focus, a center of excellence. Garrett was a businessman in the area and was very involved in the hospital. He had a great deal of future vision. He helped establish the Barnham Rehab Center, which is now the Beaumont Health and Rehabilitation Center on Coolidge Avenue. He was primarily responsible for geriatrics' being developed here. Dr. Carl Lauter, in his wisdom, actually created a separate Division of Geriatric Medicine even before my arrival.

"Beaumont had purchased a partnership in a nursing home at that time, and was in the process of developing another. Dr. Fred Arcari said to me, 'Beaumont's name is well-respected in the community. Your job is to make sure these nursing homes have Beaumont-quality patient care.'

"Beaumont has five nursing homes now. West Bloomfield Nursing Home and Convalescent Center, Evergreen Health and Living Center, Woodward Hills Nursing Center, Shelby Nursing Center, and now the Shore Pointe Nursing Center in St. Clair Shores.

"We do sub-acute short-term rehab at our facilities, probably 40% to 50%. The national average is about 10% or 11%. One of the things I'm happy to say that we did was to take some of the lessons learned from long-term care and bring them back to the hospital, specifically in regard to restraints. When I first came here it was not uncommon in any hospital to see an old person tied down to a bed. That was the norm. This was largely because they thought people would pull out lines and tubes or get up and fall. We did a project at Beaumont and found that we were lower than most others, but if a patient was 85 years of age in a hospital, he had almost a one

in four chance of being tied down in a bed. In the nursing home arena, a small group of folks out East championed the movement to get rid of restraints, and we brought that back to Beaumont. Beaumont is now the National Nursing Quality Database Benchmark for lowest use of physical restraints on general medical and surgical floors.

"What we found is that, in many case, patients didn't need all those lines and tubes, so we took them out, reducing the risk of infection, or we found other ways to keep the patients from pulling them out. For instance, with an IV, we found a way to bring it up the arm, then put a sleeve on so the patient doesn't pick at it, and have the IV come up around his shoulder, so it's not right in front of him. We found that patients were getting Foley catheters inserted if they just needed urine tests, then the catheters would stay in and there was a risk of the patients' tripping or pulling the catheters out if they got confused. We discovered we can do without those in many cases, which also diminishes risk of infection.

"We encourage exercise, sometimes as simple as resistance bands, but sometimes more complex regimens. If we could put exercise into a pill, we'd win a Nobel Prize for medicine. It markedly improves the lives of senior citizens, no matter what age. One of our colleagues, Jack Voytas, has worked with Barry Franklin to set up a program of exercise for seniors called the Optimal Aging Program that combines both resistance exercise and aerobic exercise.

"The great majority of seniors don't want to be waited on or be a burden. There's a lot that can be done to structure activities for older people to allow them to still make contributions. Even for people with cognitive impairment, we can offer choices among the simple and acceptable things that are still

Meaningful activities that incorporate exercise can benefit the majority of seniors, even those with substantial disabilities.

good for them, even if it's as basic as choosing what they want to eat. Sometimes the act of giving respect is as simple as not calling a senior by his or her first name, but rather by 'Mr.' or 'Mrs.'

"We've done some novel things, like creating a day room. We've found that demented patients can avoid restraints more often if they're in an area together with activities during the day, where we can keep an eye on them and meet their needs. We created a day room in one of the medical units where people who were at risk of pulling IVs and catheters could come together and always have a nurse to assist them. We restructured the nurses' assignments so one nurse would be twelve hours with, say, four patients, and the other nurses pick up the slack.

"At first, the nurses were leery of the new schedule, but we found that these were the patients who were causing all the problems by pulling their lines and tubes. If we kept them together and awake during the day, and kept them out of the mix and supervised, the other patients were easier to take care of. The night nurses absolutely love this, because these patients were sleeping through the night. It's simple, but not always obvious."

THE MEDICAL SCHOOL

"Wayne's niche is the urban mission. Michigan State's mission is the rural mission. University of Michigan's niche is the basic science institution. Beaumont's mission, and that of the new medical school, needs to be complex care and chronic disease. We're going to be facing a situation in the next thirty years where one out of five people will be over the age of 65, and they will have accumulated a lot of chronic disease."

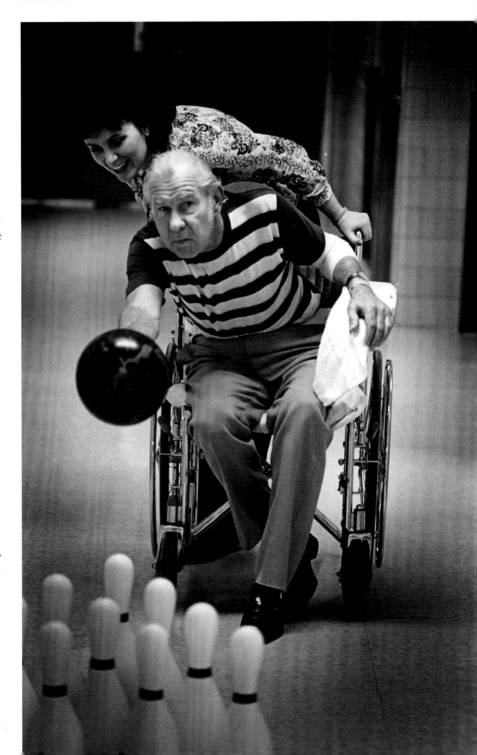

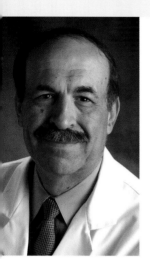

KHALID IMAM, M.D.

Associate Professor of Internal Medicine, Oakland
University William Beaumont School of Medicine
Chief, Division of Geriatrics, Department of Medicine,
Beaumont, Royal Oak

"I had my medical school in Syria,

and my inspiration is really to specialize in the United States to get more knowledge and more experience. I've been at Beaumont since July 1993.

"I did actually two fellowships: endocrinology and metabolism at Wayne State, and in my second and third year I did research on hypertension in the elderly.

"One of my associates, Dr. Michael Maddens, joined Beaumont in 1988 to establish the Division of Geriatrics. He convinced me to join him and we were able to establish a two-year geriatric fellowship at Beaumont to train physicians in the field of geriatric medicine. We take four fellows every year.

"There is a trend toward living longer, with more vibrance for the elderly, especially with preventive medicine, exercise, healthy diet, monitoring cholesterol, treating heart disease, high blood pressure, so the morbidity/mortality gap is being compressed. Our goal is for people to live in good health and as independently as they can until the end. The period between when they become acutely ill and passing away should be short, so they do not suffer, and to reflect positively on the health care costs. The last year of life people spend more money on health care than in the previous five or ten years, especially with hospital care, acute care, and intensive care units.

"Beaumont has a unique setting. We have five academic nursing homes affiliated with Beaumont, we have about 900 beds for long-term and sub-acute care after surgery or fracture, or something that makes the patient not well enough to go home yet. We have a medical director for each nursing home who is fellowship-trained and Board-certified, and they are part of the Division of Geriatric Medicine.

"We have an in-patient service where we do two types of service: other physicians consult us about their patients with geriatric syndromes or geriatric-related issues, and we have our own patients of whom we take care when they are admitted to the hospital. We also have two types of out-patient services: one is consultation in which physicians refer patients to us for geriatric-related issues, specifically memory impairment, dementia, Alzheimer's Disease, other types of dementia, falls, failure to thrive, or other conditions that are related to getting older."

ALZHEIMER'S DISEASE

"There is new information available, however we are still far away from a cure for Alzheimer's. Our knowledge now is probably 300 times more than it was five years ago. Once we know the trigger for Alzheimer's, we might have better treatment. However, normal risk factors for heart attack or stroke—high blood pressure, high cholesterol, diabetes—are the same risk factors for Alzheimer's Disease. Treating those risk factors in middle-aged people has been shown to decrease the risk of Alzheimer's.

"We are participating in Alzheimer's Disease research, trying to identify bio-markers, certain chemicals in the blood, urine, saliva, or other parts of the body. Those markers might be elevated in people with Alzheimer's and hopefully down the road might allow us to diagnose Alzheimer's with a blood test.

"The treatments available now will slow the progression of the illness, but they do not stop it. Keeping mentally active is very helpful. Research has shown that people who are mentally stimulated, doing certain exercises—crossword puzzles, ballroom dancing—and if they keep physically fit and mentally sharp at the same time, will keep more memory and cognitive function much longer.

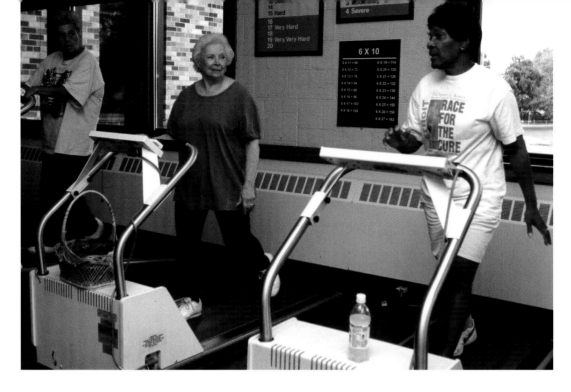

Exercise is a low cost, high return intervention for seniors.

"Also, if we take the same level of Alzheimer's Disease changes in the brain in a person with a high education level and a person with a low education level, the person with high education will have much better function, both mentally and physically. People who have higher education use their neurons more; the neurons are more stimulated. They are involved in using their mental capabilities, so neurons are functioning and active, interacting with each other. It's the same with muscles. To make them stronger, use them more. High education and mental stimulation does, first, provide some protection from Alzeimer's Disease, and, second, the symptoms of the disease are less evident."

WE REALLY ARE WHAT WE EAT

"Eating a healthy diet, especially fruits and vegetables that are high in naturally occurring anti-oxidents—oranges, apples, tomatoes, blueberries—has been shown in studies to be beneficial in working against Alzheimer's. One study suggested that people who have at least five servings a week of those fruits and vegetables have less chance of having Alzheimer's Disease as they get older. In some reports, almost 50% less. An apple a day really does keep the doctor away.

"Exercise is the other important component for physical health. Studies on people in their early 90's being put through an exercise program resulted in muscle function improvement, muscle strength improved, and the ability to remain independent improved.

"If we have retired two persons, one is active, is functioning, is volunteering, is involved in family and community, he or she will tend to maintain mental and physical function much longer than the one who sits down at home and has a sedentary lifestyle. The one who sits down will have more osteoporosis, weakness, fractures, more chance of having heart attacks, strokes, and so forth. Even an elderly person who has been sedentary, then is put to work with an exercise program, both mentally and physically, and follows healthy habits, will have amazing improvement.

"If you want to have your cognitive functions and physical health to an old age, the key is to keep working."

GERIATRICS IN THE FUTURE

"We're going to have more elderly people living longer and being more active, so there will be a huge need for more geriatricians and persons specialized in care of the aged. With 13% or 14% of our population over the age of 65, by 2050, we'll be about 20%. If we have 30 million now, it will be 60 million in 2050. We need to prepare for that.

"I am teaching faculty for the new medical school. The field of geriatrics will be one of the focuses of the Oakland University William Beaumont School of Medicine."

CHARLES SHANLEY, M.D.

Professor of Surgery, Oakland University William
Beaumont School of Medicine
Vascular Surgeon, Beaumont Hospitals

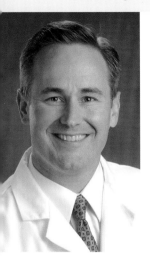

"Last year, Beaumont was the busiest

hospital in the country for acute care in terms of admissions, and we're number one, two, or three in surgeries—it fluctuates. Whenever there is a surgical enterprise that large, the risk for errors goes way up. I helped start the use of applied simulation at Beaumont. I had worked on it, but had nowhere to do it. I and others approached the administration about starting a simulation center in the department of surgery. We wanted our trainees, nurses, allied health professionals, and other members of the team to develop psycho-motor, cognitive, and interpersonal communication skills, so we created a full-emersion environment. My idea was to fully invest all the people in the department of surgery— doctors, nurses, administration, everyone."

TO LEAD THE NATION

"Beaumont is unique in terms of the passion of the people in the community and supporting its doctors, the passion of those who run the hospitals, their support of clinical and academic excellence, even the commitment and dedication of the medical staff, which is very unique with its private practice culture.

"If there ever were a place that had the potential to really lead the nation in clinical surgery, it is Beaumont. There's excellence in clinical care, clinical outcomes, quality, safety, applied clinical research, and the tremendous local brand loyalty from the community. The doctors are long-tenured. They follow their patients over the full cycle of their care.

"We started the dialogue with Oakland University to start one of the country's new medical schools. Because I was an academic doctor, I was able to participate from the beginning and influence the curriculum of the new school. Most of the significant changes in health care will happen because we'll be teaching them directly to the next generation of

doctors. It's hard to get established doctors who've been in practice for twenty years to change, but medical students come in totally on fire to do the right things."

A VISION FOR SURGERY AT BEAUMONT

"Having been in academic surgery, I saw what I believe is a disturbing trend. The shift had moved so heavily toward molecular biology, cellular and genomic research, and things like that, that some places were losing their clinical edge. A surgeon can be superb, and a superb scientist, but the level of sophistication from some of the molecular, cellular, and genomic research and the intensity of focus starts to pull people away from the bedside. Over time, if an institution's clinicians are less engaged, the reputation deteriorates. Beaumont was founded upon clinical excellence at the bedside. Surgery of all the medical disciplines, the ultimate in applied physiology and applied technology, is all about patients and patient care.

"I didn't want to lose that. We should have been using our huge clinical base to learn more about human disease, especially surgical diseases, and contributing to literature, to refining the best practices, the best safety, and other things—I thought that was our opportunity. That's where I've been focusing my vision for surgery.

"We had an enormous clinical operation, we had excellent results, and now we have the simulation component. We're shifting from the 20th Century model, with the physician as the center of the universe, to a model that embraces the physician as a kind of conductor, because now the surgical operation involves a massive team, perhaps with a surgical robot, and with several important parts. That requires focus on effectiveness and team function, not just the virtuoso musician, but with the musician in context of the orchestra. No one had really approached team-based communication or really used simulation effectively in the surgical arena. Now we're doing that."

SURGICAL LEADERS

"To expand our portfolio in complex disease and chronic disease led to the recruitment of Dr. Alan Koffron. Alan is the leading young innovator in the world in laparoscopic live-donor transplantation. That's the kind of thing a quaternary referral center must have—the stuff that's so complex it only goes on in a few places in the country. It incorporates the community hospital services with more complicated procedures. Only people like Alan Koffron can bring complicated things by virtue of their training and experience which very few others in the country or in the world are doing. We've recruited Dr. Fernando Diaz, so we're expanding our neurosurgical portfolio. Our orthopaedics department, under Dr. Harry Herkowitz, is phenomenal. In ophthalmology, we have Dr. Mike Trese, who does neonatal retinal surgery in babies from all over the world. Dr. Kenneth Peters in urology does sacral nerve re-routing. These are one-of-a-kind quaternary things whose expansion will continue in each department and division. The last thing is to bring everything into a multidisciplinary context. Can you imagine the cranial surgeon working with the ENT surgeon or the cancer surgeon, the tracheal surgeon, all in a team? And without losing what made this hospital great, which is its role as the primary place to go in the community.

"The physical plant of Beaumont is big enough. The ORs are big enough that we can actually do the quaternary care, be a referral center, and build this reputation for the medical school, while still being a very strong community hospital. We have and use a pre-operative check list, and we've done 150,000 operative debriefings. We've published it. This is the largest experience in the world employing mandatory pre-operative check lists and post-operative check lists in the OR.

"I don't like to apply a brand name to medicine, but Beaumont really is a brand name. It's the Beaumont standard around quality, a Beaumont standard in terms of outcomes. If your problem is complex, you really need to be here. But if you get a simple hernia repair, it shouldn't matter that you're at Beaumont. The place has unlimited potential."

DOCTORS UNDER PRESSURE

"Physicians are under a lot of pressure. No one is going to feel sorry for doctors, but the truth is that their incomes are under pressure and it's hard to retain the best and the brightest if you can't pay a market competitive price, so we're really focusing on trying to expand our programs and keep the resources coming to continue being the best in technology and facilities, the best in nursing, highest quality in outcomes, and making the physicians want to be here and bring their patients here. If Beaumont continues to focus on making the environment the best in quality, nursing care, the facilities, and the technologies, this will be a prestigious place for doctors to come and practice."

SUSAN CATTO, M.D.

Assistant Professor of Internal Medicine, Oakland
    University William Beaumont School of Medicine
Director, Beaumont Stroke Center
Beaumont, Royal Oak

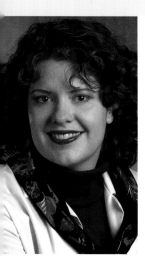

"I was born here at Beaumont Hospital

while my father was living at Belle Court as a resident in general surgery. My father has been here over forty years now. Belle Court is an apartment complex owned by Beaumont.

"My grandfather came from England and my grandmother from Scotland. My grandfather worked at the Ford factory, and my grandmother worked for Sanders Hot Fudge, right next to the old Hudson Department Store building. So my father did quite well for first-generation born in the U.S.

"As we have looked across the country to find other hospitals like Beaumont against which to benchmark ourselves, we have been unable to find a true peer. A thousand and sixty beds, suburban, private-practice, non-university until 2011... there really aren't many 1000-bed hospitals like this.

"The future for hospitals will be one of competition and financial difficulty. How can we take better care of patients, be friendlier with our outpatient physicians, streamline the entire system to reduce re-admissions, reduce complications, and better focus on utilization and safety, all while working with less money?"

MODERN STROKE CARE

"Decades ago, but in our lifetimes, people who had strokes were put in some kind of facility like a nursing home, without much pro-active therapy or intervention, or they were cared for at home by family. There was little that could be done to interrupt a stroke or make use of what we call the Golden Hour, that first hour after a stroke, heart attack, or major trauma during which we try to stop the damage and even reverse it. We do even more than that at Beaumont. We actually have an interventional program. Not only do we use the clot-busting drug, we also use a little corkscrew device called a Merci® Retriever, and something called Penumbra®, which is a little vacuum device to pull a clot out. If we can catch these within eight hours of symptom-onset in the anterior—the front arteries-- of the brain, we can get the clot out. In the posterior circulation, because the mortality rate is nearing 80% if a stroke occurs in the back of the brain, we will often treat the victim up to twenty-four hours from symptom-onset. We've bought a device called a CT Perfusion, which is a great new way to CT-scan people to find out whether there is still viable tissue we can save. We might even have somebody who's young, say 52, and has lost his ability to speak or function with the left side of his body. We can go in and remove the clot even though it's outside of the time window we would traditionally use. If the tissue is still alive when the clot comes out, the patient has a very good chance to retrieve function that might have been lost.

"So those are the two FDA-approved devices we're using. We also use stents and wing-span, and other kinds of devices. Stents are more last-ditch efforts. We really try to get the clot out first. These things were only approved since 2005, Penumbra® in 2009. Beaumont has always been very forward-looking. They've been doing Merci® and intra-arterial clot-busting from the beginning."

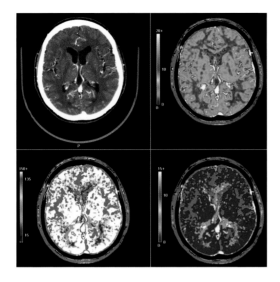

Magnetic Resonance Imaging (MRI) of the brain has revolutionized the diagnosis of treatment of many neurological conditions that in the past were difficult if not impossible to diagnose and treat.

CALL 911!

"Our biggest push is to get people to call 911. There's still too much resistance. The biggest risk factor for a stroke is having had a previous stroke. When we discharge people from the hospital, there are two things I hope to achieve with each patient: first, to at least be able to recognize and acknowledge a couple symptoms of stroke, and for family members to call without hesitation.

"'Stroke' is one of *those* words. Just hearing it causes a 'hold your breath' moment. It's a very important problem. The prognosis is terrible. Prevention and minimalization are the most effective tools—making sure strokes don't happen in the first place, then, if they do happen, recognizing what's happening and getting that person to medical care immediately. It's hard, because when we start talking about the prognosis, most people close up, because strokes are frightening. They're the leading cause of disability in the United States. In fact, the mortality rate is actually 20%. Most people don't realize that."

THE LEADING EDGE

"The future of Beaumont, with the medical school, is bright for all of us. Everyone on staff is excited to work with our community and with the medical school. We're striving to remain a community hospital while becoming a leading globally known institution We never want to lose that edge. We can take air flights of stroke patients from anywhere. Yet, we never want to lose sight of what we do best, and that's taking care of people in Oakland, Macomb, and northern Wayne Counties.

"We've always had that little bit of arrogance—the drive to always be the best, and believing we are. We want to have the greatest equipment and most modern technology, to have a great surgical department, like acquiring one of the first DaVinci robots. We have great stroke tools. We want the finest specialists, a great surgical department, a great neonatal ICU, great oncology tools for radiation like the Gamma Knife, and strive to have the financial success that lets us buy all the latest and greatest tools and attract the best physicians. We definitely want to stay on the cutting edge."

ERNEST KRUG III, M.Div, M.D.

Professor of Pediatrics, Oakland University William Beaumont
  School of Medicine
Medical Director of Clinical Bioethics, Beaumont Hospitals

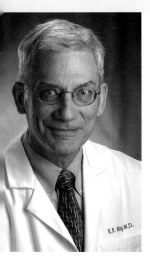

"We have a clinical ethics consultation

service at all three Beaumont hospitals. I direct the Royal Oak consultation service. Typically consults involve families struggling with end-of-life decisions about their loved ones.

"In clinical bioethics, we ensure that there is no violation of the law or of hospital policy, but ethics consultation demands a number of things. One is that we follow a good process for listening to the concerns of the patient or family members. It's not just a matter of saying, 'Well, this is the right thing to do,' then persuading someone to do it. We meet with families and listen to why their perspective is different from the medical team's. The family's understanding of the medical facts is often not the same as the medical team's. We try to build a consensus. We have to be sure our consensus is not outside the law nor outside the societal consensus— in other words, what is considered proper. We are trying to arrive at an *ethical* consensus.

"We can look to prior cases, but there are ways in which our priorities change. I also collaborate with hospital attorneys, so it really is an interdisciplinary task, while attending to the values and preferences of the patients and families.

"One issue is determining the end of a life. If a person is brain dead, he or she is dead under the law, though some people find death by neurological criteria unconvincing. The other circumstance is the persistent vegetative state. The patient is not brain dead, but possesses no cognitive function. With patients who can no longer interact with their environment, but who still have evidence of

brain function, it becomes very important for the patient to have an advance directive. In our society, we allow patients to decide whether they wish to be maintained in that state or not. Unfortunately, most people don't have advance directives in place that would guide the person who has durable power of attorney authority, or help the next of kin, to decide. If the patient's preferences are in writing, this provides the surrogate with guidelines to follow.

"But when you don't have that, the purpose of the family meeting with an ethics consultation team is to sort out exactly what this person's preferences and values are. We meet with the surrogate and/or family and with the attending physician. The focus of the meeting is, 'What would this patient want?'

"Many times, the discussions give the person with decision making authority the impression that he's deciding whether his loved one lives or dies. Preferably, physicians should make this recommendation based on medical facts, and the person with decisional authority can agree with that course of action.

"But sometimes family members say, 'You have to do everything to keep him/her alive.' They say that for a number of reasons. One might be guilt. Another reason may be the lack of trust in the medical system. They may feel they didn't do enough for the patient, or that they have to compensate at the end of life. Ultimately, family members have to gain the ability to say goodbye, to give their loved one permission to die. Some people have trouble doing that."

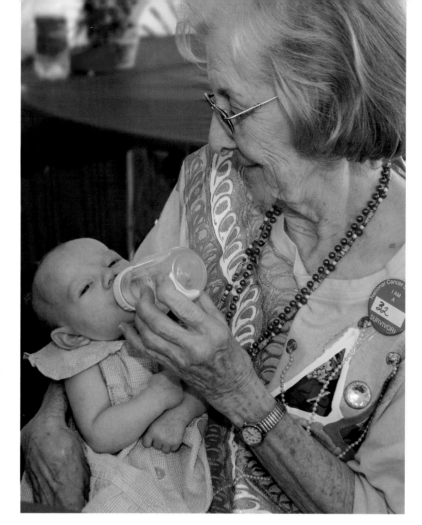

A 32 year cancer survivor with her 6 week old great-granddaughter, at Beaumont Cancer Survivor party.

"One of the things we try to introduce is the idea of *how* the family wants a person to die. Do we want the patient to die while receiving aggressive care that is uncomfortable and painful, in an intensive care unit, which isn't the most pleasant place to die, or do we want him or her to die in a hospice unit, where she can have music and low lighting, rather than people turning lights on and off, and taking blood, and all the other things that happen with aggressive medical intervention? The focus should be on comfort and peace at the end of life, but sometimes people can't accept that, and sometimes the 'H' word—Hospice—is viewed as a defeat.

"Ethics consultations and family meetings bring the focus back to the patient, because there is often argument among family members about what this person wanted. Religion is another factor, because some people have the sense that they must buy more days to give God time to do a miracle. I'm also a minister, and theologically it makes no sense to me. Obviously, my knowledge is limited about other people's belief systems, but I listen very carefully. We call in consultants, and we invite the family to bring in their pastor, rabbi, or Imam.

"You're giving people medical data, but it's not hitting the real issue. What does life mean? What is life going to mean when this person is gone, and how is the family going to deal with it?"

PARENTS AND KIDS AND DOCS AND DECISIONS

"We've had some particularly difficult cases in which parents just couldn't accept the deaths of their children. We provide as much support as we can. There are cases in which the parents refuse medical care, don't want their children to get transplants or blood transfusions, and yet we know we can do something for those children. We generally make the assumption that the parents understand the child better than anybody else and that we should respect the parents' rights as the child's guardian. On the other hand, there's a limit to parental autonomy. If the parents put a limitation on the openness of the child's future, that's a problem.

"We tend to respect keeping the child's future open, so the child can get to the point where he or she can make autonomous decisions as an adult. There's a famous Supreme Court case which involved a parent who was sending his child out to distribute religious tracts. The great statement that came out of that case was that parents can freely exercise their religion, but they don't have a right to make martyrs of their children. That particular statement has become very important in pediatric ethics.

"When a child is in danger, we want to do whatever is necessary to save that child, and give him a chance to grow up undamaged and make his own decisions eventually. If it's an emergency, we do what's necessary. If it's not an emergency and the parent rejects the standard of care, we may seek a court order, which is part of being respectful to the parents, because we're not just going to override them without a court order. If we override a parent, there are lots of consequences. It affects the way the child is going to look at the authority of the parent from then on, so we don't want to do it hastily or without good cause."

"Another important issue is how to deal with treatment options. Maybe one option is not the standard of care, but might be useful. Say it's a cancer case, and in this situation there's a treatment we can offer, but there are significant risks. Then there's another treatment with very little risk. It might not have a lot of benefit, but it has some, and the net benefit of the two treatments is about the same. Well, we could argue that it becomes a patient's choice, or a parent's.

"We in medicine have our own ethos and our own sense of what is the right thing to do. We have to step back and listen to the family or patients, and give them a fair hearing before we say, 'This is what you must do.' That's the authoritarian approach, which has risks in overriding autonomy. It's better to take what we call an 'ethics facilitation' approach, where we listen and understand and make the best decision for that particular case.

"What if a child's parents disagree with each other? That's even more difficult. When we're making a decision about medical care, we aren't required to get permission from both parents. All we need is the informed consent of one parent. If we have two parents arguing with each other, it's very difficult to proceed. We just take more time, provide more explanation. Again, we have to be sure we're not sacrificing the child's best interest while the debate goes on."

ETHICS IN ORGAN DONATION

"About 90% of organ donors are deceased. There are some living donors, but among the non-living donors, about 90% are from brain death criteria and about 7% from controlled donation after cardiac death, where a patient might come in after an accident and has severe brain damage but is not brain dead, and we determine that we can't enable this person to recover. Death is believed to be imminent without life support. A team from Gift of Life, the organ procurement organization in Michigan, can offer the family the option of organ donation. Many families believe organ donation is a way to honor their loved ones. If they decide to do it, the patient goes to the operating room and life support is withdrawn, and then we wait to see if circulation stops. Death may only be declared after a five-minute waiting period following the circulation's stopping. Upon such a declaration of death, surgical recovery of transplantable organs may commence."

THE FUTURE

"My hope is that we will eventually have a robust corporate department of clinical bioethics which can do research and training. There are many exciting things that can be done with regard to understanding patients' preferences, our process for ethics consultation, and determining best practice."

FROM DR. ARCARI

Pediatric Surgeon and former CMO of Beaumont Hospitals

"And now we have Hospice. It has been a major 'plus' in the past fifteen or twenty years, and has changed for a large number of people the environment in which they live the last three to six months, perhaps a year, of their lives.

"It has enhanced the environment for people in the last stages of life, those who are looking at dying because they have a disease incompatible with living more than a few months. It has changed the whole atmosphere of their surroundings, and changed how they function around and within their families in a manner that gives comfort and a sense of fulfillment. It relieves them to a large extent of the discomfort and loneliness that is associated with dying.

"We're usually talking about people in their 60's, 70's, 80's, or lately in their 70's, 80', and 90's. In the past fifty years, they died in hospitals. Prior to the last fifty years, they died at home, and dying at home was perhaps as ideal a circumstance as possible, but dying at home meant you had to have people in the home who could give assistance to you. In the past fifty years, families tended to spread around and there weren't always close family members in the vicinity of those who were dying, so people died in hospitals or in nursing homes. So it was that group of people who needed taking care of.

"As a pediatric surgeon, I must think about children who may be dying. Hospice could well extend to children. Children have the benefit of a mother and father, and there are people already there who are concerned about the patient and making him or her as comfortable as possible at home. And a child is better off at home.

"Hospice and other medical services are more available now in the home, but they're not the specific Hospice service that is defined, with dedicated people to serve the elderly who are dying. Hospice is not as applicable at this time to children as it is to adults. There isn't the same need for children as there is in assisting adults through those last few weeks or months.

"I haven't met a physician who hasn't felt that Hospice was a major benefit to the whole medical scene and the practice of medicine. I haven't met a family that hasn't felt that this was a positive addition to that time in life."

HOSPICE

When Beaumont Hospital was conceived in the 1940's and built in the 1950's, dying at home was normal. Human beings had died at home for uncounted thousands of years—first in their caves, later in their huts, tipis or wikiups, eventually in their own bedrooms. There were undertakers, but no funeral homes. For the western world, in Victorian times the departed were laid out in the parlor for a visitation or a wake, sometimes in a proper decorated casket on elaborately shaped iron stands, sometimes on a wooden board between two chairs. Of course, each culture around the world developed its own coping mechanism. The only inevitable consistency was death itself.

Little could be done in those ancient times, and even within living memory, to ease discomfort for the dying. But those times are not these times.

In the 1940's and '50's, just as Beaumont Hospital was establishing itself, people began more and more to die in hospitals. That is what we now regard as normal. Yet, there has been a kind of circular progress in which, in this modern age of swift advancements in medical science and instant communication, more medical help is available at home than ever before. The process of passing on has come around once again to the home, and those faced with final decisions have a choice.

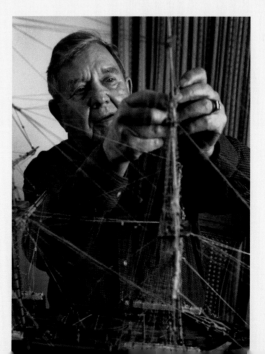

11 BEAUMONT BECOMES A THREE-HOSPITAL SYSTEM

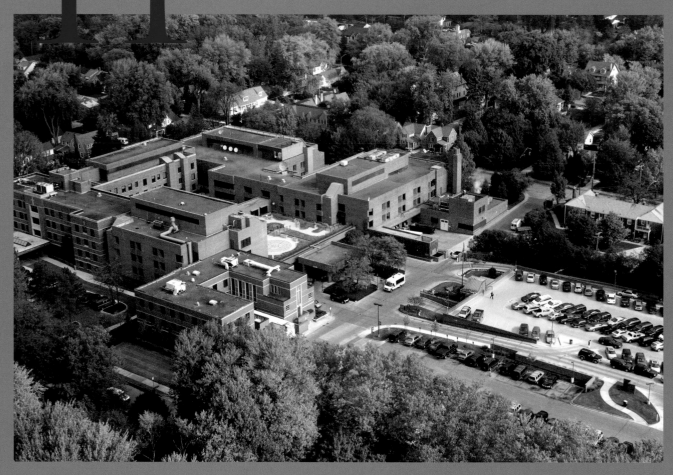

Aerial view of Beaumont, Grosse Pointe

DR. ELLIOTT ON ACQUISITION
OF BON SECOURS HOSPITAL:

"Beaumont's taking over of Bon
Secours has been wonderful."

On October 1, 2007, Beaumont expanded to become a truly regional health system when it bought the Bon Secours Health System of Michigan, located in Grosse Pointe, Michigan. The small 289-bed hospital, run by the Sisters of Bon Secours, headquartered in Maryland, would become Beaumont, Grosse Pointe.

Nestled in the lovely community of Grosse Pointe, near the shore of Lake St. Clair, the former Bon Secours Hospital is an elegant dark-brick building which is in itself almost a work of art. With the acquisition of Bon Secours, Beaumont gained a network of primary-care physicians, and affiliated nursing care and outpatient facilities on the east side of the Detroit area.

The Grosse Pointe hospital won the Governor's Award in 2004 and 2005 for excellence in ambulatory care. In 2008, a renovated pediatrics unit was unveiled, and in 2009, Dr. Dinesh Telang performed Grosse Pointe's first robotic surgery—a radical prostatectomy.

MR. MATZICK ON BEAUMONT, GROSSE POINTE and MANAGING A THREE-HOSPITAL SYSTEM

"We are a $2 billion dollar system. We had hospitals in Royal Oak and Troy, so for years we've been a two-hospital system. I had the opportunity to acquire a third hospital. If the economy shuts down and you're not growing at the same rate, you have to figure out a new path to growth. So we acquired a new hospital: Bon Secours, which is now Beaumont, Grosse Pointe.

"Bon Secours was more than just a hospital. It had a nursing home, a home health company, a physician network, and a variety of other assets which melded into our system. There were many parallels which allowed them to blend with us. The nursing home is now run by our nursing home partners, the physician network is now part of our hospital-based network, so it worked out well. Now, three hospitals create an ambulatory care division, because today's technology allows doctors to do things off campus, in their own offices, and they don't always have the capital to create the facilities, so we join with them and we both have an economic interest in their success. Their patient is our patient.

"We have maybe a dozen large clinic buildings that are usually full of private physicians who have an equity interest in the building. The developers of the building have a long-term anchor tenant called Beaumont Hospital, which helps them acquire financing for the building, and we run ancillary services like radiology and laboratories. The doctors are 'branded' and therefore more attractive in the marketplace. The brand is 'Beaumont.'

"Yet, it's complicated because the economic pressures on the doctors, with Medicare and others holding down increases in their fees, while the doctors' expenses grow, as do ours, and the margins get squeezed. They start looking for new revenue sources. Where do they look?

"Right here at the hospital. Technology allows them to move some services out of the hospital into other facilities, so we get this dynamic tension between the medical staff and the hospital. All that has to be managed."

RICHARD P. SWAINE

Senior Vice President, President,
Beaumont Hospital, Grosse Pointe

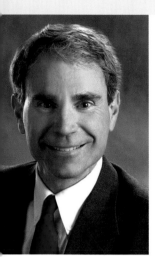

Richard P. Swaine is President of Beaumont Hospital, Grosse Pointe. In 2008, he was named Director of Beaumont's Grosse Pointe Hospital that was purchased from Bon Secours Health System, Inc.

His 26 years with Beaumont Hospitals includes a strong emphasis on operations and finance, working as vice president of Finance at Beaumont, Royal Oak and Beaumont, Troy. Swaine also held various positions including controller and assistant controller from 1985 to 2004 at Beaumont, Troy. Swaine graduated from Lawrence Institute of Technology with a Bachelor of Business Administration in Accounting in 1978 and worked as an audit manager for Hungerford Cooper Luxon and Company until 1985. He joined Beaumont in 1985 as an assistant controller. Swaine became a Certified Public Accountant in 1983 and earned his Master of Science in Finance in 1993.

RICK SWAINE ON THE ACQUISITION OF BON SECOURS HOSPITAL

"The former Bon Secours Hospital, which was purchased in October of 2007, was operationally and financially stressed. The physicians and community had begun to abandon the hospital seeking their healthcare services at competing facilities. The collective vision of the administrative team was to create an environment that would draw the community back to the now, Beaumont, Grosse Pointe Hospital, by emphasizing high clinical quality, exceptional customer service and nursing care second to none."

RICK SWAINE'S VISION FOR BEAUMONT GROSSE POINTE

"Based on our successes over the last three years and envisioning the next five years, we foresee Beaumont, Grosse Pointe as the community hospital that provides personalized healthcare services specializing in women's health, orthopaedic care, minimally invasive surgical procedures and a facility in which the community can obtain exceptional emergency services. Individuals will choose Beaumont, Grosse Pointe for their healthcare needs because of its reputation as a caring environment and one in which the physicians and hospital staff work together as a team to coordinate care during and after their hospital stay…it will be the hospital of choice on the east side."

DONNA HOBAN, M.D.

Assistant Professor of Family Medicine, Oakland
University William Beaumont School of Medicine
Senior Vice-President and Physician in Chief
Beaumont, Grosse Pointe

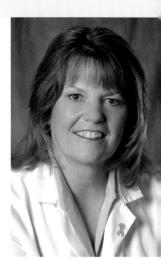

"This hospital was started by the

Sisters of Bon Secours. That order of sisters was originally in Paris, France, then came to Baltimore, Maryland, where they have many health care facilities, then stretching along the East Coast from New York to Florida. They came to Michigan 100 years ago. We celebrated their centennial in October of 2009. Their purpose at that time was to take care of people in their own homes, so they were essentially home-care nurses. They were nurses by education.

"They lived here down on McClellan in Detroit, and there's a cornerstone on the house where they lived. They continued and grew, and finally realized they couldn't take care of everyone in the patients' own homes, so they bought a house where they could take care of sick people around the clock. They bought a cottage at Cadieux and Jefferson and that became the first Bon Secours Hospital. We have many pictures over the years of how the hospital grew into what it was about twenty years ago. We're licensed for 289 beds here, and up until ten years ago our average census was in the range of 220 or 230, so it was a busy place.

"It's a small community hospital, very much supported by the community, the only hospital in Grosse Pointe. The sisters still lived and worked here, in a set of condominiums right on the edge of the parking lot, up until the hospital was sold to Beaumont. The Chairman of the Board was a sister, and another sister, Sister Ann Lutz, who came here from Baltimore, was the 'Sister-President.' They were all sisters, all trained as nurses, and they became relatively savvy businesswomen.

"Then, seven or eight years ago, there was accounting fraud. It had gone on for a couple of years before it was noticed. By the books, people thought the hospital was making $8 million to $10 million a year, but in reality it was probably losing $10 million a year. That caused a tumbledown effect. There was no capital expenditure in the building. By then, the sisters had joined into an agreement with Henry Ford Health System called Bon Secours Cottage, so Henry Ford had entered into a contract thinking they had one

set of income statements, which in fact were incorrect. The real statements were quite different. Even the outside auditing firms had entirely missed it.

"There was no capital spent in the hospital and we really fell on hard times. We lost a lot of the medical staff, the patient census dropped to about 120, and we were losing $17 or $18 million a year. It's a terrible story after so many years of honest service to the community.

"The sisters decided to put the hospital up for sale, and there was brisk competition. St. John's Health System, only two miles away, was very interested, as was the Detroit Medical Center from downtown, Oakwood, which is on the west side, and then there was Beaumont, a surprise to everyone because Beaumont was always a very successful health system. People here were very happy that Beaumont was interested. There was a sense that St. John's interest wasn't really out of passion to acquire Bon Secours, but was generated out of trying to keep a competitor from acquiring it. There was a fear that St. John's would make it a specialty hospital, maybe mother-baby, or make it a senior center, or close it completely, but keep it from being a full-service hospital. The physicians and the community worried about that.

"It came down to St. John's or Beaumont, and Beaumont was the successful bidder. They were most wanted by the physicians and the community. People were delighted to see Beaumont purchase the hospital.

"Then came the process of building a team that would take this hospital that had fallen on such hard times and turn it into 'a Beaumont Hospital.'

"When Beaumont knew it was the successful bidder for purchasing Bon Secours, Ken Matzick and Dr. Diokno asked me to have dinner with them. I couldn't imagine why. They asked me whether I would be interested in a job, and my initial response was no. I really wanted to remain taking care of patients; I like taking care of patients. They wanted me because I'd been around here a long time, and since so many of the new staff were from Beaumont rather than Bon Secours, they needed 'Bon Secours DNA', as Ken put it. I had been the president of the medical staff, so I knew the doctors. At the first dinner, it was a 'no.' By the second dinner, it was a 'yes.' Dr. Diokno is a very convincing man.

"The Sisters actually had to get permission from the Cardinal of Detroit, Cardinal Adam Maida, in order to sell the hospital, because it was a Catholic facility located within his Arch-Diocese. I've been here for twenty years and I didn't even know that at the time. Ken Matzick and Sister Ann Lutz together had to meet with the Cardinal of Detroit and get his blessing. I never would've known that he had authority over the hospital.

"The whole thing was fascinating. The purchase was effective on October 1 of 2007. About a week later, the Cardinal came and had a huge Catholic mass in one of the churches near here. All of the nuns and all the leadership from Beaumont, the Boards of both hospitals all came for this Catholic/secular kind of service, and in the middle they had a candle service. The sisters came forward with candles and talked about their mission here as a Bon Secours Hospital, and one by one they handed their candles over to their counterparts from Beaumont's staff like Ken Matzick and Gene Michalski and Dr. Diokno. The experience was actually very moving and lovely. We were used to having all the Sisters around and the Catholic aura, but I'm sure the Beaumont people were a little amazed. It was a ceremonial passing of the torch."

MAKING A BEAUMONT HOSPITAL, BUT NOT FROM SCRATCH

"When Beaumont took over, the first thing they did was invest a great deal of money for a facelift for the hospital. The front lobby was completely redone. The outside was still pretty, so very little was done other than some landscaping. We still have the lingering touch of the sisters—stained glass windows, the Labyrinth, and other reminders of the Catholic roots.

"Then we went about discovering what the physicians needed in the O. R., and a lot of money was spent on new equipment to bring the doctors back. If you're going to attract the best physicians, you need the best equipment for them to work with. Once we had the best tools and the best physicians, we needed to provide the best patient safety, patient quality, and customer satisfaction.

"During one of the saving-money times of Bon Secours, the nursing ratios became far too low, so we raised them to Beaumont standards. Nurses had fewer patients to take care of, which improves patient satisfaction and safety.

"It really has been remarkably successful. We had customer satisfaction scores that were in the 10th percentile, and now they're in the 90th percentile. We're actually as high or higher than Troy or Royal Oak. All our graphs are just beautiful. The physicians are happy, the community has embraced us and we've been the beneficiaries of multiple millions of foundation dollars from people who saw the hospital coming back. We were budgeted to continue losing money for a couple of years, but we've actually exceeded our budget.

"Now we are going about the process of finding new doctors and new things to do. Part of the reason Beaumont bought this facility was the new medical school. They need an additional spot to train the students. They needed a community setting and this is one, and broadens the footprint of Beaumont in the whole metropolitan Detroit area."

TOP NOTCH

"Beaumont, Grosse Pointe is known for its top-notch nursing care, which also attracts doctors to this nice community setting. With these great safety scores, people are very happy getting their care here, and they know we won't do things that would be better treated somewhere else. If you're here, you know this is the best place for you.

"The decision to keep the hospital full-service was also a Beaumont commitment. We have a beautiful pediatric unit and labor and delivery unit.

"We have just recruited a neurosurgeon, which, for us, is really terrific. It's hard to find a neurosurgeon, especially for a small hospital. There just aren't enough of them. We found one. He's an M.D. Ph. D. in his early 30's who just finished his fellowship, a young doc who does lots of research and innovative things. He has many innovations that have not been done here before. He does a lot of cranial—skull-based—surgeries. In all of medicine, we need young doctors to build programs and see into the future.

"We always have to battle—why should he come to Grosse Pointe? Well, with the medical school coming and our being part of the Beaumont system makes us much more attractive. He came to meet with us not expecting to be working here, but once again Dr. Diokno was very convincing at dinner."

THE FUTURE

"The future here at Beaumont, Grosse Pointe is very positive. We're different from the other two hospitals because of the economic crisis, pay cuts, and so on, but the doctors here are so happy with everything Beaumont has brought them and brought this hospital that they're thankful every day to be part of Beaumont. As one of the doctors recently told me, 'It's like Christmas every day here.'"

LUKE ELLIOTT, M.D.

Assistant Professor of Family Medicine, Oakland
University William Beaumont School of Medicine
President of the Medical Staff,
Beaumont, Grosse Pointe

"I always wanted to be a physician.

I got a Master's degree in physiology, then went to Wayne State's medical school, and applied for two residencies—one in orthopaedics and one in family practice. My mentor, Dr. Charles Lucas, asked why I was applying to two residencies, and said, 'You have to make up your mind about what you're going to do with your life.

"I felt called to family practice, so I gave up my applications to orthopaedics. The family practice residency was for Bon Secours Hospital here in Grosse Pointe. I came here for a three-year residency, and I've remained here ever since.

"In January of 2007, the Sisters of Bon Secours announced that they were selling Bon Secours to Beaumont Hospitals. I had just become president of the medical staff; I represent the medical staff in administative issues. My first month of president was to help figure out who would buy us. There were five hospitals with bids in, and the medical staff recommended that the Sisters sell to Beaumont, and ultimately they did.

"I love taking care of people. There's an intimacy that doesn't exist anywhere else. I always tell my patients that they have to trust their pastor, their lawyer, and their doctor. If they don't trust those three, they have to get new ones. Doctors and administrators have to work together too, with the doctors leading the way because they're the ones who understand health care, supported by administration. The Board of Directors have been urged to get more physician input. They've put the president of the medical staff on the Board on a rotating basis. Dr. Gary Chmielewski from Royal Oak was the first medical staff president ever to be put on the Board. This year it's Dr. Betty Chu from Troy, and next year it will be my turn, then it rotates again. The president of the medical staff is an elected position.

"Bridging the gap between business and medicine is crucial. Physicians know how health care works, and should be able to lead in a way that is professional and business-minded. My goal in life is to bridge that gap. That's why I've gone back to school to get a Master's in Business Administration."

BRAND NEW EVERYTHING

"Beaumont's taking over of Bon Secours has been wonderful. They've changed the hospital. Many things needed updating, and Beaumont turned the place around. We have everything that's brand new. We have the latest and greatest MRI, the greatest CT, called the Flash CT. We have the latest and greatest non-invasive surgery. We have the da Vinci robot. We have a new vascular lab in which we can do cardiac interventions and cardiac caths.

"Rick Swain, our hospital director, is very keen on keeping things looking nice. Even the walls are pretty now."

"Beaumont doctors will be advanced. They'll keep up with both their medical knowledge and also knowledge of how to work with the new systems, like electronic medical records. Instead of the doctor's black bag, I carry an iPad. The system is changing whether we like it or not.

"The Grosse Pointe system has a unique culture of collaboration between the doctors. When I was a resident, I could float a Swan-Ganze catheter with cardiologists—that means put a catheter in a heart in the ICU. There was a resident there who invented it. At the time, it was very advanced technology. I was able to go to anyone's office, stop anyone in the hallway, talk to them at the supermarket, because it was a small and very open community. It still is. The Beaumont family is friendly. It's a bit more formal and I've had to get used to that, but we all have to understand what I'm trying to instill in all the doctors. Who is Beaumont? *We* are Beaumont. It's *we*, not *they*."

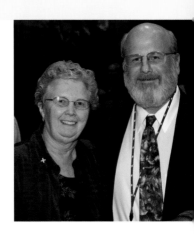

Dr. Elliott with Sister Patricia Heath, SUSC, senior vice president of sponsorship for Bon Secours Hampton Roads Healthy Communities, Bon Secours Hampton Roads Health System.

THE **LABYRINTH**

You're a patient in a hospital. You're surrounded by the old brown brick edifice of the former Sister of Bon Secours Hospital, now Beaumont, Grosse Pointe, and you're not feeling well. Under the proprietorship of Beaumont Hospitals, the interior of the third Beaumont is quickly becoming ultra-modern, stocked with the latest equipment in medical science and staffed by the best doctors and nurses. However comforting this may be, being in a hospital has an element of the scary. It's hard to relax and calm down just because everyone is telling you to relax and calm down. You need a little help.

Look outside.

Set on the elegant grounds of Beaumont Hospital, Grosse Pointe, is a spiritual doorway, even in its silence echoing a human need from the deep past. In the midst of this three-hospital citadel of modern medical science is an ancient portal–a small mosaic patio surrounded by park benches. It is the Labyrinth at Beaumont, Grosse Pointe.

Founded somewhere in the depths of Minoan mythology, even older than Greek mythology, labyrinths have been popular for millennia as artwork—tattoos, basket decoration, wall carvings, fine art, and mosaics. Their most proper use is as floors, something to be walked upon. And there are reasons for that.

There are labyrinths all over the world, many very similar to the flori-centered labyrinth at Beaumont, Grosse Pointe, formerly the Sisters of Bon Secours. There is a labyrinth in the Trappist Abbey of Our Lady of Saint-Remy in Wallonia, Belgium. There is one at St. George Square Gardens in Edinburgh, another at the Basilica of St-Quentin in Aisne, France, and a 9/11 memorial labyrinth at Boston College. There is an ancient one carved on a cave wall at Tintagel Castle in Cornwall, and terraced into the hill at Glastonbury Tor in Somerset, England. While embraced by Christianity and often found in churches and cathedrals, labyrinths are far older than Christianity, rooted in the deep artistic and spiritual past, beyond the Romans, well into the Iron Age and Neolithic periods. They are messages from ages before writing. Or are they lessons? Or guides?

If you were to walk the path at Glastonbury Tor, for instance, you would be led along a shallow route around the oblong mound on seven symmetrical terraces, and at times would seem to be nearing the top, only to be piloted down again in frustration. The top, at 158 meters high, is reached only by knightly discipline in not climbing straight up the hill. Is the frustration a lesson in patience?

The word "labyrinth" is often incorrectly used interchangeably with "maze," but they are not the same. A maze has a cunning system of pathways that branch from one another and have dead ends. A maze calls for choices, guesses, uncertainty, and the very real possibility of getting lost.

A labyrinth has only one path, one beginning, and one end point—in the center—as if a long ribbon has been coiled flat in an elaborate pattern. In fact, a labyrinth allows us to see the way in, see the whole route, and see the goal—the center. Navigation is easy; just stay on the path. Nobody gets lost in a labyrinth. That's because labyrinths are meant for *finding*.

Although they're pretty, labyrinths are not meant to be simply gazed upon. They are meant to be traveled, by eye or by footstep. A labyrinth forces discipline upon the walker, for the advanced path is only a sideways step away, but we're not supposed to take that step. You're supposed to continue on the path, even if it leads away from the center. In a maze, you're supposed to walk between the lines. In a labyrinth, you walk *on* the line. The mind becomes gradually more focussed by the calmness of ritual.

On the Bon Secours Labyrinth, you walk from the entrance toward the center—there it is, right in front of you—but halfway there you're forced to turn sharply left and embark on a long circuitous route that takes you farther and farther from the center. You can see the point of victory—it's right there–but you're not allowed to get there. Not yet.

And don't hurry—that's no help.

A labyrinth offers a road to security. The physical movement provides a theraputic sense of taking action, going forward. You're moving, have a goal, and you will never go wrong as long as you stay the course and continue. Speed isn't important. In fact, moving slowly actually helps. There's time to think, to meditate, to relax, perhaps to clear your head.

Labyrinths are contemplative, meditative. Labyrinths are theraputic. It's impossible to walk a labyrinth with your eyes up. You must gaze downward, keep your balance and control yourself, and that takes a state of calmness. Breathe evenly. Suspend worries. Conquer fears. Concentrate. The labyrinth forces self-discipline and quietude as related to healing. A labyrinth is a pilgrimage to a physical and spiritual center. At the center, there is a sudden turn, a point of decision and accomplishment.

That's when you clearly see the way out again.

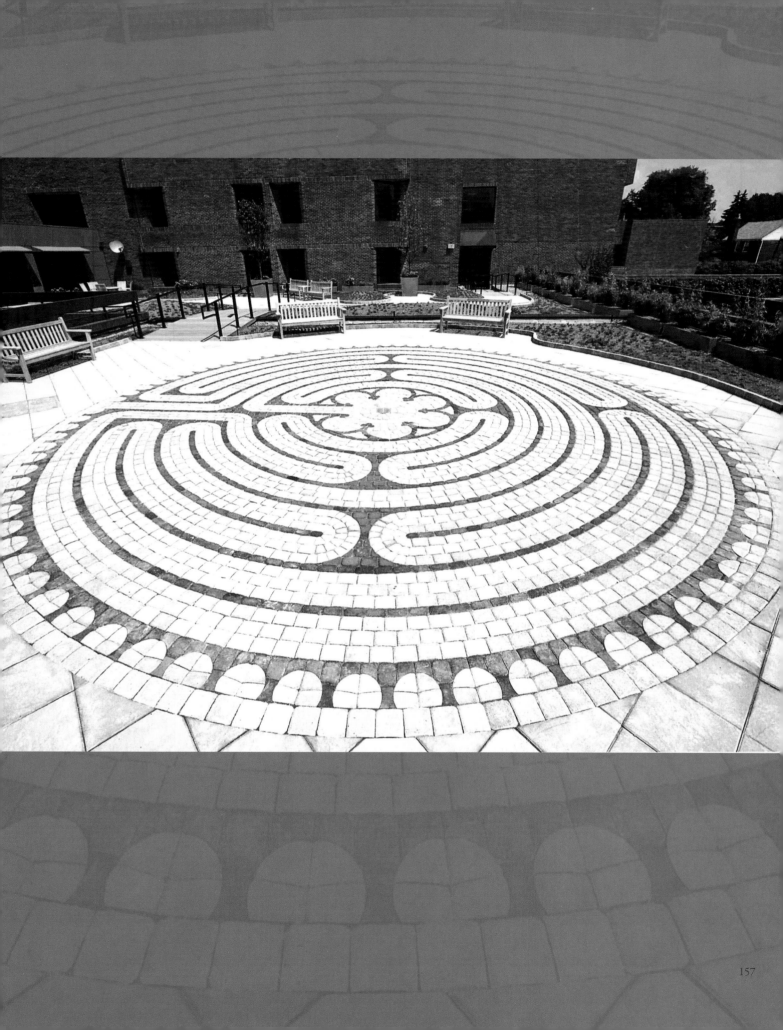

To E.R. is Human

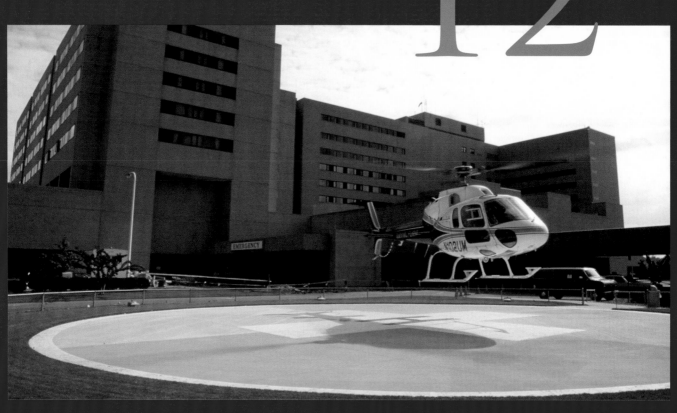

12

Beaumont, Royal Oak heliport, conveniently located adjacent to the Emergency Center entrance.

JEDD ROE, M.D.

Professor and Chair of Emergency Medicine, Oakland University William Beaumont School of Medicine and Beaumont, Royal Oak, 2006–2011

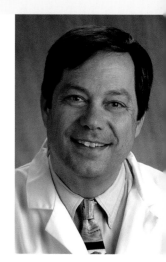

"Emergency Medicine is one of the newest

and most vibrant medical specialties. Most of us are attracted to the specialty by the variety of medical conditions we face and the chance to immediately see the results of our actions for acutely ill or injured patients.

"I grew up in the mountains of Colorado. I'm an avid skier, and when I gave up ski racing in college, I became a ski instructor and ski patrolman. To be a patrolman, I had to become an Emergency Medical Technician (EMT), and my first exposure to medicine was treating and bringing ill and injured patients off the mountain.

"While I waited to get into medical school, I worked on a first-response ambulance in the northwest Denver area, so when I entered the Royal College of surgeons in Ireland, I had a pretty good idea of the kind of medicine I wanted to practice. I pursued my specialty training at a large trauma center in Bakersfield, California. Later, as a faculty member in emergency medicine, I was responsible for the Denver EMS system, directing a large emergency department in Portland, Oregon, a residency program in emergency medicine at the University of Alabama at Birmingham, and ultimately became Chair of Emergency Medicine at William Beaumont Hospitals.

"The early ideas for emergency medicine as we know it were probably born during the French Revolution in the late 1700's, when Dominique Jean Larrey, a French military surgeon, observed the maneuvering of artillery carriages on the battlefield. He got an idea of 'flying carriages,' a precursor of ambulances, to take patients directly to field hospitals.

"The United States used ideas generated by military emergency plans and aggressive M.A.S.H.

units of the Korean and Vietnam conflicts and brought them to civilian application. Still, even in the mid-'60's, many hospitals didn't have emergency departments, and patients were brought to hospitals in hearses. As the number of emergency department visits tripled in that decade, it became apparent that there were drastic deficiencies and that the practice of emergency medicine required unique skills and training.

"In 1968, a long-time resident of Lansing, Michigan and seven other founding physicians came together to form the American College of Emergency Physicians (ACEP) with the goal of establishing standards, training, and structure for emergency care. The first national ACEP meeting in Denver, Colorado in 1969 had 128 attendees, and in 1970 Dr. Bruce Janiak became the first resident to be trained in emergency medicine."

FROM HEARSES TO ROLLING EMERGENCY ROOMS

"The first ambulances were mostly just transport services. There were no medically trained personnel, but just drivers and aides. Ambulances were usually Cadillacs, because everyone thought a soft ride was the most important factor. The general public was introduced to the idea of trained paramedics, EMT's, and rescue specialists in TV shows like '*Emergency*' and '*Rescue 911*,' which also featured ambulance units that were faster, tougher, roomy enough to treat a patient in the back, and loaded with medical and rescue equipment, virtually mini-ER's. They've become more and more sophisticated over the years, and so have the medically trained personnel manning them."

EMERGENCY CARE AT BEAUMONT

"There's a rich and storied tradition in emergency medicine at William Beaumont Hospitals that demonstrates an early commitment to emergency patients. In 1978, Dr. Ken Gray came here to recruit Board-certified emergency physicians to Beaumont to deliver the highest standard of care to the community. In 1984, two of the 'giants' of our specialty came to Beaumont—Dr. Ronald Krome, the first academic chair, and Dr. Judith Tintanelli, the first resident director. They established our emergency medical residency program in 1985. Since then, our department has become a respected national leader in emergency medicine education and research, and produced almost 200 residency graduates. Many of them have risen to prominence in the emergency medicine field by making notable contributions as national and regional leaders."

"Today, there are 74 Board-certified emergency medical faculty and 42 residents providing care in the three William Beaumont Hospital emergency centers.

"The Emergency Center at Beaumont, Royal Oak is the second largest in Michigan, and one of the largest in the United States. We see over 116,000 patients per year, so to handle this demand we have areas dedicated for resuscitation, for low acuity patients, pediatrics, and emergency observations, with all the latest technology to provide cutting-edge emergency care. That includes two dedicated high-speed CT scanners. In our pediatric emergency center alone we see almost 30,000 patients annually, and they're cared for by physicians and nurses with specialized pediatric emergency expertise, and subspecialty consultation is always available through the Beaumont Children's Hospital."

"Our Emergency Center has had a mission not just to treat, but to advance the management of emergency cardiac patients, and with our partners in the cardiology department, the vast majority of our patients experiencing myocardial infarctions are treated in our catheterization labs in under 90 minutes. We've continually advanced the science of emergency medicine by being among the first to report on and use hypothermia in the management of cardiac arrests, which results in improved neurological outcomes for these patients. We're the national's leader in using CT angiography to achieve more accurate visualization of coronary artery anatomy, which enhances our diagnostic abilities for cardiac patients. All of our emergency centers are accreditied by the Society of Chest Pain Centers, which validates the very high standard of care our patients receive."

LEVEL ONE TRAUMA CENTER

"As the only Level 1 trauma center in Oakland County, we embrace the mission to treat critically injured patients with our colleagues in trauma surgery. Our use of bedside ultrasound devices lets us identify problems and intervene in minutes to correct life-threatening injuries. We provide substantial medical direction and education to our local EMT agencies, which builds a tight bond between the pre-hospital care and our emergency centers. Whether through Beaumont Medical Transportation or our partnership with Midwest Med-Flight, we receive patients from all over the Mid-West who require advanced quaternary medical care.

DR. ARCARI ON THE TRAUMA CENTER

"One of the additions in surgery became quite important—the trauma center. Beaumont's is a Level One trauma center and has been for over the past ten-plus years. Category One is an identification of the capacity of an institution to look after the worst kind of trauma there is."

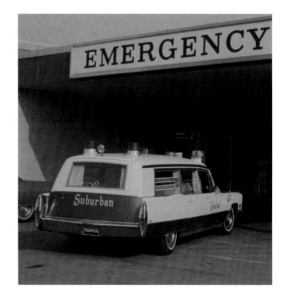

"We have one of the largest emergency observation units in the country and our research has allowed us to provide advanced diagnostic and therapeutic options for such diseases as transient ischemic attacks (TIA), chest pain, kidney stones, abdominal pain, and dehydrations. These strategies provide more rapid, cost-effective diagnostic options than are possible during a typical inpatient admission.

"Our multidisciplinary stoke team also deserves to be recognized. The team is available 24/7 and provides rapid intervention for patients showing evidence of strokes. We bring together emergency medical specialists, interventional radiologists and neurologists to choose the most appropriate evidence-based intervention for each stroke patient, and our outcomes have led to our being accredited by the Joint Commission as a Comprehensive Stroke Center."

EMERGENCY MEDICINE IN THE NEW MEDICAL SCHOOL

"Our national leadership in emergency medicine graduate education means that we're well-positioned to become a full Department of Emergency Medicine at the Oakland University William Beaumont School of Medicine. We already make extensive use of medical simulation technology in our core curriculum, and we look forward to supporting the mission of our new medical school from its inception in the fall of 2011."

THE FUTURE

"What does the future hold for the Emergency Center at William Beaumont Hospital? We've already moved to a completely Electronic Medical Record system, and use of computers and other information technology will only grow. There will be greater access to, and enhanced techniques for, bio-imaging. Use of bedside laboratory testing will increase, as will enhanced information flow to the patient and other physicians in the community.

"We know the numbers of emergency department (ED) visits have risen every decade since the 1950's, and EDs are the principal sources of care for over 45 million Americans. Primary care physician offices are referring more people each year to the diagnostic center that EDs have become. The U.S. baby boomer population is aging, and use of emergency department increases with age. The impact of health care reform remains to be seen, but we do know that while national ED visits have been increasing, the number of inpatient beds have been declining, so more and more patients are waiting in the ED for their inpatient beds.

"These data demonstrate the stress on the whole health care system. Our department uses the latest operations management techniques to improve processes and patient flow. We're nationally known for our innovations, like triage redesigning, the use of queuing theory, and new methods to optimize the patient experience in one of the most stressful environments imaginable."

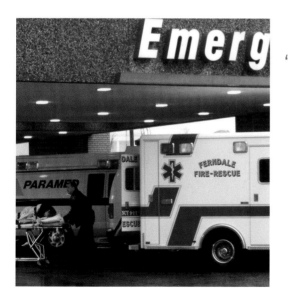

DR. HOBAN ON PATIENT SAFETY

"While Beaumont focuses on having the best surgeons, the best doctors we can find, as much time as we spend on those things, we really are focused on patient safety. We're focused on the littlest things—making sure a patient doesn't fall, on medical safety, and all the things that can happen in a hospital. You would think those things would come automatically, but I've learned that it doesn't unless it's really drilled into everyone's head every moment, that we want patient safety. We're going to spend as much time talking about how we're going to protect the little old lady who comes in for pneumonia, to make sure she doesn't fall on her way to the bathroom, because she is just as important as that headline-making innovative surgery.

GREG HOWELLS, M.D.

Associate Professor of Surgery, Oakland University William
 Beaumont School of Medicine
Chief of Trauma Surgery and Acute Care Surgery
Director of Beaumont Access Center, Beaumont, Royal Oak

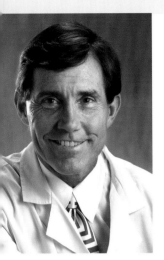

"The Access Center is a new hospital initiative

to facilitate the transfer of complex patients into the hospital. It emanated out of the trauma service, because we were moving patients without any infrastructure and things were becoming complicated. The trauma nurse coordinator, Holly Bair, suggested that we institute the same kind of pattern for the whole hospital rather than just the trauma department. This is for patients who are not in our system and are at another hospital, a particularly complex case, perhaps a person with a bad case of pancreatitis, some type of cardiac problem, or maybe a pediatric case at another hospital that doesn't have the facilities to deal with that kind of patient.

"The Access Center acts as the go-between for the referring physician and the accepting physicians at Beaumont. It takes care of all the phone calls, the infrastructure elements, like summoning a helicopter if one is needed. It's expanded in its scope from being a sort of dispatching service to much more than that. It also runs the in-patient bed system, so it's much bigger than we originally conceived it to be three or four years ago.

"I was first asked by Dr. John Glover, who used to be the Chief of Surgery here, whether I would like to take on the job of making our hospital a level-one trauma center. That was in 1993 or '94. The impetus for that was two-fold: first, to provide state-of-the-art care for injured patients, and second, to provide experience for our residents, predominantly in orthopaedic surgery and general surgery, in caring for patients with severe injuries. There was very limited trauma experience in our residency program prior to 1993, and we wanted to enhance our residents' experience. This was the answer.

"We had to transform from a busy surgical hospital into a trauma center, which took about four years of intense work, going through every department in the hospital and affecting the way care was given, so that the requirements for a level-one trauma center could be met. Those requirements are set by the American College of Surgeon's Committee on Trauma. We were first awarded the level-one verification in 1993, and we have to re-verify every three years."

ANY INJURY, ANY TIME

"A level-one trauma center is the ultimate organization for the care of all injuries. In addition to caring for trauma patients, we also have requirements for outreach to physicians, nurses, EMS for educational process for our hospital and other hospitals. We have to publish twenty papers in trauma-related literature every three years. We also serve as a resource for other hospitals, either providing advice, or as a referral hospital for patients who are brought to other hospitals."

"When a severe injury occurs in the vicinity of a level-one or level-two trauma center, EMS responders go to the scene, then call the emergency center with what they find on the scene. There are criteria that the ER has for the activation of the surgeons. The criteria are very strict. They involve blood pressure, or the Glasgow Coma Scale, a scale used to measure the severity of head injuries, and other evaluations.

"There are about sixteen beepers that go off in the hospital, and everybody who needs to be there converges on the ER—all the things necessary for this patient from the time he enters the ER to the time he's done with his urgent care needs. Surgeons have 15 minutes to respond, so we're usually here by the time the patient arrives.

"People often think I'm an ER doctor, but I'm a trauma surgeon. Trauma centers have surgeons at their trauma stations; that's one of the big differences between trauma centers and non-trauma centers.

"I've been around long enough that I was here

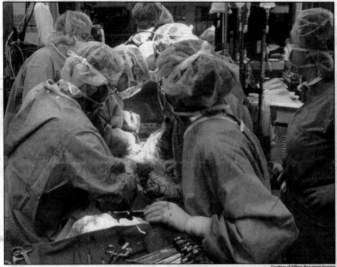

ER Excellence

Beaumont Hospital's trauma center designated 'level-one' accreditation

By Catherine Kavanaugh
Daily Tribune Staff Writer

ROYAL OAK — When being in the wrong place at the wrong time leads to a medical emergency, William Beaumont Hospital is the place you want to end up next.

One of the best hospitals in the United States now is one of the top trauma care centers in North America.

Beaumont has been designated a "level-one" trauma center by the American College of Surgeons, making it the first hospital in Oakland County, the sixth in Michigan and the 76th in North America to obtain the prestigious accreditation.

What does that mean for patients who have complex injuries and need immediate medical attention, and perhaps emergency surgery?

"It means we offer nationally recognized care from the time of impact through rehabilitation," said Dr. Greg Howells, chief of trauma services. "Patients will find no better care under any circumstances anywhere than at Beaumont."

More than 1,000 employees worked 5 1/2 years to meet the ACS criteria. Their goal is to provide trauma patients with the best treatment in the shortest amount time.

To that end, Beaumont has hired more personnel, bought new equipment, developed a database for records and research and added community education programs.

The trauma bay was expanded to handle six patients needing resuscitation at one time. And, an operating room can be fully prepped and staffed in 10 minutes compared to an hour in the past.

If the medical staff on duty is busy,

See BEAUMONT, Page 4A

DR. HOWELLS

Courtesy of William Beaumont Hospital

With scalpel in hand, Dr. Greg Howells, chief of trauma services, performs an emergency surgery at William Beaumont Hospital, which now ranks among the top trauma centers in North America.

---

before there was the CT scanner. That revolutionized everything I do as a general surgeon and as a trauma surgeon. We used to fix the thoracic aortic transections through open thoracotomies. Now the peripheral vascular surgeons repair them with percutaneous stents. The improvement in survival has been phenomenal. We were among the first hospitals to use that technology."

THE WHOLE-HOSPITAL APPROACH

"The most important thing about Beaumont is the whole-hospital commitment. It's not about a person or a department, but about the whole place. As surgeons, we can't do anything alone. The EMS people are much more effective on the scene than we are. We need a massive institution around us with all the capabilities of this hospital and all the people who are here to help with all the things that are done. That's the challenge to creating and maintaining a level-one trauma center: keeping all the people pulling in the same direction. It's like an orchestra— all the people are here, but all their energies must be directed toward the one goal. My job, as Chief of Trauma Surgery, is to get them directed at the trauma patient and keep that level of interest and expertise. That's why it took four years to become a level-one trauma center. This was a busy surgical hospital long before it was a trauma center.

"To actually transform a busy surgical hospital into a trauma center means that all the departments have to be enlisted and actually buy in, and enthusiastically support the whole mission of a trauma center. Far and away the people who bear the responsibility of a trauma center are the surgical residents. If we were not a trauma center, their lives would be completely different. Also, the orthopaedic, neurosurgical department, and the surgical intensive care units are greatly affected by the fact that we're a trauma center. The operating rooms, the radiology department, nursing, the ER...the whole hospital.

"The 'trauma center' is not a place. It's a system rather than a location. We do start out in the trauma room, in the ER, and we're there for a while, but the patient may spend three months in the hospital. The 'trauma center' isn't anywhere in the hospital. It is the whole hospital."

JAMES M. ROBBINS, M.D.

Associate Professor, Department of Surgery, Oakland
University William Beaumont School of Medicine
Executive Director, Applebaum Surgical Learning Center
Beaumont, Royal Oak

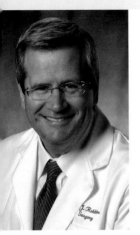

"I first stepped in the doors of Beaumont

when I was about ten years old. My father was the Chief of Anatomic Pathology at Beaumont. I grew up a Navy brat. The Navy sent us all over the world while my brothers and I were growing up, and the last assignment he had was at Bethesda Naval Hospital. He was recruited to come to Beaumont by the then-Chief of Pathology, Dr. Jay Bernstein, who was a world-renowned kidney pathologist. My father became Chief when Dr. Bernstein retired. My father came to Beaumont in 1970, so in many ways I grew up here.

"I wear several hats and have different titles. I'm the general surgeon here in private practice and a trauma surgeon as part of our trauma team. I'm a surgical intensivist, one of seven Board-certified surgical intensivists, certified to run intensive care units. And I'm the Director of Education at the Applebaum Surgical Learning Center.

"I'm also one of the elected representatives of the medical staff. I'm a member at large of the staff at Royal Oak. The last hat I wear is that of General Surgery at the GI Tumor Board.

"I absolutely fell in love with general surgery. I was inspired by Dr. Robert Lucas, the best surgeon I ever knew. He was Chief of Surgery at Beaumont for many years and generations of Beaumont surgical trainees aspired to grow up to be Robert Lucas. He was, and is, a brilliant man, a brilliant surgeon, incredibly talented and fearless. He read voraciously, knew everything in surgical literature, and would tackle any problem with incredible skill and extraordinary judgment. He was a tough, no-nonsense surgeon who got the job done. And there were many others here who were inspiring to us and instrumental in the early days of Beaumont.

"I loved critical care, the excitement and the rewards of taking care of people with multiple injuries or who were severely sick. I loved the idea that surgeons have to be 'doctors' in the truest sense of the word—surgeons are not technicians. Surgeons are the ones who figure out how to prioritize and care for the sickest of patients. At a time when many residents were being told that general surgery was dead and that everything was going to become sub-specialty based, I have for the past 16 years had an absolutely wonderful, fulfilling, exciting, broad-based general surgery career, practicing many different types of surgery."

STARTING THE TRAUMA CENTER

"Shortly after I went into practice here, Dr. Greg Howells was tasked with starting the trauma service at Beaumont. He had been told by many of the wise senior people that this was not a realistic goal because there were so many logistical barriers in this environment. There are rigid and strenuous rules dictated by the American College of Surgeons as they sanction trauma centers. All trauma patients have to be admitted to a surgical service. Many people said that orthopaedic surgeons wouldn't want to admit old ladies with hip fractures or that neurosurgeons wouldn't want to admit old men with minor traumatic bleeds. Those practices were deeply entrenched here and at most hospitals, and in direct violation to the rules of the American College of Surgeons. The College stipulated, and still does, that patients who come in severely injured needed a team assembled in fifteen minutes, with an attending surgeon on site in the ER. Who was going to put surgeons on a fifteen-minute leash, to stand around during a fifteen-minute resuscitation, whether the patient was going to the operating room or not? That wasn't something that could realistically be asked of private practice surgeons.

"There are lengthy research requirements, publishing requirements that are quality intitiatives or quality markers that have to be met. Patients must have quick access to CT scanners without delay. The blood bank has to be prepared to respond to multiply-injured patients. Anesthesia, neurosurgery, cardiac surgery, the operating room—all these must be worked out. The goal was considered unrealistic and impractical.

"Greg Howells said, 'Anybody who doesn't think it's going to happen should get out of the way and watch, because it's going to happen.'

"By shear will and his determination, he approached a few of us and told us he thought we were the ones to do this and that it was right to do. Oakland County needed a level-one trauma center, and Beaumont was the only place in the region capable of fulfilling this need.

"For the first year, Greg came to the trauma center every day. He put himself on call seven days a week, twenty-four hours a day, 365 days a year. He lived across the street. He came in for everything. He's one of my great role models, so when he asked me to be a trauma surgeon for the ER, I couldn't say no.

"Now there are three of us sharing the trauma surgery duties—Dr. Howells, Dr. Mark Frikker, and I—and Beaumont has a Level-One Trauma Center with at least one surgeon available in 15 minutes."

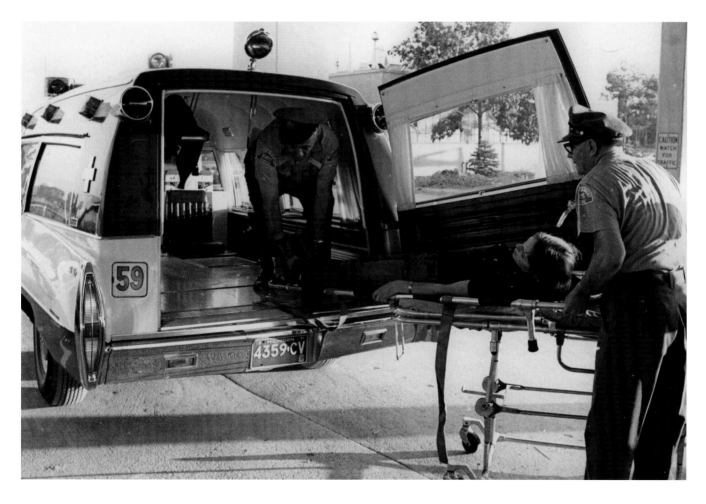

13

DOES YOUR CHILD HAVE A BEAUMONT DOCTOR?

"The Children's Hospital is not a separate building. The physicians at Beaumont can now provide the specialty services required for a 'children's hospital.' There is also a floor in the new building donated by the Carls Foundation."

Robert Reid, M.D.
Obstetrics and Gynecology

INNOVATIONS IN PEDIATRIC SURGERY

by Federico Arcari, M.D., Pediatric Surgeon

"When I first saw this hospital, I thought this might be the place to be. And thus with my coming here as a pediatric surgeon, this may have been the only private hospital in the state that had a pediatric surgeon.

"It's a relatively new field. At the time I started, there were only about 50 of us who had this specific area of concentration. There weren't very many hospitals that had training programs in pediatric surgery, so we were doing the learning as we went, and developing the field, then passing it on. When I arrived, this was fairly unusual. It meant that more and more patients from the surrounding area came to Beaumont instead of Children's Hospital of Detroit for surgery.

"The *raison d'etre* of pediatric surgeons is the newborn and the first year of life—the newborn with congenital anomalies that are incompatible with life, and the surgical problems present in the first year of life. That's what distinguishes the pediatric surgeon from the general surgeon.

"As time went by, the pediatric surgeon came to look after babies and children up to the ages of 14, 15, even 16. Then, adult surgeons looked after them. After I was here about five years, I recognized a young surgeon in training with whom I was impressed, and I asked whether he would consider becoming a pediatric surgeon. He said yes, so I arranged for him to go Children's Hospital in Glasgow, Scotland to train. He did so, then came back and joined me in pediatric surgery, so then there were two of us here at Beaumont. That made a fairly strong surgical activity in that small specialty.

As a result of our being here, a pediatric radiologist came on the staff to help in diagnosing medical problems in children, a very necessary part of the process. Then we got a pediatric anesthesiologist. Previously, we had an anesthesiologist for adults giving care to all ages of patients. Soon we had a pediatric intensivist. We developed a newborn intensive care unit, and that was new—incubators and so on.

"Gradually, as our specialty developed, so these other areas developed specialties in pediatrics. Over a period of ten or fifteen years, we acquired and developed enough that Beaumont could be identified as having a pediatric specialty area—pediatric pulmonology, pediatric urology, pediatric orthopaedics, pediatric neurosurgeons, pediatric oncology, pediatric hematology, and all the sub-specialties with all that support. It became a substantial activity here.

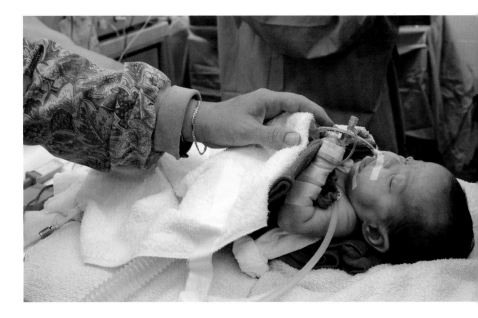

TOM THOMPSON ON
BEAUMONT CHILDREN'S HOSPITAL

" In the '50's and '60's, pediatrics were done on one floor. We didn't have a neonatal intensive care unit. We did have three or four very good pediatric surgeons in the mid-'60's, which was very rare for a small hospital. We just kept growing. Since then, we've acquired pediatric intensive care, neonatal intensive care, sub-specialists in pediatrics in almost every sub-specialty. Right now, the pediatric division is as good as anywhere else for the vast majority of services. In other words, they have everything they need including pediatric coverage in emergency medicine, which is important. Not many hospitals are able to take care of kids who come into the emergency area. That's important, because kids aren't just little adults."

"Then, we got the present Chief of Pediatrics, Jeffrey Maisels. He's first-class, and along with him came other people, and in 2009 we obtained the identification of a Children's Hospital here.

"I like to think that a major part of that might have been the establishment of pediatric surgery here, thus giving Beaumont a different view in that it was a hospital that was interested in taking care of children."

"Working with newborns and children presents special challengers. Diseases of the intestinal tract where some babies are born with a paralysis of the large intestine, for instance, and we have to create a new intestinal transit from that which existed before. Or children born without an anus, with nothing between the skin and the intestine, requires us to create a new anus. Or creating a new esophagus—we have to bring up a remnant from below the diaphragm to meet the upper portion at the level of the trachia and larnyx. It then grows with the child and usually requires no further surgery. Maybe twenty years ago there would've been some further surgery, but we have enough information and science and enough knowledge of technique to do the procedure successfully in eighty-five or ninety percent of the cases. So babies who died without question before now will live full lives. We started off doing these operations at two years of age, and now we're doing them on two-month-olds, or even newborns.

"Cardiac surgery on the newborn is another advancement. The first big one was "patent ductus arteriosis," a channel between the artery and the veins, and at the exit of the stomach into the intestine there would be an absence of gut there and surgeons have to create a junction. Another problem might be extrophy of the bladder, in which the whole bladder of the newborn is lying open on the abdominal wall, and surgeons must create a bladder and try to ensure that there is a controlled sphincter there.

"Now there's a movement to do intra-uterine surgery, for instance when a babies are about to be born with congenital renal disease or with abdominal hernias—born without an abdominal wall. The surgery is done while the baby is still living off the placenta, before the anomaly or abnormality of development gets too far along, so we can interrupt that process. The correlation is in-utero ultrasound—the whole science of imaging is in its infancy. This is all very aggressive."

JEFFREY MAISELS, M.D., CHAIR OF THE DEPARTMENT OF PEDIATRICS, ON BEAUMONT CHILDREN'S HOSPITAL, LAUNCHED MARCH 2009

"We love the Children's Hospital. We've just acquired the name. We are a children's hospital within a hospital. We do all of the things that are required to be considered a children's hospital. There are about 70 hospitals in the country that are classified as being children's hospitals within hospitals. The classification requires us to submit to the National Association for Children's Hospitals and Related Institutions (NCHRI).

"When I first came here, the department was relatively small. We had only maybe 10 or 12 full-time employed doctors. Over the last 23 years, that number has dramatically increased. Now there are 250 pediatricians who admit patients to us, and we have about 40 employed physicians.

"We must have certain criteria in order to be a member of this group, which offers a certain status. "We have available specialists like a pediatric pulmonologist, a pediatric cardiologist, a pediatric geneticist, a pediatric endocrinologist, gastro-enterologist, neonatologist—and so on. We must have a certain number of beds, and a certain number of full-time faculty employed who provide care. We have to have a certain range of sub-specialty care. We have to be a teaching hospital. We have to have a certain number of patients. Once we met all these criteria, we could become a member of NCHRI."

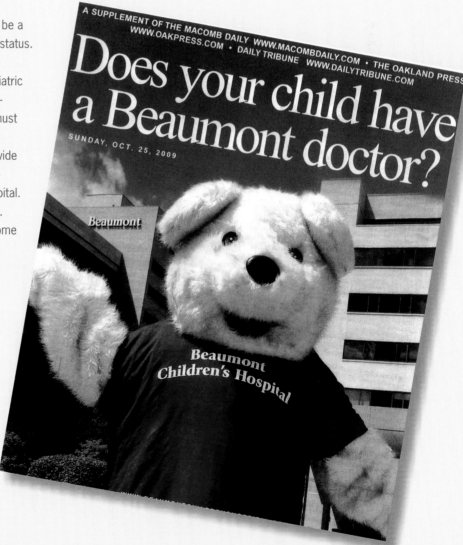

STANLEY M. BERRY, M.D.

Professor and Chair, Obstetrics and Gynecology, Oakland University
William Beaumont School of Medicine and Beaumont Hospitals

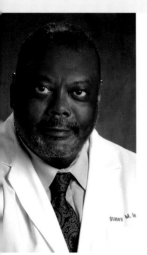

"I'm a medical doctor, an obstetrician/

gynecologist who specializes in caring for high-risk pregnancies. The specialty is actually called 'Maternal/Fetal Medicine.' I've been here since 2004. I'm a full-time employee of the hospital, and also provide patient care to keep my hand in it, which gives me insight as an administrator. My view on administration is that my job is to make life easier for the people who are here taking care of patients and to ensure safety and quality.

"I only knew Beaumont from afar. I was at Hutzel Hospital for a total of fourteen years, so I'd always heard about Beaumont, but when I began to read about it, I was shocked at how little I knew. About ten years ago I got privileges to come here for one day, to do an intra-uterine fetal transfusion. They treated me like an absolute king.

"I remember coming back and telling my chairman, jokingly, 'Y'know, I think I might want to just stay there.' I never had a clue what would be coming in the future. Much later, the wife of one of my former residents, who is herself an OB/GYN, asked whether I'd be interested in interviewing for the Chair position here. That was great—I'd fallen in love with Michigan, my kids were here, and it was perfect.

"I've been very pleased, because I was so unhappy in the position I had at the time, which was Chief of Service of an OB/GYN department in Atlanta, that if I could have afforded it I might have quit medicine right then and there. So Beaumont has been excellent because it rejuvenated me. I inherited a great department, but all great departments have challenges and this has been no exception. I've had a mostly glorious, fun time trying to meet the challenges and make things better. I must say that it probably took Beaumont some getting used to me.

"The first challenge I had here was to rejuvenate, not to initiate, but to rejuvenate the patient safety initiatives in our Family Birth Center, which is our labor and delivery unit. That work is constantly in progress, but we've made remarkable changes in terms of establishing team training between physicians and nurses, bettering communication, and bettering patient service to the extent that we now have the numbers to show we have made inroads into making labor and delivery safer."

"I've worked in three major academic centers since graduating, and by far Beaumont confronts its problems head-on more so than the other centers. Things don't get done in a snap, but the mentality is that we have to change, to keep up. There's not a mentality ingrained in the culture about how we've always done things a certain way and we have to keep doing them that way. There definitely isn't an ingrained psyche that we don't have problems we have to confront and solve, and that's refreshing. We don't stop at the meetings, we're goal and achievement-oriented."

MIDWIVES

"I can proudly say I've hired the first midwives at Beaumont, Royal Oak Hospital. There are about ten. They are not working in a traditional midwifery practice, but they're actually working in the triage area, which is the pre-admission care area for pregnant women. Hopefully someday we'll have midwives practicing and delivering babies here. I've always admired midwives and actually that was one of the things that got me in trouble in Atlanta. They had fired all the midwives before I got there. I managed, with help from several people in the system, to get them all re-hired. The administrators at the top of the pyramid were not too happy with me. That was one of the mistakes I've made that if I had to do over I would do the exact same way.

"Midwifes give women a greater choice, and often structure their practices so they can spend a great deal of one-on-one time with their patients. There's a developing trend for certified nurse-midwives to work in practices with doctors so there's always a back-up if trouble arises."

. . . AND NURSES

"When I came here, Dr. Robert Lorenz was the Director of the Division of Maternal/Fetal Medicine. Dr. Lorenz had done a lot to initiate the original team training, which is the core part of our safety program in the Family Birth Center. I was amazed that during rounds in the morning, the nurses on the unit participated by presenting their patients. I had never seen that before.

"Even before we started our simulation program, we bought a high-tech $20,000 training doll. The problem with these dolls is that they are great teaching tools *if* they're used. The majority of training programs get the doll, use it for maybe three or four months, then the doll sits in the closet collecting dust. Here, we took one of our delivery rooms off line and set it up as a simulation training room for the doll. We installed cameras and put all our residents and many of the attendings who work on labor and delivery through the simulation training with the doll. The residents go through three modules a year to learn how to function in obstetrical emergencies before the problems happen in real life.

"We're far ahead of the curve, because most places get the doll, it's fun, it's nouveau, then they lose interest in it. We've had the doll now for three years and every year we're writing new training modules and putting residents and physicians through simulation drills. It's very much a part of what we do here."

"I am a professor in the Oakland University William Beaumont School of Medicine, and we're looking forward to our first class' metriculating in 2011. Believe me, we will give these young medical students a superior education.

"Beaumont is a place that has allowed me to be 'me.' It has allowed me to be creative and to bring ideas to fruition. There was a position open at a medical school for department chair—the school shall remain nameless—and a number of people asked me whether I'd be interested in applying, I said no. After six years here, I'm too used to people's saying 'yes' to me. 'Yes' is appreciation and validation."

DR. DIOKNO ON THE CHILDREN'S HOSPITAL

"The children's service at Beaumont is one of the well-kept secrets in Michigan. We have outstanding pediatricians, some recognized, many not yet, and their contributions deserve to be recognized. One of the best ways to recognize them is to develop a unit they can call their own. So it's always difficult to build another building, especially nowadays with expenses, yet we have a group of pediatricians here who are managing and treating patients. It's not new to have a 'hospital within a hospital,' but it is new at Beaumont.

"This is truly an autonomous organization within our main organization. We can consider the Children's Hospital as a true division. We have the Division of Royal Oak, the Division of Troy, the Division of Grosse Pointe, the Division of Ambulatory Services, and this could be the Children's Hospital Division. There could be a Board of Directors, a physician chief who will be running the Division, and its own administrative structure. By grouping all those responsible for children's care under one leadership and one administration will help us focus more on the needs of the doctors and the patients and raise the level of care and service culture at this hospital."

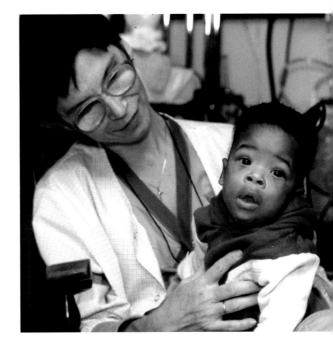

BETTY CHU, M.D.

Associate Professor, Obstetrics and Gynecology, Oakland
   University William Beaumont School of Medicine
President of the Medical Staff,
Beaumont, Troy

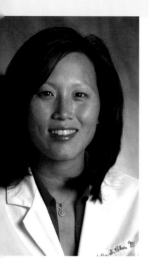

"My family moved to the Rochester

area when I was five. My father worked for GM and my mother was a nurse at Crittenton Hospital. I went to the University of Michigan for undergraduate studies and medical school, spending seven years there as part of a program called Inteflex, which combined pre-medical and medical education. It combines three years of undergrad with four years of medical school.

"When I came to Beaumont, it was my third year of medical school for a clinical rotation. It's much harder to decide which kind of doctor you want to be than it is to decide to be a doctor. There are so many specialties and sub-specialties, and you're picking a lifestyle. My last rotation was OB/GYN, and during that I had a great time in surgery and delivering babies. I came to realize that OB/GYN was a sort of combination of all the things that interested me. I would be able to see patients in an office, be a primary care physician, see people over the spectrum of their lives, and get to do surgery. Labor and delivery is a unique experience that I felt privileged to be a part of.

"I also really liked the fact that OB/GYN has moral and ethical dilemmas intrinsic to the specialty, about fertility and all the emotions and ethics about getting pregnant or not getting pregnant, who should be pregnant and how many babies a woman should have. Contraception can be a contentious issue, abortion, family planning—all this was interesting to me, as the social aspects of OB/GYN.

"Again, the surgical part was interesting too. GYN surgeons do hysterectomies, which now are geared toward miminal invasion, using laparoscopic or robotic removal, and we also do that for other problems such as fibroids, pelvic diseases and cancers. For large fibroids, we use a device called a morcellator, which breaks up the tissue. We use multiple ports—one is a camera, one a manipulator, one a suction device, and so on.

"I looked at different programs, mostly in Michigan, and Beaumont rose to the top because of the amount of clinical experience. Nothing can really prepare a doctor for a complication in obstetrics, and most of obstetrics is normal. We have to do a lot of normal to get to the abnormal, so volume of experience makes a big difference. We want to know how to manage the abnormal, so it was important for me to do lots of deliveries and surgeries in a hands-on clinical environment. At the end of my four-year residency, I went into practice with a colleague who had started his own practice in Clarkston. We've been there for twelve years."

DEFINE "SENIOR"

"We've changed our minds about what a 50-year-old is. Society has changed. We consider a 50-year-old a young person. A 60-year-old is still young. In past generations, a 60-year-old was a senior citizen, and would act that way. We don't think that way anymore, especially for women. If you're a 50- or 60-year-old, the level of expectation is higher—for activity, for work life, for everything. The problem now is to marry expectation with what our bodies are doing. Part of being a physician is to help people define what's 'normal' and what is 'disease.'

Test-tube baby clinic opening at Beaumont Hospital

By MARYANNE GEORGE
Free Press Staff Writer

Three hundred couples are on a waiting list at Royal Oak's William Beaumont Hospital in hopes Dr. S. Jan Behrman and his team of fertility specialists can make their dreams come true.

The couples have turned to Behrman, who is chief of obstetrics and gynecology at Beaumont, and his eight-member team for help in conceiving a child through "in vitro fertilization" — more commonly known as making a test-tube baby.

The process costs about $3,500 and involves fertilizing a woman's egg in a laboratory. The fertilized embryo is kept about two days in a special incubator and returned to the woman's uterus.

The success rate for the procedure is between 20 and 30 percent, Behrman said, while natural conception rates are about 31 percent. Worldwide, an estimated 300 babies have been born after in vitro fertilization. Behrman anticipates the clinic, about to handle its first case, soon will do two procedures a day.

are six other in vitro clinics in the country.

A spokesman at Pontiac's St. Joseph Mercy Hospital said ethical and moral questions may preclude opening a clinic there.

Among other things, "in vitro fertilization bypasses normal sexual relations of a man and a woman," a spokesman said.

INITIALLY, the fertilization procedure at Beaumont will be limited to couples under age 40 where the woman either has blocked or missing fallopian tubes.

Of the 300 couples on Beaumont's list, 90 percent are from the six-county area. They range in age from 23 to 40.

To avoid moral and legal problems, Behrman and his team treat only married couples. "I've already had one letter saying that I'm discriminating against single women," he said.

The clinic includes one lab, where the husband donates his sperm, a second lab, where fertilization takes place, and a specially equipped operating room where eggs are harvested from follicles in the ovaries. Three or four eggs are harvested with each attempt.

Behrman said the process begins with a

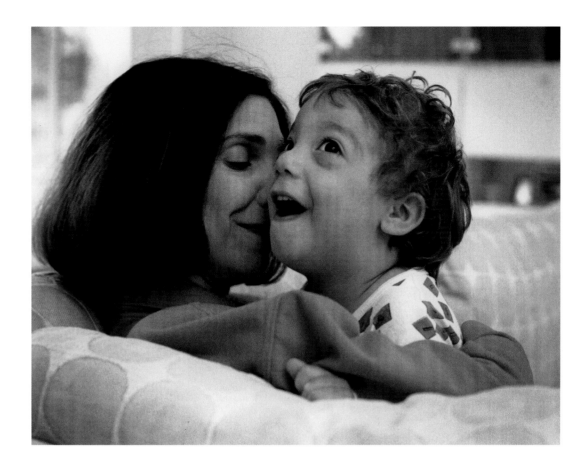

"For instance, there are many changes in how we're handling hormone therapy. It has changed how we manage abnormal bleeding in women and the menopause. For the last 15 years, we've been able to burn the lining of the uterus to reduce heavy menstrual bleeding. I have patients who have no periods anymore because we've done a minor surgical procedure lasting thirty minutes. It permanently burns the tissue so it doesn't regenerate every month. This is typically a 40-year-old lady who's done having kids, has heavy periods, doesn't want to take medication, and just wants to be done with periods. This doesn't disturb the ovaries, maintains the hormonal balance, but removes the end product—the lining of the uterus. The patient will still go through menopause, but won't have the bleeding problem."

PHYSICIANS INVOLVED IN THE COMMUNITY

"I firmly believe that physicians should be leaders in their communities as well as leaders in their own businesses and relationships. As part of that, I got involved in physician leadership organizations. As a resident I was involved in the American College of OB/GYN. I started a leadership role there as a representative in the state. My true love ended up being legislative advocacy and health policy advocacy. I got involved with the Michigan State Medical Society and the Oakland County Medical Society. I became the county treasurer and the president, and am currently sitting on the Board of the State Society. I spent four years chairing the State Legislation and Regulation Committee and watched the health care landscape change dramatically. I also began my involvement with the American Medical Association and am now one of the elected representatives from Michigan advocating for policies set forth by Michigan physicians.

"I'm very interested in our local community and how the environment affects people's lives. In Bloomfield Hills, where I live, we don't have bike paths. I spent two and a half years trying to get bike paths funded in Oakland county. That kind of initiative has allowed me to develop an understanding of community advocacy, tied to health care, tied to public policies, because I feel strongly that Beaumont as a non-profit hospital benefits the community and really should engage the community, and that the physicians should collaborate with the community, because it benefits our patients."

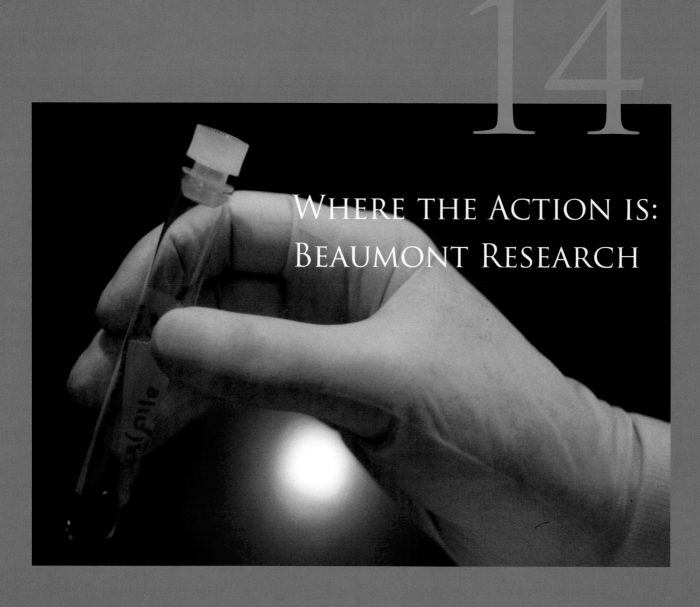

14

Where the Action is: Beaumont Research

DAVID FELTEN, M.D., PH.D. ON THE
BEAUMONT RESEARCH INSTITUTE

"I think that Beaumont can end up with one of the most productive Bio Banks in the country, with truly significant biomarker studies and clinical translational research."

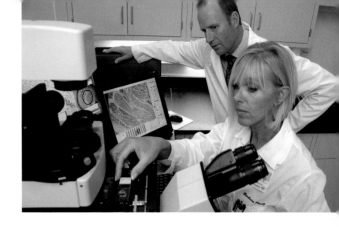

The Erb Family Molecular and Genetics Laboratory, Beaumont Research Institute. Here, under the watchful eye of Jan Akervall, M.D.. Ph.D.

Researchers have come a long way since Dr. Frankenstein. That enduring tale had its anchors in reality and a high demand for a lowly subject—cadavers desperately needed by physicians for examination and instruction. In Victorian Britain, there was a fair living to be had for grave-robbers. Grim careers for grim times.

Sadly, that's how history goes—huge leaps in medical knowledge have usually coincided with periods of violence or deprivation. Nothing advances knowledge like a war. Civilization plods along, generally static, until some upheaval causes a great leap forward. During the Korean War, M.A.S.H. units—Mobile Army Surgical Hospitals—invented the practice of "get in and look," "meatball surgery," which evolved into today's on-the-spot paramedic and EMT practices, and the always-ready trauma unit. The United States' Civil War resulted in field doctors with vast experience in saving the lives of men whose limbs had been blown to shreds. During the appalling Black Plague, which killed almost half the population of Europe, physicians who survived planted the seeds of scholarship about infectious disease. The sudden drop in population gave poor serfs and farmers an economic edge because manual laborers were so desperately needed, and society changed again.

Throughout much of history, women had a low chance of surviving childbirth, but midwives practicing in dark huts learned which herbs, roots, and teas would have an effect for mother and child, and for common illnesses as well. They memorized their medicinal recipies by creating chants, which morphed into what the paranoid and power-crazed called "witches' spells." The flower foxglove carries digitalis, and anti-rhythmatic agent. Dill soothes the stomach. Aspirin comes from a plant called meadowsweet. Ginger eases nausea. Belladonna, or Deadly Nightshade, has a long history as both a remedy and a poison. Woodland pharmacology was passed on to apprentices, who memorized those spells and conjurings in an age when few were literate. Throughout the Dark Ages, little aromatic huts of witches and wizards were the purest of laboratories, where medical knowledge gathered over generations was protected and nurtured.

In ancient Rome, circa A.D. 150, Galen of Pergamon carried out experiments in anatomy, physiology, pathology, pharmacology, neurology, brain control of muscles, and the circulatory system with such workmanlike methods that his theories and discoveries influenced medical science for two thousand years. During the Black Plague epidemic in Avignon in 1348, master physician Guy de Chauliac relentlessly documented Plague symptoms and treated victims, despite grave personal danger.

And, of course, in the mid-1800's there was our own Dr. William Beaumont, who turned a gunshot victim's stomach into his own private laboratory. One does research where one can find it, apparently.

DAVID FELTEN, M.D., PHD

Associate Dean for Research and Professor of Biomedical Sciences,
  Oakland University William Beaumont School of Medicine
Vice President for Research
Medical Director of the Research , Beaumont Hospitals

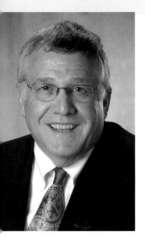

"I grew up in a middle class environment

in Wisconsin. I learned about the real life manifestations of neurological disease early on; my mother was crippled with polio from the age of 8, and my father, an accountant and a minister, provided wonderful care and a great home environment for our family.

"I always greatly enjoyed science and math, and became enamored with neuroscience while I was an undergraduate at MIT.

"I had the privilege of studying in a neurosciences research laboratory under one of the greatest neuroscientists of the 20th century, MIT Institute Professor Walle J.H. Nauta, M.D., Ph.D., a pioneer in defining the connections and functional role of the limbic system, the "emotional brain." Dr. Nauta taught me neurosciences one-on-one at the microscope, and provided didactic instruction using Dr. Frank Netters Atlas, "Nervous System" from the incomparable "CIBA Collection" of medical illustrations, used worldwide. This "Green Book" collection was the best selling set of medical illustrations in the world. I learned neurosciences at the feet of two great masters, Dr. Netter's illustrations and Professor Nauta's astonishing and insightful depth and breadth of knowledge. At a senior phase of my career, I was asked to revise the Netter's Atlas of Human Neuroscience as primary author, now (2010) in a second edition (Netter's Atlas of Neuroscience), with many new illustrations, Netter's classic illustrations with new figure legends, and a host of clinical points and explanations to bring neurosciences to the level of patient application for the student. Coming full circle, from using the Netter atlas to initially learn neurosciences to becoming the author is a very moving experience, perhaps one of the greatest honors I have ever had."

"When I engaged in neurosciences research early in my career, at Indiana University School of Medicine, I was fascinated with chemically specific systems of the brain, which I had studied under Professor Nauta. I carried out some of the first mappings of the norepinephrine, dopamine, and serotonin systems of the primate brain, using new chemically specific techniques and new anterograde and retrograde tracing techniques. These studies confirmed that just a small number of neurons possessed incredibly widespread connections throughout every subdivision of the central nervous system, and acted as 'set point regulators' or 'thermostat' neurons to control the excitability of a vast range of other neural systems and functions. This work occurred just as we were discovering the wide range of applications for pharmaceutical agents that were being used in affective and cognitive psychiatric disorders and in neurological disorders."

PSYCHO…NEURO…IMMUNOLOGY
SAY IT FIVE TIMES, REALLY FAST

"I believe that the initial significance of this first evidence of direct connections between the nervous system and immune system was the stark, hard-core demonstration of direct synaptic-like connections with chemically specific wiring. One could argue about stressors and altered immune responses, but the anatomical and molecular evidence was both substantive and thoroughly repeatable and documentable with microscopic techniques."

SELF-STRESS…WE ALL KNOW
THESE PEOPLE

"High levels of stress can profoundly affect a person's health and physiology of virtually every organ system. The laundry list is huge, so we focused on how the neurotransmitters and hormones of the major axes (norepinephrine, epinephrine, cortisol, and some inflammatory cytokines) interplayed with the immune system. Of course, the demonstration of detrimental effects of chronic stress hormones has a long history, even before we realized that the nervous system has direct connections with cells of the immune system in the bone marrow, thymus, spleen, lymph nodes, gut-associated lymphoid tissue, pulmonary-associated lymphoid tissue, and skin-associated lymphoid tissue.

"The important question that was raised is 'How do you treat the problems associated with chronic stressors?' The glib response is to reduce the stress. But the practical answer is to employ the triad of western integrative medicine—exercise, nutrition, and stress management. This should be done in addition to the outstanding conventional medical approaches we now have. There are opportunities to use pharmacologic agents in some instances (e.g. beta blockers) to counter the effects of some stress hormones, but integrative medicine embraces the use of this triad to be used side-by-side with the conventional treatments of Western medicine. This has been shown to be particularly effective in the integrative, whole-person care of oncology patients, who often alter their lifestyles, nutrition, and exercise, and actively take control over their own lives and health care choices. This falls back on the basic premise of preventive medicine, how you choose to live your life. You can't change your genes, but you can change your lifestyle and habits. It should be a major goal of medicine, especially in this new era, to help patients focus on just that."

AND ALONG CAME BEAUMONT

"This is a wonderful gem of an institution with many doctors who are extraordinary physicians who take care of patients for a living, and yet have great intellectual curiosity and great ideas for how to move forward in research. The doctors here do not have the luxury of taking 75% effort for three years in order to learn how to do cell sorting or gene chip analysis. At the Research Institute, we can provide the infrastructure to make that happen. It is an exciting opportunity to develop a truly full-service Research Institute.

"At Beaumont, my job is to help make research move more smoothly. We brought in a grant-writing and support team, expanded our coordinating center to encompass studies in all disciplines, strengthened our support in education, grants and contracts, financial support, outcomes research, and many other areas. And importantly, we built a core molecular laboratory with the generous support of the Erb family (Erb Family Core Molecular and Genetics Laboratory), and then a BioBank."

I hold all of our personnel and researchers to the highest of integrity and ethical standards, and do not tolerate anything less.

"First, we brought in 20-plus pieces of the latest, most technologically sophisticated equipment for biomedical research, especially for genomic, proteomic, cell sorting, imaging, small molecule discovery, and other components of state-of-the-art clinical translational research, bringing basic sciences findings directly to the patient's bedside. We have the latest Affymetrix genomics system, a cell sorting system that can sort 70,000 cells/second based on multiple parameters simultaneously, a laser-capture microdissection system that can remove single cells (e.g. a cancer cell, a transitional cell, and a normal cell) from a single section of tissue and then carry out detailed gene analysis. We have a micro-array system that lets us take blocks of tissue, punch small samples from up to 300 different specimens or blocks, then reassemble them into a single block of tissue, and stain it, prepare it, analyze it, and do side-by-side comparisons of samples from up to 300 patients in one set of observations. The technology is wonderful.

"But, you might ask, don't all the other universities have a similar set up?" The answer is, for the most part, yes, they have the equipment, but it is often scattered in multiple laboratories at multiple and distant sites, under the direction of multiple lab directors, being used by multiple principal investigators who may zealously guard their use of the specific equipment. Many institutions have this "silo mentality" which is not conducive to a clinical investigator delving into the use of sophisticated but highly useful technology to answer burning clinical questions. So under the leadership of Drs. Jan

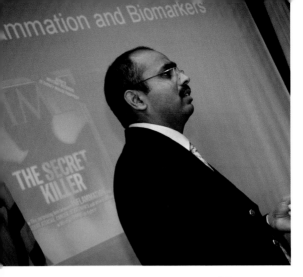

Pradeep Tyagi, Ph.D. presenting at the 2010 Biobank symposium on inflammation and biomarkers.

Akervall and George Wilson, we built a full-service BioBank at the Research Institute, integrated with the Erb Family Core Molecular Laboratory, with the intention of making this facility available to all of our investigators. We have all of the equipment and the bar-coded system for the BioBank in the same facility on the 4th floor of the Research Institute. It is under one roof, one set of Scientific and Clinical Directors, with Research Institute oversight of Ph.D. level and other technical support, and full support of service contracts and maintenance.

"As part of our full service, we can help investigators with the generation and write up of their hypotheses and specific aims, we can help them plan the application to our IRB, we can help them write the protocol, we provide full research nurse support for tissue sample collection in the OR to provide minimal disruption to the surgeon, we help to prepare and sort/store the tissue specimens for the specific study at hand, and we provide technical assistance for use of the sophisticated equipment. This has allowed several outstanding clinicians who thought that such sophisticated research was beyond their reach to launch important clinical translational research studies that have resulted in significant findings and publications. We are helping to bring investigators into the realm of academic medicine as we build the Oakland University William Beaumont School of Medicine. This is an incredible service-based core facility unlike anything I have seen at other Schools of Medicine in which I have worked.

"In a collaborative effort with Oakland University faculty and graduate students, we have built our own IT platform for research, where we can integrate data from our clinical electronic medical record system (EPIC), our clinical trials data base (Crossbreak), our BioBank software (Big R), and the individual data from the many pieces of sophisticated equipment whose output varies with its function (graphs, data arrays, HPLC traces, gene array data, etc.). We are particularly focused on identifying biomarkers related to specific diseases, specific

types of tumors, specific risk factors, key decision making about choice of therapeutic approaches and risks, and other important components of tailoring diagnosis and treatment for each individual using the best information possible.

"Many people wouldn't think that Beaumont Hospital could pull this off. The reason we can is that we make our efforts a truly cooperative endeavor. This is a team effort where we help the physician take ideas all the way through to completion of a study. We also assist physicians with the every-increasing complexity of the regulatory and compliance world. I hold all of our personnel and researchers to the highest of integrity and ethical standards, and do not tolerate anything less.

"I think that Beaumont can end up with one of the most productive BioBanks in the country, with truly significant biomarker studies and clinical translational research. I can see this enterprise 10 years from now being an incredible engine for clinically significant findings, for intellectual property development, and for identifying biomarkers that aid in early diagnosis or decision-making regarding diagnoses, treatments, and prognosis.

"I enjoy working in a hospital research environment. This is a business, and must be run in a business-like fashion. The kinds of services and capabilities and support that we are building for research through the Research Institute do not happen by accident. This requires planning, thoughtful focus on core strengths, unremitting support for grants and projects, and financial support."

As a pioneer in the field of psychoneuroimmunology, Dr. Felten received a John D. and Catherine T. MacArthur Foundation fellowship, dubbed "the genius award" by the press. He was also recognized by the National Institute of Health with double MERIT awards, one from the National Institute on Aging, and one from the National Institute of Mental Health.

NUTRITION AND PREVENTIVE MEDICINE RESEARCH

The Division of Nutrition and Preventive Medicine is the home of one of the nation's largest and most sophisticated weight control centers. A multidisciplinary team of physicians, currently led by the interim chief, Wendy Miller, M.D., mid-level providers, psychologists, dietitians, and exercise physiologists care for approximately 2,000 patients per year. Patients are referred for obesity and its related problems including dyslipidemia, diabetes, hypertension, coronary heart disease, sleep apnea, and a multitude of other comorbidities.

A broad focus of our research centers on commonality of obesity and cardiovascular diseases in our current populations. Epidemiological studies, studies of clinical decision-making and randomized trials involving preventive and therapeutic interventions are considered. The overlapping interests and patients of Nutrition and Preventive Medicine with Cardiology allows for a natural synergy to pursue collaborative projects.

KEY RESEARCH AREAS

Investigation into the underlying clinical science of obesity including studies on epidemiology and secular trends; the genetic, physiologic, psychological and sociocultural pathogenesis; associated comorbidities including Type 2 diabetes, cardiovascular disease, osteoarthritis, surgical issues (e.g. gallbladder disease and abdominal hernias), sleep disorders, and malignancies (breast, colon, prostate, uterus) and the abnormal circulatory physiology of obesity. The goal is to take results from such research studies and integrate them into novel treatments for obesity. We focus on both pediatric and adult multi-disciplinary approaches to weight control and promoting healthy lifestyles. Adult interventions include food, diets and exercise; meal replacements; medical therapies; and bariatric surgery.

NOTABLE DIVISION RESEARCH ACCOMPLISHMENTS INCLUDE:

- Dr. Nori, Director of Nutritional Medicine, demonstrated a breakthrough in the treatment of type 2 diabetes. Using interventional (nonsurgical) weight loss approaches, she has demonstrated that remission of type 2 diabetes is possible. Her study patients have normal measure of blood sugar control and no longer require insulin or other diabetic medications. Dr. Nori is currently studying micronutrient status of obese patients and bariatric surgery patients.

- Dr. Zalesin, Director of Bariatric Medicine, has completed a project in morbidly obese patients with diabetes undergoing bariatric surgery and has also shown reduction in Framingham Risk Score in the bariatric surgery population. Her research has focused on remission and improvement of obesity-specific comorbidities and post-operative complications in bariatric surgery patients.

- Dr. Franklin represented Beaumont Hospitals on the American Heart Association Council on Clinical Cardiology, Subcommittee on Exercise, Cardiac Rehabilitation, and Prevention; the Council on Cardiovascular Nursing; the Council on Nutrition, Physical Activity, and Metabolism; and the Stroke Council, producing the published scientific position statements on exercise and heart disease.

- Dr. Miller was recognized by the Michigan State Surgeon General as leading one of the top, innovative programs (Beaumont Healthy Kids Program) for improving health behavior in the State of Michigan in 2005 and also received the National Kidney Foundation of Michigan 2007 Innovations in Healthcare Award. She was appointed to the Governor's Childhood Obesity Prevention Workgroup in 2007 and also serves on the Michigan Healthy Weight Partnership Committee. She has published outcomes on the Beaumont Healthy Kids Program as well as the adult Beaumont Weight Control Program.

THE FOUNDATION, PHILANTHROPISTS, AND THE ART

15

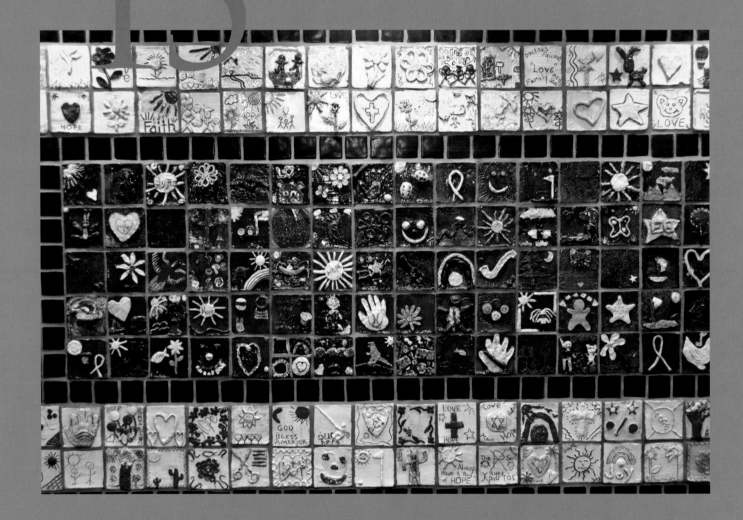

"Americans as a society are generous. It is important for the public to know that we researchers are grateful."

Alvaro Martinez, M.D.
Radiation Oncology

MARGARET CASEY
President, The Beaumont Foundation

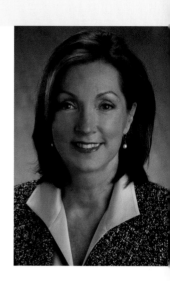

"So much of giving is the question,

'Am I giving to something worthwhile?'"

"Our mission and purpose is to raise funds for all three William Beaumont Hospitals, and to support the capital needs, the clinical needs, the program needs, and the research needs. We're now in the last components of a capital campaign for $170 million, of which we have $155 million pledged to date, and that will conclude, we hope, by next year.

"We're also in the beginnings of a medical school campaign that we're doing jointly with Oakland University. Beaumont's component of that goal is $125 million, and that is to raise money for program needs, clinical support, faculty support and scholarships, along with some new or renovated facilities to house and teach the physicians and medical students. We're looking at developing a new auditorium, a number of new classrooms, and a conference center that is also a teaching arena.

"We have a number of ways we go out into the community for fund-raising. First of all, we have a Foundation Board, and their sole responsibility is to help Beaumont raise philanthropic funds. To be a member of the Board, each must make a minimum pledge of $100,000, which can be paid over five years. They must have given, and must be able to ask for donations.

"The Foundation began in the early 1980's, and I came on board in 2000. During the late '80's to '90's, the health care revenue was so positive that the Foundation didn't put much effort into philanthropy. They did a few special events, created a presidents' club, created some giving societies, but I think the annual amount of philanthropic funds in 1999 was about $4 million. We also ran federal grants through the Foundation at that time, and that

has changed. All the federal grants go through the Research Institute since 2003. Most development offices or foundations handle philanthropy from private foundations, corporate foundations and from individuals. Federal research grants take a different training and science background, so they go through the Research Institute.

"Our philanthropy, because there was no strong need for it, was only a few million a year, so the Foundation had a small staff. After I arrived, we did a strategic plan in 2001, analyzed the needs, knew our Foundation was understaffed based on comparable health care systems, and did benchmarking for hospitals of our size, knowing that Beaumont is one of the largest teaching medical centers in the country that isn't aligned with a university. We have medical students and teach about 400 residents a year, who come from Wayne State, Michigan State, U of M, as well as outside Michigan. This is a huge graduate medical education program. Those students needed research and education money. There was very significant reimbursement from the federal government in the early 2000's for graduate medical education. With all the changes in health care, Medicare, Medicaid, that reimbursement began to evaporate.

"We made a presentation to the Board of a strategic planning process, and got permission to invest more money for a growing staff, and laid out a five to ten-year goal if the proper investments were made, and they were. We now have a team of about 45 people, and at our peak we raised $40 million in one year, but our budget is determined on a three-year rolling average. That is cash and pledges. Ninety-nine percent of the money we raise goes

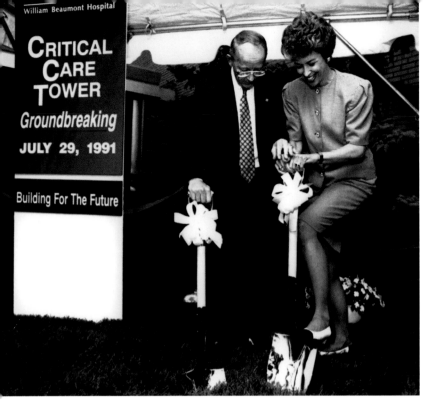

William Beaumont Hospital

CRITICAL CARE TOWER

Groundbreaking

JULY 29, 1991

Building For The Future

DR. MARTINEZ, RADIATION ONCOLOGY, ON PHILANTHROPY

"One thing that people need to recognize more is that Americans as a society are generous. Americans don't mind contributing to philanthropic funds. If all they can give is $20, they give $20. If they can give $10, they give $10. The wealthy can give a million dollars, and they do. But in general, as a society, medical science is where it is because they have been donating money to us so we can do research.

"I think it's important that the public knows that we researchers are grateful. That's a very important message for the public. We are sensitive, we are grateful, we value their contributions highly. Without their contributions we would not be anywhere close to where we are."

Ken Myers, CEO and Caroline Davis, Chairperson for the Board of Directors, breaks the ground for the additional Critical Care Tower at William Beaumont Hospital, Royal Oak, July 29, 1991.

into restricted funds, which means that the donor is presented with a number of options and has chosen one of them to which he or she will donate.

"Physicians are sometimes reluctant to get involved in fund-raising because they don't like to have to ask for money, and I tell them that they don't have to. They just talk about what they're doing and lay out their visions. Our physicians are very involved in the philanthropic process, as are our administrators. When I first started here in 2000, none of them were involved. They didn't need to be, but they were beginning to realize they should have more philanthropy, with the way health care was headed. They knew they had to invest in a Foundation that could raise philanthropic funds. How health care is paid for is a contantly changing dynamic and getting worse. Getting scary."

GREAT NEEDS, GREAT PROJECTS

"There's a tremendous need for additional philanthropy. We had a small campaign in 2002 to raise $15 million for the neuroscience center at the time they were building the South Tower. That brought people in to see other areas of the South Tower. One of the things we do is to analyze the hospital and develop proposals, have physicians involved, doing lectures, and host tours so potential

donors can get to know the hospital, and of course the Foundation Board's role is to identify those people who have the capacity to give. When people came in to see the new South Tower, we got a $5 million donor for the pediatric center, several donors for neurosciences, a donor for the surgical waiting area, so you'll see a lot of donor recognition in the South Tower, because it was a focused effort. When that was accomplished, we updated our strategic plan and designed a comprehensive campaign that started in 2005."

ENGAGING THE COMMUNITY

"In fundraising, you're almost always in a campaign. You're either planning one, executing it, winding it down, and studying and planning the next one. We've recruited a Campaign Executive Committee and created a number of sub-committees. The people on the Campaign Executive Committee have to be very active to talk to people in the community, engage them, have them learn about Beaumont, to get the story and mission out. We carefully recruit people to serve on our many committees and sub-committees, mostly from the community, as a way to get people involved. We now have about 200 volunteers who work with us in fundraising.

"Before we started these campaigns, we had only

a few million-dollar donors. Now we have 27 one-million-or-above gifts that have come in through a major campaign. Those range from one-million through thirty-million.

"We've come up with $300 million in needs to take out to the community. We have to develop feasibility studies to see what the community wants us to do and what they would like funded. Those studies give us an idea of who has the wealth and who among those people might be willing to give, and in what range of donation."

QUICK CHANGES

"Needs change in health care rapidly, so we have to constantly develop proposals to identify projects and why someone would want to donate to that project. We bundle many aspects into projects, and present them as 'centers,' so the donor is providing capital dollars, program support and often research dollars, rather than just trying to raise money for equipment or something separate. It's more attractive and donors can see the bigger picture and the impact of what they're providing. For instance, in heart and vascular right now, there is a donation of $3 million recently for a heart assessment center which is now being built. We're looking for $2.5 to $3 million to renovate and upgrade a cath center so all our cath labs have the latest equipment. We had a commitment of $5 million that created the Women's Heart Center and also developed the capability to buy the first MRI research machine for the study of the heart, which later developed into CT, a 64-slice CT, and now we have the Flash CT. All of that funding came from philanthropy.

"We got the money for our fabulous and successful Surgical Learning Center from a donor, Gene Applebaum, $2.4 million to establish it, and we hope to expand it with more money from that donor, to have more simulators. We're one of the few places in the country that has a surgical learning center on the scale of ours, right in the middle of a clinical environment, set up as an education center. Plans to expand include more ORs to do more training, more classroom space, distance learning—it's very impressive and will be important to the medical school.

"Beaumont was in a good financial position in the '70's and '80's. It's much more challenging now. Back then, we developed a financial plan to generate a bottom line net income of 6½ %. The only reason to generate that was to put it back into the hospital for the benefit of the patients. We managed to achieve this goal well into the 1980's, until the Medicare and Blue Cross programs started ratcheting down reimbursements. We were increasingly limited in our ability to generate funds ourselves. Therefore, we had to recognize that the growth and development vision for Beaumont required us to turn to the community to continue building.

"In the early '70's, we recognized that we would need a fund-raising entity, but we put pressure on ourselves to generate the money from operations to support the growth of the hospital. By 1985, we could see that it was going to be more and more difficult, so we set up the Beaumont Foundation.

"I got a good object lesson early on, when a patient came in to see the Foundation President. She said, 'I had such a wonderful experience here that I'd like to contribute some money.'

"That was music to our ears. The Foundation President always had a menu of options, and went over those, then asked how much money she had in mind. She wanted to donate $50,000. There were two items on the list that she liked and she couldn't choose between them. She finally said, 'I'll do both of them for $50,000 each.'

"She eventually gave us several million dollars. We realized we should have been doing this long before, because there are plenty of people in our community who want to be part of what we're doing. All we had to do was give them the opportunity. If somebody wants to give us a dollar or a million dollars, it doesn't matter. If anyone wants to be part of what we're doing, we welcome that.

"Everybody wants to be sure that whatever they're donating doesn't go down a bottomless pit. Too often when people donate to charities, they have no idea where the money is going or how its being spent. At Beaumont, we give people targeted choices and they know how their money is being used."

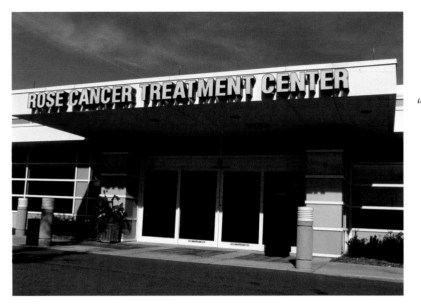

DR. PETERS ON PHILANTHROPY

"We at Beaumont Urology have been fortunate in that people have recognized what we do. We have a donor, Peter Ministrelli, who has given our department a million dollars a year for the past five years as an infrastructure for research. It has really allowed us to hire the right people and write for an National Institute of Health grant and get new funding for the department. Without that, in this economy, we would have much more trouble advancing. Research isn't glamorous and doesn't attract much money, but it's absolutely critical."

Rose Cancer Center. The generous gift from the Rose Family Support Foundation made the Rose Cancer Treatment Center a reality.

"These kinds of research and projects can't be done without philanthropy. New technologies and machines are developed, and the manufacturer needs to test it, and they want the testing done at centers with the best physicians and teams of nurse researchers and physicists all of whom understand the protocols, and also a place with a large volume of patients who will use that technology in a relatively short time. Beaumont has the largest in-patient volume of anywhere in the country.

"In clinical trials, the patients can't be charged, yet physicians, nurses, and others have to be there administering the tests. That takes money."

DONATIONS REALLY DO WORK

"There are so many stories—Beaumont has, I think, the highest rated radiation oncology department in the country. Dr. Alvaro Martinez, who heads that, has research that has defined new treatment methods that are now the standard of care. He developed a lot of oncology imaging. He has created the ABC breathing machine, a way to manage the heart during chemotherapy. We have a family named Rose who have been very generous with the cancer center. Not only do we have the Rose Cancer Center, but in the last three or four years they've given us $1 million to $2 million a year to invest in radiation oncology, to help with purchase of the Omni Beam, the Gamma Knife, a new PET/CT scanner, some of the research tools, because they're invested and they believe in the quality of the team that Martinez has, and they see what it does to improve patient care. Radiation

treatments used to take six months; they've gotten it down to one week because of how they can deliver the beam so close to the tumor. In just the time I've been here, ten years, it's remarkable to see the advances that have been made."

"It's relationships that bring in money. There has to be a good product, which Beaumont is. There have to be physicians who are willing to talk about what they're doing, be passionate and give their vision, and explain the impact philanthropy has on the patients and their families. Then, we need key community leaders who can open doors. It's that level of high-quality community people who feel a desire to participate, who know it takes time and effort and work, who understand philanthropy and are willing to do it. The Board members, we say, 'have to be able to give and get.'

DR. MAIN ON PHILANTHROPY, VOLUNTEERS, AND PRIVATE SOLUTIONS

"One of the patients' fathers came to me about twenty years ago and said, 'The merchants of Birmingham are going to have a big fashion show, and we might raise some money. If we gave you the money, what would you do with it?'

"One of the things that had always bothered me is that sometimes the children who finish chemotherapy still don't feel like they're finished. They still feel like patients, feel restricted, didn't get very good grades because they missed so much school, and their parents have spent a lot of their savings, so it's extremely difficult for these kids to go to college. I told the Birmingham merchants that I wanted to give one or two of our children a scholarship, to help them think of themselves as college material.

"The first year, we gave the money to a girl whose dad was a minister in Birmingham. We then decided it wasn't good for us to make the decision, so we picked a company to give out Beaumont scholarships; last year they gave out over $125,000 in scholarships.

"When we were rounding eight or ten years of the scholarship, we had done well with the money we raised and had given out quite a few scholarships, but it turned out that we weren't awarding as many as we wanted to. I called the scholarship company, they said they were giving out all they could. I asked who decided how many we could give out.

"The answer was, 'The Internal Revenue Service decides. We can only give out four scholarships for every ten applications, or it becomes a "gift" and they have to pay taxes on it.'

"That just didn't seem fair. These kids have already paid their dues and been through their life trials. So I called my Congressman, who at that time was Bloomfield. He agreed that it didn't make sense. About four days later, the scholarship company called and said, 'We don't know how you did this, but the IRS just called to tell us that your scholarship can now be given to six out of ten applicants.'

"This year we have forty kids in college. They get $2000 per year for every year they're in school. Some people say, 'Why don't you just give out one or two full scholarships instead of several small ones?' My answer is that giving out big scholarships means you're only helping the 'stars'–kids who are going to win scholarships anyway. I want to help the kid who doesn't think of himself as college material. We've had kids come back and say, 'Until you gave me that scholarship, I never even thought about going to college. Then they announced my name at the honors assembly—somebody thought I was smart enough to go to college!'"

PRIVATE SECTOR SOLUTIONS

"About three years ago, at Costco, I ran into a former patient. I asked, 'Why don't you come back and see us? We should be looking at you to see what damage we did with the chemotherapy and checking your condition.'

"He said, 'I can't. I don't have insurance. I have a pre-existing condition, so I can't get any.'

"The next time we had a meeting here, I said, 'In addition to giving college scholarships, I'd like to give health scholarships to kids who are off our programs, who are too old to get state initiative help, and who are off their parents' insurance. They can come in and get thorough examinations, X-rays, be seen by learning and development specialists, dieticians, social workers, and leave the building without receiving a bill.'

They said yes, and asked how many I thought we would see. I guessed two or three a month. Now we're seeing over twelve a month. That takes a lot of fundraising. Everyone is a volunteer; no one is paid. Our fundraisers are 'Stars Guitars.' The volunteers go out and get guitars autographed by famous people, famous entertainers. The two requirements are that the events are casual-dress, and that the admission is low enough that anyone can go. We recently had an event—it was a stroll-around dinner, and our volunteers collected fifty-five guitars, which we then auctioned. We also auctioned a Lebron James all-star jersey, Curtis Granderson signed baseballs and jersey, and friends made donations. We cleared over $110,000.

"It's been so satisfying . . . many winners, many hugs and many thank-yous whispered into my ear. I'd like to take all those thank-yous and give them to each one of the volunteers."

THE ROLE OF **PHILANTHROPY** AT BEAUMONT

Philanthropy has been the cornerstone of the Beaumont story from its very beginning. It is in large part responsible for our being consistently ranked among the finest hospital systems in the country. For more than five decades, Beaumont has been providing excellent health care services to patients and families who live in our communities and who come to us from across the state and around the world.

The respect that Beaumont has gained as a health care provider of choice is due to the exceptional skill and talent of our physicians, nurses and clinical staff. Philanthropic support from this community has also been critical to our success, allowing us to remain on the leading edge of medicine. Our donors' charitable gifts have helped us to continually enhance our programs, build our buildings, and fund research and the latest technologies—all for the benefit of our patients.

We would like to especially recognize those donors whose leadership gifts have exceeded $1 million. Their exceptional generosity has had, and will continue to have, a profound impact on the delivery of patient care, and the advancement of clinical knowledge and research.

A gift from **Marcia and Eugene Applebaum** to establish the *Marcia & Eugene Applebaum Surgical Learning Center* allowed Beaumont to shift the learning curve for surgical procedures and technologies out of the operating room and into a highly sophisticated simulation laboratory, thus improving patient safety and outcomes. In 2007, the center became the 10th facility in the United States to receive accreditation from the American College of Surgeons.

A gift from **The Carls Foundation** to establish the *William & Marie Carls Children's Medical Center* at Beaumont, Royal Oak allowed us to greatly enhance and expand our pediatric and neonatal programs. The foundation's exceptional gift was crucial to our achieving membership in the National Association of Children's Hospitals and Related Institutions and led to the creation of the Beaumont Children's Hospital.

Long-time Hospital and Foundation board member and local philanthropist **Susan E. Cooper** made a very significant gift to create a Women's Urology Center at Beaumont, Royal Oak, the first of its kind in the Midwest. Her gift funded construction, equipment and furnishings for the center, and will also underwrite ongoing research in the field of female urology.

Jon, Michael and Sean Cotton made a very generous gift, creating the *Shery L. & David B. Cotton, M.D., Family Birth Center* at Beaumont Hospital, Grosse Pointe in honor of their parents. Their support has established a beautifully appointed facility for new parents and their babies.

Barbara and Harry "Kirk" Denler made an exceptionally generous bequest to establish the *Harry "Kirk" & Barbara Denler Leukemia Research Fund*. Their gift will support research initiatives in the care and treatment of leukemia patients.

The creation of the *Erb Family Molecular and Genetics Laboratory for the Assessment and Prevention of Chronic Diseases* at Beaumont, Royal Oak was made possible by the generosity of **Frederick and Barbara Erb**. This gift is advancing our understanding of the genetic and molecular causes of a broad range of diseases.

A very significant gift from **Max and Debra Ernst and Family** established the *Ernst Cardiovascular Center in memory of Ellen Ernst*. Featuring six multidisciplinary clinics, the center is dedicated to the diagnosis, treatment and care of people with cardiovascular disease and provides community-wide screening and assessments of young student athletes to identify potentially life-threatening heart conditions.

Beaumont Hospitals has received an exceptional gift from **Madeline and Sidney Forbes** of Bloomfield Hills to name the *Madeline & Sidney Forbes Family Orthopaedic Center* at Beaumont Hospital, Royal Oak. This gift provides support for programs and services within the center and will fund innovative research initiatives in orthopaedic medicine.

Ford Motor Company has provided exceptional support since the very beginnings of Beaumont with substantial gifts to help fund the Critical Care Expansion and Neuroscience Center of Excellence campaigns as well as offering major sponsorship support for the Vattikuti Invitational.

Very significant gifts from **General Motors Corporation** have funded the Critical Care Expansion Campaign and provided sponsorship support for numerous events that have benefited our Oncology Services at Beaumont.

Combined gifts from **Richard Hough, David and Bonnie Hough**, and **The Hough Family Foundation** have very generously established *The Hough Center for Eating Disorders* at Beaumont, Royal Oak. Their kindness has allowed Beaumont to offer a comprehensive eating disorder treatment program to patients and their families.

Florine and J. Peter Ministrelli have made numerous gifts that have transformed our Cardiovascular Medicine and Urology Services programs, including establishing the first Women's Heart Center in the state of Michigan. Their extraordinary generosity has permitted Beaumont to create and endow multiple centers and funds within these two programs, advancing physician education and research, and developing groundbreaking technologies and procedures to address cardiovascular disease and urological disorders.

Generous gifts from **Jo Anne and Donald E. Petersen** established the *Donald & Jo Anne Petersen Breast Care Support Endowment Fund*, initiating Beaumont's Sharing & Caring Program, and helped establish the *John A. Ingold, M.D., Distinguished Fellowship in Breast Surgery*.

Stephen and Roberta Polk generously established the *Polk Family Endowed Chair in Developmental-Behavioral Pediatrics* at the Center for Human Development (CHD). Their gift will support physician recruitment, programs and services at the center.

An exceptionally generous gift from **Harold and Marian Poling** was the lead gift in a $15 million capital campaign and established the *Harold & Marian Poling Neuroscience Center* at Beaumont, Royal Oak. The center is dedicated to meeting the needs of neurology and neurosurgery patients.

For more than two decades, the **Rose Family** has made significant gifts in support of Oncology Services at Beaumont. A bequest from the **Estate of Edward and Lillian Rose** established *The Rose Cancer Center* at Beaumont, Royal Oak. Additional significant gifts from

Irving and Audrey Rose; Sheldon and Joan Rose; Leslie Rose; and Warren and Carol Ann Rose have supported the development of new radiation oncology diagnostic and treatment technologies, and established *The Rose Family Adaptive Oncology Imaging Suite.*

A gift from **Shirley K. Schlafer** established the *Schlafer Cardiology Institute* within the Beaumont Heart Center. Mrs. Schlafer's very significant generosity was instrumental in creating a dedicated Heart Center at Beaumont, Royal Oak.

A very significant gift from **Rajendra and Padma Vattikuti** established the *Vattikuti Digital Breast Diagnostic Center* at Beaumont, Royal Oak and funded the purchase of digital mammography equipment at Beaumont, Troy and the Beaumont Medical Center, West Bloomfield. Their gift helped set a new standard for breast imaging.

South Oakland Anesthesia Associates, P.C., has been exemplary in its giving, supporting numerous campaigns and establishing the *South Oakland Anesthesia Physicians Fund* to underwrite anesthesia research initiatives and respond to emerging patient care and medical education needs across the health care system.

The **Wayne and Joan Webber Foundation** made an exceptional gift to establish the *Wayne & Joan Webber Imaging Center* at the Beaumont Medical Center, Macomb Township and name the Cardiac Progressive Care Center at Beaumont, Troy.

A most generous gift from **Walter and Marilyn Wolpin** established the *Marilyn & Walter Wolpin Comprehensive Breast Care Center* at Beaumont, Royal Oak and will create the *Marilyn & Walter Wolpin Endowed Fund for Breast Care Research.*

Beaumont's Additional Leadership Donors

The following are other individuals, foundations, corporations and organizations have, over the years, made exceptional gifts to Beaumont of $1 million. These generous donors have chosen to partner with us in our efforts to improve the lives of our patients and their families, helping Beaumont to fulfill its Mission "to provide the highest quality health care services – delivered efficiently, effectively and compassionately."

Individuals

John A. and Marlene L. Boll Foundation — Gift to establish the *John A. & Marlene L. Boll Center for Human Development* at the Neighborhood Club in Grosse Pointe

Borgo Sisters: Frances and Virginia — Bequest to create a Speech & Language Endowment Fund

William M. Davidson Foundation — Gift to establish the *Sandor H. Shoichet, M.D., & William M. Davidson Endowment for Excellence in Internal Medicine*

Barbara and Tom Denomme — Gift to establish the *Thomas & Barbara Denomme Neuroscience Patient Care Center*

Miss Charlotte S. Dey — Gift in support of the Grosse Pointe Legacy Fund

Amber K. and David B. Flint — Gift to establish the *Amber K. and David B. Flint Breast and Prostate Research Fund*

Dr. and Mrs. William S. Floyd — Bequest in support of Beaumont, Royal Oak

Mr. and Mrs. H. Richard Fruehauf Jr. — Gift to establish the *Janet A. & H. Richard Fruehauf Jr. Center for Orthopaedic Medicine* at Beaumont, Grosse Pointe

Barbara and Charles Ghesquiere — Gift to establish the *Ghesquiere Family Center for Children's Surgery*

Robert C. and June H. Gurwin — Gift to establish the *June H. and Robert C. Gurwin Family Endowment Fund* in support of Surgical Resident Education

Mr. David A. Hagelstein — Bequest in support of the Cancer Treatment Program at Beaumont, Royal Oak

Mrs. Edward J. LeVoir — Bequest in support of Beaumont, Royal Oak

Cis Maisel Kellman — Gift to establish the *Cis Maisel Kellman Endowed Fund for Women's Heart Health*

Edward Mardigian Family — Gift to establish *The Edward Mardigian Family Surgery Center in Memory of Marilynn Mardigian Varbedian*

Mr. and Mrs. F. James McDonald — Gift in support of the Critical Care Expansion at Beaumont, Royal Oak

Ben D. Mills Trust — Bequest in support of Beaumont, Royal Oak

Frances and Dominic Moceri Sr. — Gift to establish the *Dominic & Frances Moceri Heart Rhythm Research and Education Fund*

Mr. and Mrs. Garrett H. Mouw — Bequest in support of Beaumont, Royal Oak

Roncelli Family: Carol and David Roncelli, Sharon and Gary Roncelli, Lisa and Scott Roncelli; Linda and Thomas Wickersham — Gift to establish the *Roncelli Family Orthopedic Center* at Beaumont, Troy

Edward and Lillian Rose — Bequest to establish *The Rose Cancer Center*

David W. Salisbury — Gift to establish the *Debra Saber-Salisbury Memorial Garden*

Ms. Constance Sczesny — Bequest in support of the *Von Reis Breast Cancer Research Fund*

Mr. and Mrs. John R. Secrest — Bequest in support of Cancer Research at Beaumont, Royal Oak

Elizabeth A. and G. John Stevens — Gift to establish the *Elizabeth A. and G. John Stevens Center for Minimally Invasive Surgery*

Suzanne and Herbert Tyner — Gift in support of programs at Beaumont, Royal Oak

Barbara and Sam Williams — Gift to establish the *Barbara & Sam Williams Acute Cerebrovascular Center*

Malcolm Yerkes Unitrust — Bequest in support of Beaumont, Grosse Pointe

Corporations

ALICE 106.7 FM — Gifts in support of the Beaumont Children's Hospital

Costco Wholesale — Ongoing support of the Beaumont Children's Hospital

Forum Capital — Gift of property to Beaumont, Royal Oak

Rite Aid Corporation — Ongoing support of the Beaumont Children's Hospital

Speedway SuperAmerica LLC — Ongoing support of the Beaumont Children's Hospital

Unisys Corporation — Gifts in support of the Critical Care Expansion, the Beaumont Children's Hospital and the Beaumont Drive to Beat Breast Cancer

Wal-Mart/Sam's Club — Ongoing support of the Beaumont Children's Hospital

WKBD UPN50 — Gifts in support of the Beaumont Children's Hospital

WYCD-FM 99.5 — Gifts in support of the Beaumont Children's Hospital

Foundations

The Kresge Foundation — Gift in support of the Critical Care Expansion at Beaumont, Royal Oak

The Ravitz Foundation — Bequest in support of Beaumont, Royal Oak

Respiratory Foundation of Southeast Michigan — Ongoing grant support for Respiratory Services at Beaumont, Royal Oak, Troy and Grosse Pointe

Organizations

Beaumont Hospital Grosse Pointe Assistance League — Gifts to support ongoing needs at Beaumont, Grosse Pointe

Ford Senior Players Championship — Gift in support of the Critical Care Expansion at Beaumont, Royal Oak

Michigan Heart Group, PC — Bequest in support of Beaumont, Royal Oak

United Way Community Services — Gifts in support of programs at Beaumont, Royal Oak

A MESSAGE OF **APPRECIATION**

"Beaumont has always been able to rely on the generosity of this community. The gifts listed here send a wonderful message of confidence and trust in our mission as a health care institution. Now, more than ever, we must seek opportunities to partner with individuals, corporations and foundations to ensure that we can sustain our commitment to providing the highest quality healthcare services to all those who come to us for care.

On behalf of the Beaumont Foundation, I extend my deepest gratitude and appreciation to every single donor who, over the years, has included Beaumont in their charitable giving. We welcome your continued generosity."

— Margaret Cooney Casey

THE BEAUMONT ART COMMITTEE

The Art Committee was established in 1992, following conversations between Myron Laban and the then-CEO, Kenneth Myers. Dr. Laban and his wife, Joyce, were asked to form a committee to bring art to the hospital. The committee would include representatives of the hospital staff as well as art-informed volunteers from the community. This happened because hospitals around the world are beginning to recognize the importance of art in the process of healing, and its positive effect in humanizing the otherwise sterile and institutionalized atmosphere of medical environments.

Art serves as a way-finding device in a place where the corridors are multiple and alike. It is also a pleasant distraction for those waiting in the hospital, and carries a sensation of hope and community involvement. The Art Committee includes an in-house architect who helps resolve the technical aspects of art placement.

Since Beaumont is a private hospital, it does not have an art fund. The committee includes a member of the Beaumont Foundation, an umbrella organization under which the Art Committee functions. There are also several physicians, a member of the Board, and there also might be an interior design manager for a specific project.

The committee's responsibilities are limited to placing permanent art in public spaces of the hospital. It is not involved with patient rooms, offices, or internal departments. All the selected art is privately funded. The committee selects locations, artists and donors for each permanent site. Whenever possible, Michigan artists are considered first.

In the early years of the committee, sites were selected in the existing buildings. Once the new hospital was being developed, the committee was able to work with the architects from the blueprints. The mandate is to determine what kind of art will live well in a given location, considering lighting, presence, size, and colors in the environment. Then, artists are identified who might be abe to execute the work, and are invited to make proposals. The selected artist will receive a stipend for creative

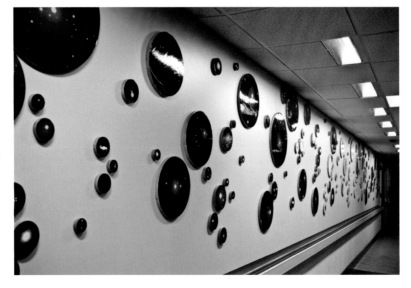

Celestial Walk, an installation of hand-painted images on wood, is the work of artist Beverly Fishman, and located on the first floor of the South Tower at Beaumont, Royal Oak. This artwork was a gift of multiple donors.

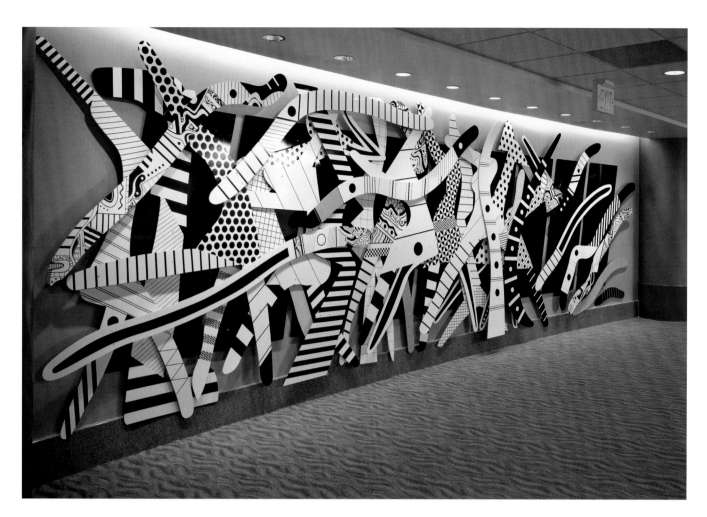

contribution, and once a proposal is in its final form, the Foundation actively helps to locate potential donors.

The first five works were completed by 1995. At that time, the East Tower was the main entrance to the hospital. Several works are mounted in this area. Glazed carved bricks were installed into existing walls of the reception area. As an example of donor involvement, we solicited help from Belden brick, who supply all the hospital's bricks. The other four initial installments include a tapestry of Michigan flora and fauna, a fused glass cascade of color at the head of the reflecting pool in the employee garden, a 26-part installment between the new intensive care unit and the patient rooms of the original hospital, and a lovely colorful abstract canvas, commissioned by a major hospital donor.

From the beginning, the Art Committee has enjoyed the encouragement of the hospital and sponsorship from many clinical departments. The department of Anesthesiology, Oncology, Orthopaedic Surgery, Cardiology, Pediatrics and Urology have all supported commissioned pieces of art. In addition, private donors such as Dr. Todd Wilkinson and the Wilkinson Family Foundation, Dr. Myron Laban, and Susan Cooper have embraced the Art Committee's mission. Ms. Cooper represents the hospital's Board and quickly became a valued supporter and donor.

Over the last seventeen years, the committee members have learned about the technical aspects of lighting and installation, which are major portions of the overall cost. With new construction, placement and lighting can be considered in advance, though reality often causes changes.

Those who pass through William Beaumont Hospital are often surprised and amazed to encounter the artworks. Art is more than pretty pictures, but touches us emotionally and offers enjoyment and reflection over and over. The Art Committee is devoted to adding to the collection, as time and economics permit, adding more healing touches of beauty and creativity to the surroundings at William Beaumont Hospitals.

Black and white cut aluminum wall sculpture by Detroit Artist, Charles McGee, shows 12 organic forms interacting with 14 amorphous human-like figures in clockwise formation. This gift is just one of the many sponsored art work pieces.

DR. DIOKNO ON VOLUNTEERS

TOM BRISSE, PRESIDENT OF
BEAUMONT TROY ON VOLUNTEERS

" We would not be where we are without the millions of hours of service contributed by our volunteers, hours that normally would require a paid employee: manning the reception areas and family areas at the operating rooms checking people in and out, transporting patients, way-finding, support during events, delivering food and helping the Foundation in fund raising, and providing scripted information from the administration. We have wonderful volunteers at Beaumont, some who have been here for forty or fifty years. Some started as candy-stripers and have made the hospital a major part of their lives and are very devoted. Just by their willingness to offer a voluntary service, they save the hospital large amounts of money that can go directly to research, technology or patient care, which we would otherwise not be able to provide. We would have great difficulty trying to succeed without our volunteers."

" The key to our success rests in people like you, who embody the spirit of greatness. You have given countless hours to make sure our patients are comforted, their families kept informed, and anyone who needs a helping hand gets just that. I could not imagine a more dedicated group, and words cannot express how grateful we all are to have you as part of our team. It is a genuine pleasure and privilege to work with you.

Again, please accept my sincere and heartfelt appreciation for the exceptional work you do every day. It is because of people like you that Beaumont, Troy is able to provide the highest quality of care and service to all of our patients. Thank you for your inspiring dedication and tremendous example."

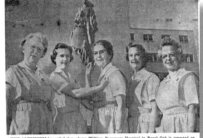

THE ALUMINUM bas-relief that adorns William Beaumont Hospital in Royal Oak is repeated on the gold pins which were awarded six Women's Service Committee members in recognition of their 1,000 hours of volunteer work. Proud wearers are (left to right) Mrs. Walter A. Plumb, Mrs. LeRoy W. Gilger, Mrs. Daniel E. Ford, Mrs. Maynard Mayo and Mrs. Merrill C. White. Mrs. Howard S. Christie was traveling in the East, so she missed the presentation ceremony.—News Photo.

6 Win Pins for Hospital Work

Six women share honors for being the first to chalk up 1,000 hours of volunteer service at William Beaumont Hospital in Royal Oak. They are members of the Women's Service Committee, which was organized four years ago.

The six may now wear special gold pins on their starched aqua pinafores. The face of the oval pin is replica of the aluminum bas relief sculptured by Marshall Fredericks which fronts the hospital. It is of a family.

The six winners are: Mrs. Daniel E. Ford, Mrs. LeRoy W. Gilger, Mrs. Maynard Mayo, Mrs. Walter A. Plumb, Mrs. Merrill C. White and Women's Service Committee president Mrs. Howard S. Christie.

Irving B. Babcock, president of the hospital board of trustees, made the awards at a service committee meeting in the hospital cafeteria. He also presented silver pins for 500-service hours to 28 volunteers. One hundred and forty-seven others earned the right to wear a scarlet stripe on their blouses, in recognition of 100 hours of work.

Mr. J. H. Spiller, chairman of the awards committee, announced that the 300-member auxiliary last year contributed 33,135 hours to the hospital.

[The Beaumont group is devoted exclusively to volunteering their services to the hospital. It never stages fund raisers. Members work on 18 projects there ranging from visitors' information booths to gift carts

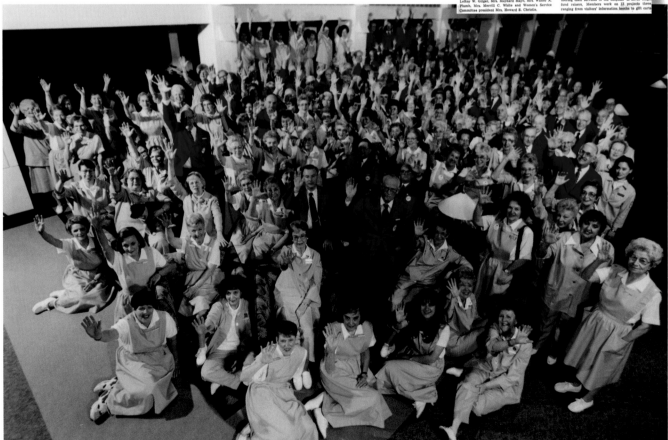

16 THE FAST, THE FURIOUS, THE FAMOUS, AND THE FIRSTS

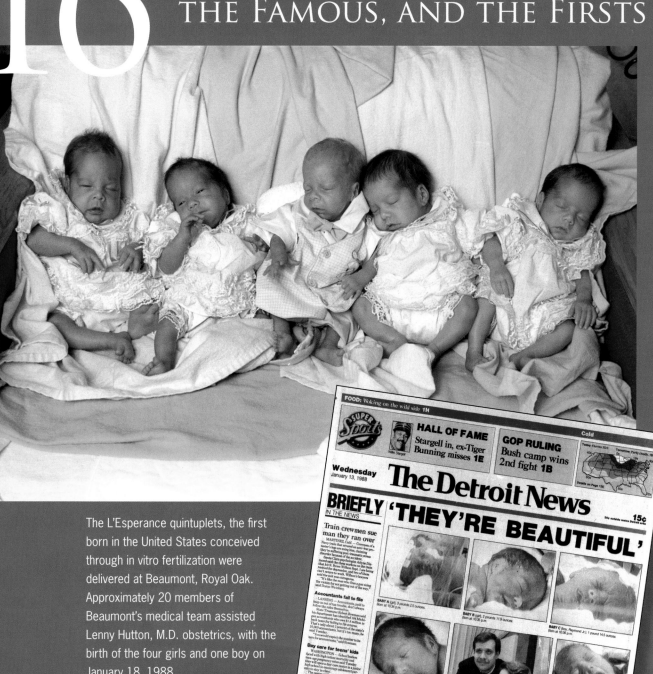

The L'Esperance quintuplets, the first born in the United States conceived through in vitro fertilization were delivered at Beaumont, Royal Oak. Approximately 20 members of Beaumont's medical team assisted Lenny Hutton, M.D. obstetrics, with the birth of the four girls and one boy on January 18, 1988.

(newspaper reproduction in photo — The Detroit News, Wednesday January 13, 1988, "THEY'RE BEAUTIFUL")

193

DR. ROBBINS ON THE RED WINGS CRASH

"I was thrust into a bit of a limelight in 1997 when the Red Wings got into their crash. I was on call at home on Friday the thirteenth when I got a level-one trauma activation. I had just walked in the door, turned around and walked out again. As I raced down Woodward Avenue, I passed a crash scene. There was a demolished car in the median, several police cars and ambulances. I rushed past to get to the ER, and was told there were multiple injuries from a bad crash. Two of the victims were already in bays and a third was coming. Somebody whispered that they might be the Red Wings.

"It was a week after they had won the first Stanley Cup in about fifty years and they were having their end-of-season golf outing. They had hired limousines. Several of the Russian players weren't golfers and had left early.

"Detroit is a great hockey town. Along the way, the Red Wings had recruited several Russian players. The first Russian to play for the National Hockey League was Viacheslav Fetisov, nicknamed 'Slava.' He was a captain of the Red Army team in Russia during the Gorbachev days of Perestroika and Glasnost. There were public pronouncements that the Soviet Union had become an open society, but nobody believed it inside or outside of Russia. Fetisov had a close friend, a chess player, who told him, 'You need to call their bluff. Leave Russia and every year the premier Russian players will get drafted to the NHL on a chance that they might be able to defect.'

"So Fetisov announced that he was going to America to play in the NHL. He woke up the next morning to find a public announcement in the paper that Fetisov had been suspended from the Red Army team and banned from every hockey rink in Russia, and that his crime was beating up a decorated World War II veteran in a drunken brawl. The only people more revered in Russia than hockey players were the decorated WWII vets, so that was the story that was concocted. His friends all stopped calling and he got death threats.

"There was a younger Red Army star player named Igor Larianov, who gathered some of the players together and said, 'If Slava doesn't play, we don't play.' So he was allowed to play in the World Championships and they won a Gold Medal. Then Fetisov upped the stakes by saying publicly that he was going to play for the NHL. His commanding officer then further upped the stakes. Fetisov was pulled into the Ministry of Defense to be confronted by the second most powerful man in the country, the Minister of Defense, who threatened and harangued him. He was told he would be sent to Siberia for the remainder of his Army commitment, which was 20 years, and that his whole family would be sent there. Publicly, they said he could leave the country if he wanted to.

"He called their bluff. He kept insisting he was going to go to America. Eventually he did get out of the country, by walking out the front door rather than defecting out the back door. His wife came with him, and his father came to visit.

"The Red Wings had recruited other Russians. Sergei Fedorov was a star player, and Vladimir Konstantinov was one of the great defensive players. They got Slava from the New Jersey Devils, and a couple more. In 1997, the Red Wings had five players on the ice who were Russian, and they won the Stanley Cup for the first time since the 1950's. Detroit went crazy with celebration.

"A week later, they had this big crash in which Fetisov was injured. It was a horrendous crash. Their limousine hit a tree in the median on Woodward Avenue and the vehicle was demolished. The passengers weren't wearing seat belts. The driver was eventually found to be impaired on some substance and did not even have a valid driver's license. When he was released later, he had to sneak out of the hospital because there were so many threats on his life.

"My patients were the limo driver, the two star players, and the Russian masseur. I had all of them in the Intensive Care Unit. I was up all night managing their care and the hospital was surrounded by media, camped around the emergency room and in front of the hospital. Reporters were grabbing anybody in a Beaumont jacket, trying to find out what was happening. The Red Wings team and the whole management of the

Dr. James Robbins, trauma surgeon, along with Red Wings teammates (left to right) Steve Yzerman, Brendan Shanahan, and Chris Draper, speak to the news media about injured Detroit Red Wings player Vladimir Konstantinov and team masseur Sergei Mnatsakanov during a press conference at Beaumont Hospital, Royal Oak, in June 1997.

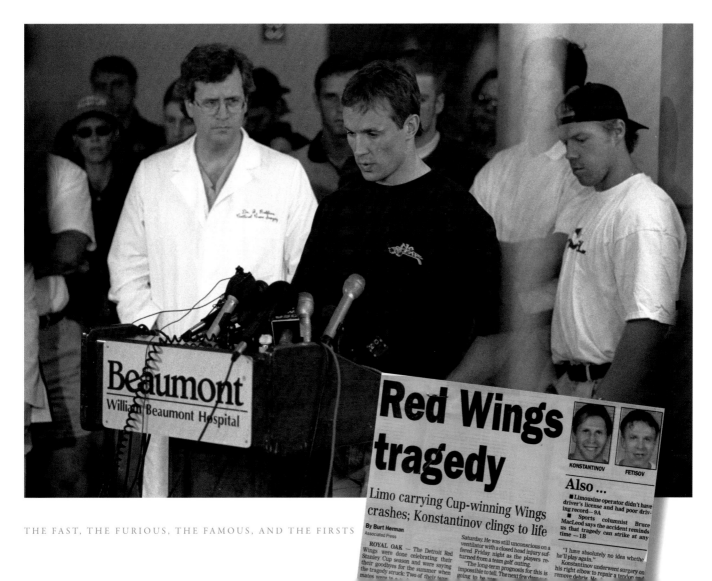

Red Wings tragedy

KONSTANTINOV   FETISOV

Also ...

■ Limousine operator didn't have driver's license and had poor driving record— 9A
■ Sports columnist Bruce MacLeod says the accident reminds us that tragedy can strike at any time —1B

Limo carrying Cup-winning Wings crashes; Konstantinov clings to life

By Burt Herman
Associated Press

ROYAL OAK — The Detroit Red Wings were done celebrating their Stanley Cup season and were saying their goodbyes for the summer when the tragedy struck. Two of their teammates were in a limo that...

Saturday. He was still unconscious on a ventilator with a closed head injury suffered Friday night as the players returned from a team golf outing.

"The long-term prognosis for this is impossible to tell. The next few days is going to be...

"I have absolutely no idea whether he'll play again."

Konstantinov underwent surgery on his right elbow to repair a tendon and remove debris. He...

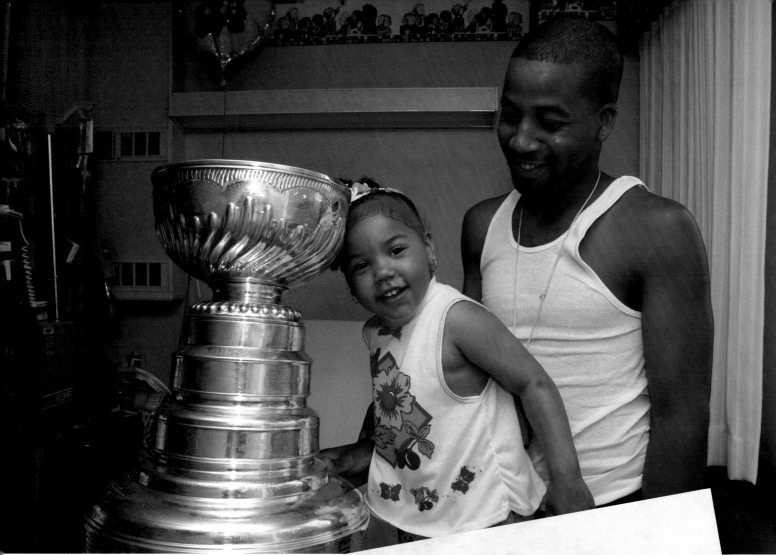

Yes, that is the real Stanley Cup! The Detroit Red Wings delighted Beaumont's pediatric patients and their families by bringing Stanley to the hospital the evening of July 1, 1997.

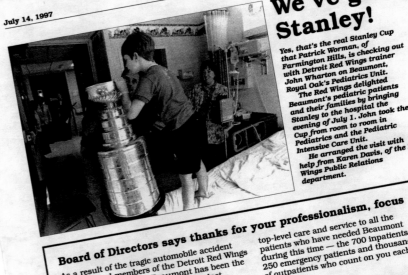

Pipeline

News and events for employees, medical staff and volunteers at Beaumont, Royal Oak

July 14, 1997

We've got Stanley!

Yes, that's the real Stanley Cup that Patrick Worman, of Farmington Hills, is checking out with Detroit Red Wings trainer John Wharton on Beaumont, Royal Oak's Pediatrics Unit.

The Red Wings delighted Beaumont's pediatric patients and their families by bringing Stanley to the hospital the evening of July 1. John took the Cup from room to room in Pediatrics and the Pediatric Intensive Care Unit.

He arranged the visit with help from Karen Davis, of the Red Wings Public Relations department.

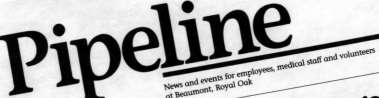

Board of Directors says thanks for your professionalism, focus

As a result of the tragic automobile accident that involved members of the Detroit Red Wings hockey team June 13, Beaumont has been the focus of extraordinary attention this last month. This, I'm sure, has brought more stress to your daily work, but it has also provided the opportunity for you to demonstrate the superior quality, caring and dedication for which Beaumont has become known.

~~half of the Board of Directors, I would like ~~~~medical staff, employees~~

top-level care and service to all the patients who have needed Beaumont during this time — the 700 inpatients, 250 emergency patients and thousands of outpatients who count on you each day.

Your continuing commitment to every patient is truly what sets Beaumont apart.

We, the Board of Directors, thank you and we applaud you.

~~William R. James~~
~~of Directors~~

team were there. Beaumont's public relations people and attorneys were there, and the Red Wings' public relations people were there. Rumors were rampant. Misinformation was being disseminated about who was injured and that some had even died. The only way to keep control was to promise a press conference and release some information.

"I refused to announce the conditions of the players. It was private information. I needed to talk to the wives of Konstaninov and Mnatsakanov, to Fetisov himself, and ask permission to disclose information and get some parameters about what could be said.

"We assembled a group of reporters. The next morning, I appeared before them in scrubs, unshaven, having been up all night, standing shoulder to shoulder with team owner Mike Ilitch, team captain Steve Yzerman, and Brendan Shanahan and all the Red Wings, and their team physician. We were locked in the lobby of the Administration Building, in a surrealistic theatre of flood lights, microphones, and popping cameras.

"Konstantinov, whom many considered the best defense player in the NHL, was severely brain-damaged; his ultimate prognosis was unclear. The team masseur, Sergei Mnatsakanov, was severely brain-damaged and paralyzed. Slava Fetisov was in fair condition, with a bruised lung and chest injury. The limo driver was also in fair condition.

"I started getting phone calls from relatives and hearing from colleagues that my press conferences, which went on for days, were being broadcast internationally. A colleague traveling in Russia said he was in an airport and saw me on TV, talking to a press corp, speaking Russian. For a short period I was being quoted in *Sports Illustrated*, on ESPN and in the *New York Times*. It was bizarre. I developed a relationship with them and especially Slava Fetisov, who is an iconic sports hero, one of the most loved and revered people in all of Russia, because he stood up to the regime. I was a hockey fan and I knew all this.

"One day after he was discharged, he called and said he was getting pain in his chest and his leg was swollen. I was concerned he had a blood clot and maybe it had traveled to his lung. There was still a media blitz. I was concerned about him being seen returning to the hospital. I picked him up in my car, drove him through a descrete entrance to the hospital and had someone from the vascular lab meet us, so Slava could get a Doppler test to see if he had a clot. Along the way, he told me the story of his departure from Russia. He talked about his conflicts with his coach and the Red Army team, the Minister of Defense, and how he was unsure he would ever be able to leave Russia. We developed a friendship. During Slava's hospitalization I operated on his wife, for appendicitis, and put her in the room next to his.

"He did have a blood clot in his calf, which we kept secret at the time, because he was in contract negotiations with the Red Wings. He was 39 and had been in a severe car crash. The general manager of the Red Wings called me to ask whether the injuries would preclude Fetisov's playing. We treated the clot with medication, walking and repeated Doppler tests to make sure it didn't travel out of his calf. He did play the next year.

"He's a remarkable role model and pioneer, revered by the other Russians in the NHL because he made their lives in freedom possible."

The "C" Word:
Cardiology

17

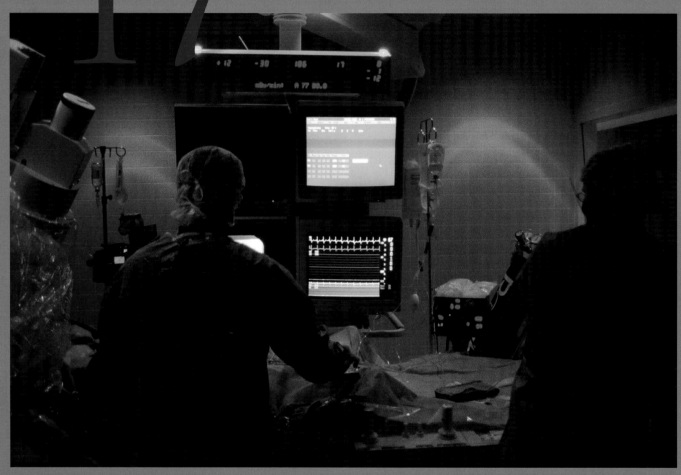

GERALD TIMMIS, M.D.

Emeritus Director of Cardiology Research,
Beaumont, Royal Oak

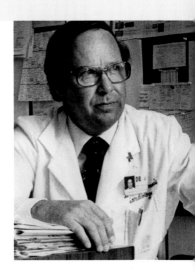

"The heart is three things:

it's a pump, it's a muscle, and it's an electrical system. Cardiology began here at Beaumont in the late 1960's, when I came from downtown. I began at Children's Hospital in Detroit, then went to the Detroit Medical Center. In pursuit of what I was trained for, I finally found my way out to Beaumont.

"My time at Children's was a very exciting period in my life. I started the heart lab there, and did the same kind of thing with babies and children as we've done with adults, all at a time when the mortality rate of fixing a hole in the heart was about 50%. The mortality rate now is about 0.5% or less.

"When I came to Beaumont, the Division of Cardiology consisted of a room with seven or eight electro-cardiographic machines with a bathroom next door. There was an abject absence of anything remotely serviceable in terms of practicing cardiology, so Dr. Seymour Gordon and I began to put an organization together. We began the more modern phase of cardiology, prior to which cardiology was a feel/touch/hear/think method, diagnose by physical and historical means, that is, to listen to the patient as to what ails him or her, putting together a diagnosis from those rudimentary tools, and armed with an electro-cardiogram, the only technology which existed then.

"Eventually we put together a heart lab in 1973. Prior to that, we used some obsolete X-ray equipment to put catheters in the heart. Finally we got into relatively high technology, for that time, which was an image-intensifier, which reduced the dose of X-rays by a factor of 8,000. Before that, the exposure was malignancy-generating. The image-intensifier radiation system was housed in a special laboratory for doing invasive cardiac diagnostic procedures.

"In the mean time, we developed an intensive care unit for heart attack patients, called a Coronary Care Unit. We introduced the use of monitoring catheters, the so-called Swan-Ganz catheter, which isn't used anymore.

"We incorporated echo-cardiography into the diagnostic armory. It was completely non-invasive. The quality and dimensions in terms of 2-D, 3-D, and 4-D echo-cardiac studies, color-flow mapping evolved enormously. We were hand-maidens to this progress, with the generous collaboration of the hospital administration obtaining the costly tools that allowed us to do this work.

"We added another lab for cardiac catheterization, and from that point the volume of diagnostic and therapeutic cardiology grew immeasurably. One of the more important developments has been the use of clot-dissolving enzymes, which we instill directly into the coronary artery through a catheter that we would snake, at first from the arm, and later through the groin. We would pass the catheter up the aorta and through into the root of the aorta where the coronary arteries arise, and enter both major coronary arteries and instill this medicine into that culpable vessel harboring the clot. This all followed the more diffuse introduction of these enzymes, things like streptokinase (SK) and tissue plasminogen activator-inhibitor (TPA). We used to inject it intravenously, but thought it was more effective when we did it directly into the coronary arteries.

"We did many studies, published a good deal, and began to participate on a broader scale. Oxford

University asked me to head a study for the United States called the Isis Trial, named after the Isis River that runs through Oxford University. This was a broad-scale trial of some 17,000 people comparing streptokinase to aspirin, to both, to neither. We found that the combination of streptokinase and aspirin hugely reduced mortality from heart attacks. Those were exciting times."

THE NOT-SO-GOOD OLD DAYS

"Back in those days, there were no such things as heart muscle biopsies, so we would use a liver biopsy needle and stick it right into the chest into the heart muscle to get a piece of muscle. Then pacemakers came and really added to the enzyme story, referred to as thrombolitic enzymes—'thrombo' meaning 'clot,' and 'litic' meaning 'dissolving.' We experimented with new pacemaker leads; a battery is embedded subcutaneously into the chest wall, then connected via a specially insulated wire that is introduced into the heart. One of the problems with that system was that the wire would lose its position in the heart, so a company called Medtronics supplied me—the only doctor in the world—with a special wire we called 'leads,' because they were complex things, requiring insulation and conductive material on the inside, and the tip of the wire was configured into the shape of a screw. We would screw these things in, doing research at night, on live dogs, which we would transport from the animal lab to our cardiac lab in an ice cream cart. We would do this from 10:00 PM to 1:00 AM and spent a lot of time on this device, which we called the 'endocardial screw.'

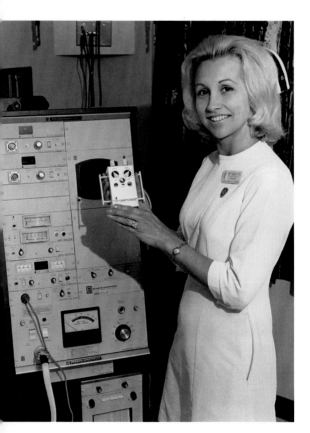

Nurse with an early version of a pacemaker.

"Finally I presented my results in Tokyo in 1976. I presented my paper with 42 dogs and 32 patients. And the very next presentation was Jacques Nugica from Paris, discussing the same device. I hated this guy for a long time because Medtronics had told me I was the only one in the world who had this device. So here I am in Tokyo, supposedly having the only report on this device. Nugica came right after me on the same device. He hadn't done any research on dogs and had a smaller number of humans.

"I got to be very fond of Jacques. He was a big shooter in Europe. He would have me over every other year to Monaco or Nice to do talks. I made about twelve or thirteen trips to Southern France as his guest. We got to be fast friends."

"In the mean time, I was asked to edit a new journal on interventional cardiology, which I did for eighteen years. The publication was sired from the loins of Beaumont Hospital and still exists. I had a group of seven cardiologists with whom I worked. We would water and grow these little buds that would eventually blossom into cardiologists and the group became seven strong. I was asked to disengage from the group and become Chief of Cardiology, which I was already, but I was asked to be uninfluenced by the travails and distractions of private practice and dedicate my full time to being Chief. So I went from being a private practitioner, self-employed, to being an employed doctor. I ultimately became one of the four Vice-Chiefs of Staff here."

"I had a wonderful marriage to a fabulous woman for forty-two years and twenty-two days. I lost her about six years ago. We have six sons. The eldest is an investment banker. I have three lawyers, a business man, and my baby is a cardiologist. He's on the staff here at Beaumont—Steve Timmis.

"Because of my research in pacing and electrophysiology, I was inducted into the North American Society of Pacing and Electrophysiology, which now has its own fellowship. I became president in 1993. They now call it the Heart Rhythm Society.

"That same year I stopped seeing patients and taking night calls, and took a job with Beaumont as an employee, and I remain so. They refer to me as 'Emeritus Director of Research,' and I did run the research activities in cardiology for the better part of fifteen years. I had about fourteen research nurses who worked for me and we did many studies, brought in a lot of research dollars. They made me Director of the Research Institute, which is now run by Dr. David Felten.

"I'm going to be 80, and I'm thrilled to still be working. We can't afford for people to retire at 65 anymore. We're retiring our most experienced people. Activity is a wonderful thing. There's no question that your brain stays sharper."

NEWFANGLED GADGETS—LIKE COMPUTERS

"Last year I did 67,000 electrocardiogram units, so I'm still working. I used to work four days a week, but now I work seven days a week, because I'm at my laptop at the crack of dawn every day, reading electrocardiograms.

"All computerized ECG's have to be over-read by cardiologists, because the computer is good, but not perfect. The computer can't have experience. Well, I've come to love it. The computer goes with me everywhere.

"What's happened in my medical lifetime is awe-inspiring. We were indicted many times as being overly aggressive. We were powerpuffs compared to what's going on now, compared to what my son does. We can put in a heart valve without opening the chest. We can stop lethal rhythm abnormalities with a device that is implanted permanently with minimal invasion. So much has been accomplished in cardiology, and the epidemiologist would say that we have reduced the mortality of a heart attack, or more generically of coronary artery disease, and still more generically by atherosclerotic arterial disease, by a factor of 30% in the last three or four decades. My mother died when I was a junior in medical school of rheumatic aortic valvular disease, which today they could manage with one arm tied behind their backs."

MY GREATEST SATISFACTION

"Beaumont evolved from its inception in 1955 when it was a 238-bed family hospital into an academic center through a great deal of effort by everybody connected with this organization, and that's my greatest satisfaction. Now we're going to have our own medical school.

"Beaumont is representative of the very best in American medicine. It has fulfilled its obligation to the community in an elegant way. It has fulfilled its obligation to the art and science of medicine, in that we have been sufficiently academically curious, energetic and inventive, trying to add something to the toolbox we were first given, and have done so effectively and well. We have many young superstars now."

WILLIAM O'NEILL, M.D.

Chief Division of Cardiology, 1987–2006

Vice-Chair of Medicine, 2001–2006

Beaumont, Royal Oak

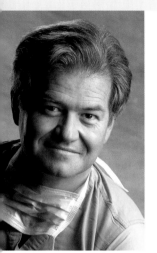

"I graduated from Wayne State University

in 1977, then went to the University of Wisconsin for an internal medical internship, then returned to Wayne State in 1978 for a medical residency. Dr. Arnold Weissler was the Chairman of Medicine at Wayne State and a pre-eminent non-invasive cardiologist. I became interested in doing non-invasive evaluations of heart functions.

"In 1978, there was no way to assess how well a heart was functioning other than a cardiac catheterization. Dr. Weissler invented 'systolic timed intervals' (STI), which were popular and I did some research with using STI after heart attacks. We found that if patients had severe impairment of heart function after a heart attack, they had very poor 5-year survival. This led me to think about how heart damage after heart attacks could be prevented.

"I became a cardiology fellow under Dr. Bertram Pitt at the University of Michigan during an incredibly exciting time in cardiology. The University had begun collaborating with Henry Ford Hospital, and we performed the first randomized trial of intracoronary streptokinase administration. Streptokinase is a thrombolytic (clot-busting) drug that opens an occluded coronary artery in the early stages of acute myocardial infarction, which is a heart attack. I was a first-year cardiology fellow in May of 1980, when a patient presented with an acute inferior-wall mild cardiac infarction. I took the patient from the ER to the cath lab, and with Dr. Joseph Walton performed the first intercoronary streptokinase administration.

"I still remember that first patient. It was dramatic, and we could visualize in the angiogram that the right intracoronary artery was completely occluded. We put the medication into the patient's vessel, and about thirty minutes later his chest pain diminished and the electrocardiogram started to normalize. The angiogram showed that the artery was now open.

"That was really the first demonstration, and it really changed my career and my life."

WHERE THE ACTION IS

"The study was published in the New England Journal of Medicine. I had planned to go into private practice, but was persuaded to stay on the faculty at U of M, while also becoming an attending at the V. A. in Ann Arbor with a chance to develop a coronary angioplasty program. I was extremely interested in this new field, and also in continuing my studies of emergency treatment of heart attacks.

"After a year and a half, I was offered the position of Director of the Cardiac Catheterization Lab, and I started the original randomized trial of balloon angioplasty compared to intracoronary streptokinase for the treatment of heart attack. So two years into my career, I was consumed in doing work on emergency treatment of cardiogenic shock. Both of these clinical works brought me in contact with Dr. Gerald Timmis at Beaumont Hospital.

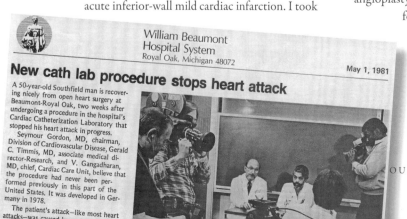

William Beaumont
Hospital System
Royal Oak, Michigan 48072

May 1, 1981

New cath lab procedure stops heart attack

A 50-year-old Southfield man is recovering nicely from open heart surgery at Beaumont-Royal Oak, two weeks after undergoing a procedure in the hospital's Cardiac Catheterization Laboratory that stopped his heart attack in progress.

Seymour Gordon, MD, chairman, Division of Cardiovascular Disease, Gerald C. Timmis, MD, associate medical director-Research, and V. Gangadharan, MD, chief, Cardiac Care Unit, believe that the procedure had never been performed previously in this part of the United States. It was developed in Germany in 1978.

The patient's attack—like most heart attacks—was caused

OU HAVE A BEAUMONT DOCTOR?

"Drs. Timmis and Seymour Gordon were both leaders in cardiology at Beaumont and very academically oriented. They wanted to collaborate with us on treatment of emergency heart attacks. During the next two years, I would perform the very first randomized trial of balloon angioplasty compared to intracoronary streptokinase, and this article also was published in 1985 in the New England Journal of Medicine.

"It was the first article that demonstrated the superiority of angioplasty over thrombolytic therapy. Dr. Carl Lauter approached me to join the Department of Medicine at Beaumont and become the Director of Cardiology. He had been a mentor of mine at Wayne State University. In December of 1987, I switched over to Beaumont.

"Through my collaboration with Dr. Timmis, I had come to recognize that Beaumont was a fantastic place to do myocardial infarction research because of the large emergency room and the large catchment area of Beaumont Hospital and the many heart attacks coming into the ER. I realized that in order to do proper heart attack research, I had to go where the action was."

A GOLDEN ERA AT BEAUMONT

"In the 1990's, the entire world was treating heart attack patients with intravenous thrombolytic therapy. At Beaumont, we started studying heart attacks, and I brought the concept of doing angioplasty as the primary emergency method of treating heart attacks, but there was still a great deal of resistance. We decided to do a randomized trial. I recruited Dr. Cindy Grines and Dr. Robert Safian, both gifted interventional cardiologists with well-established track records. Both were interested in establishing clinical trials at Beaumont.

"The 1990's were a golden era for cardiology at William Beaumont Hospital. In addition to Drs. Grines and Safian, I recruited Dr. Jim Goldstein from Barnes Hospital in Washington University in St. Louis. This group began numerous clinical trials and the most important study was the PAMI study, headed by Dr. Grines, the very first major multi-center randomized trial of angioplasty compared to thrombolytic therapy. It remains the cornerstone of this entire field.

"Other investigators at the Mayo Clinic and in the Netherlands found similar results, and these three original studies demonstrated that angioplasty was superior to thrombolytic therapy. Based on

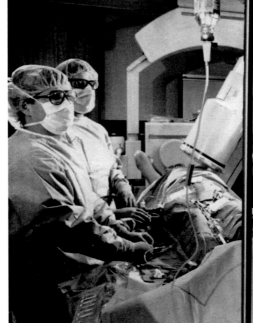
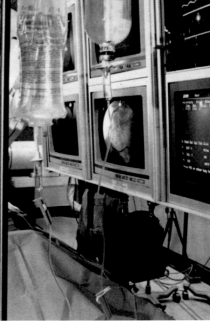

the work we did at Beaumont, the entire practice of treating heart attacks was changed throughout the country, and the world. Currently angioplasty therapy is accepted as the treatment for heart attacks, largely based on the scientific evidence from the PAMI group study. I believe this is probably the most important scientific work that the Division of Cardiology ever conducted, and will remain one of the high water marks for academic practice at William Beaumont Hospital."

MORE 'FIRSTS'

"We started many other pioneering observations during my time at Beaumont. We performed balloon valvuloplasty to stretch narrow aortic valves, and published a manuscript in 1990 looking at the use of aortic balloon valvuloplasty. This is a very important field of observation, and we found that although the balloon stretched the aortic valve, the valves almost always became narrow again within six months, so this wasn't a good long-term strategy. On the basis of the study we did in the early 1990's, I was chosen to be the primary investigator for the Edwards Percutaneous Heart Valve, and in 2002 Beaumont was the first hospital in North America to implant a Percutaneous Aortic Valve, and the first in the country to start doing implantations of valves in people with aortic stenosis.

"The entire field has exploded, and this will be another high water mark for Beaumont, the pioneering institution in using balloon expandable valves to treat stenotic heart valves."

Dr. William O'Neill performing the very first randomized trial of balloon angioplasty compared to intracoronary streptokinase. This article was published in the New England Journal of Medicine in 1985.

TURBULENCE AND TRIUMPH

"When I came to Beaumont in 1987, the only method of treating stenosis coronary artery was with a balloon. Other devices were developed at Beaumont, which became the first hospital to use rotational atherectomy with a rotoblator. Atherectomy is the removal of plaque clogging an artery, and a rotoblator is a type of rotating spool mounted on a catheter that grinds away the plaque. Beaumont was the first hospital to use this procedure. We performed the first study in 1989, and subsequently this has become a widely accepted technique.

"Dr. Safian pioneered the use of directional atherectomy, and I pioneered the work of a transluminal extraction catheter, or TEC, as another atherectomy device.

"Dr. Timmis was the Chief of Cardiology and Dr. Renato Ramos was Chief of the Cath Lab, and both these doctors were wonderful friends and colleagues with whom I enjoyed an incredibly warm and collaborative relationship. Carl Lauter was Chair of Medicine and the one who approached me to come to Beaumont; he had been in charge of the residency program at Wayne State, so I knew him also as a warm friend, wonderful colleague, and trusted leader. Dr. Fred Arcari was at that time the Medical Director for Beaumont, and a wonderful mentor who stood by me during amazing and turbulent times, and was very influential in helping us make the transition to the Beaumont Heart Center.

"I'd like to acknowledge the leadership of Mr. Ken Matzick, who had the confidence in the Division of Cardiology and was the one who ultimately persuaded the Board of Trustees to build the Beaumont Heart Center into the strong unit it is today—one of the strongest in the world."

Dr. William O'Neill is currently the Executive Dean for Clinical Affairs, Chief Medical Officer and Professor of Medicine and Cardiology for the University of Miami Health System.

Simon Dixon, M.D., Health System Professor and Chair, Department of Cardiovascular Medicine at Beaumont Hospitals meeting with the first United States patient treated with the IMPELLA (device), a ventricular assisted device, for percutaneous high risk angioplasty.

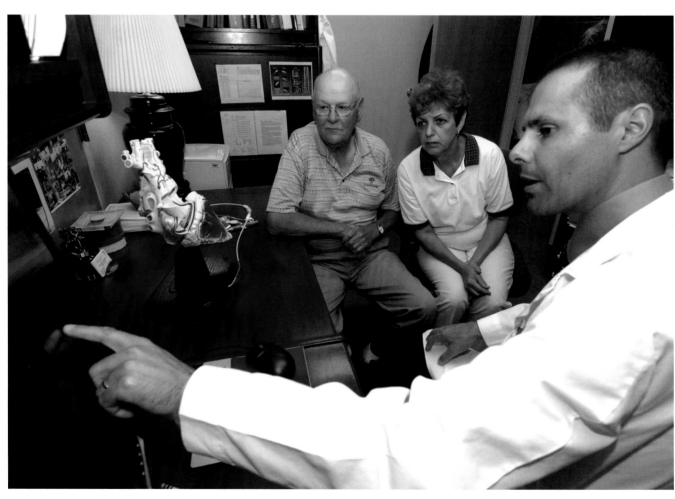

DAVID HAINES, M.D.

Professor, Internal Medicine, Oakland University William
Beaumont School of Medicine
Medical Director, Electrophysiology Laboratory and Program
Director, Electrophysiology Fellowship in the Department
of Cardiovascular Medicine, Beaumont, Royal Oak

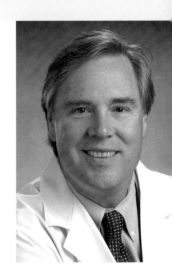

"I did cardiology training at the

University of Virginia, then stayed on faculty and
was there for a total of twenty years. I certainly knew
Beaumont by its growing reputation, which was
driven by Dr. William O'Neill, who founded the
Cardiology Department, and Dr. Cindy Grines, who
is one of the luminaries of research and clinical care.
They were leading the nation in terms of advanced
interventional care with cardiac patients. I was always
highly impressed with Beaumont. I sent a couple of
fellows to Beaumont for interventional training from
the U of V program.

"I'm employed full-time here at Beaumont.
I came as the Director of the Heart-Rhythm Center.
Then Bill O'Neill had a great opportunity at the
University of Miami and I was asked to step into
the role of the Interim Chief of Cardiology. It was a
daunting task, because there were so many moving
parts within the division. I'm one of the new kids at
Beaumont, which gives me a unique perspective.

"I worked to change the structure to make us a
free-standing department. We used to be a subsidiary
of the Department of Medicine. We are now the
Department of Cardiovascular Medicine, a broader,
more comprehensive, and better descriptor of what
we do here. It reflects the institution's understanding
of the importance of our work and our system,
nationally and world-wide, in advancing the health
and survival of our patients.

"I have a tremendous team working with me. We
have some of the top researchers in the world in their
respective fields. We continue to do cutting-edge
research in a wide variety of areas and are recognized
as one of the leading cardiovascular centers in the
country."

CT ANGIOGRAPHY

"One of the research programs is headed by Dr.
Gilbert Raff, in the area of CT angiography as well
as MRI, non-invasive tests that give us exquisite
anatomical insight into what's going on in the heart
with three-dimensional high-detailed picture. There
are new multi-slice scanners and it seems there's one
on every street corner now. As utilization of this test
ramps up exponentially, what's the real value of the
test for the care of the patient? The test is not free.
It costs cash-dollars for the system and also exposes
the patient to radiation. There's a big push to lower
patients' radiation risk exposure. Beaumont has been
one of the leaders of the world for both determining
appropriate use of the tests, and dosage reduction
with the test.

"Radiation is measured in millisieverts. When
CT angiography first started, patients were getting
twenty millisieverts for one test, which is equivalent
to 200 chest X-rays. We're getting better information
with newer scanners. We're down to ten millisieverts,
which equals about ten chest X-rays. Not a bad
trade-off.

"Gil was awarded a grant from Blue Cross/
Blue Shield of Michigan to prospectively monitor
the utilization and outcomes of Blue Cross patients
who get the CT angiography for assessment of
heart disease. He was doing such a good job of it
that four or five other states have requested that he
manage their database as well. So now Beaumont is
the repository for the largest CTA database in the
world."

"I'm a heart-rhythm person, very involved in
the area called 'atrial fibrillation catheter ablation.'
The most common abnormal rhythm in the world
requiring treatment is the rhythm called atrial

fibrillation. Atrial fibrillation is not a very serious rhythm; the phrase we hear is 'Atrial fibrillation won't kill you, but it'll just ruin your life.' Many people live with it and if they're asymptomatic they can live well for decades, but it does often present with palpitations, jumping of the heart, shortness of breath and general ill-feeling.

"We continue to do cutting-edge research in a wide variety of areas and are recognized as one of the leading cardiovascular centers in the country."

"We are actively developing tools to identify the hot-spots where the atrial fibrillation is coming from, and deliver certain types of energy to burn out or 'ablate' the hot-spot, to destroy the heart muscle that is allowing the rhythm to propagate. Though still not perfect, it's very gratifying and we're comfortable offering this procedure as opposed to lifetime medication. The medications, anti-arrhythmic drug therapy, are very strong, associated with a roster of potential risks and side-effects, so they're a double-edged sword. If we can fix the rhythm with a catheter, so these people never have to take drugs again, that's a good option. It's estimated that about six million Americans have this arrhythmia right now."

MY BEAUTIFUL BALLOON

"We have a research protocol using a laser balloon to do the catheter ablation. The balloon is inflated in the heart at the end of the catheter, then there's actually a small scope to look into the balloon and see where it's touching the heart muscle, and aim a laser at that point and burn those areas. There's a hot balloon being developed by a medical company in Japan.

"I'm actually the inventor of a technology for ablating on the outside surface of the heart, being developed by another company. It accomplishes the same things we do with the catheter on the inside surface of the heart. We can ablate with that tool and create the same pattern to burn out the hot-spots that are causing the arrhythmia. We're working on a 'convergent procedure,' in which the surgeon does one part of it from the outside of the heart and the cardiologist finishes from the inside of the heart.

VULNERABLE PLAQUE

"One other area that is the future of coronary disease management is examination of what's called 'vulnerable plaque.' This is a program that Dr. Simon Dixon, the cath lab director, and Dr. Jim Goldstein, one of the core academic group members, are working on. Vulnerable plaque is a cholesterol-loaded abnormal region in the coronary artery that sometimes will continue to accumulate, bulge into the artery, narrow the artery, and start impeding the flow of blood through the artery to the heart tissue. If that narrowing gets severe enough, people get chest pain when they exert themselves. If it closes off completely, the heart muscle dies. That's what a heart attack is. About 50% of heart attacks can be accounted for by this severe narrowing caused by cholesterol build-up in the artery.

"But the other half turn out to have cholesterol-not enough to impede blood flow through the artery, but if it has a thin cap, a covering of this blob of cholesterol, the cap is subject to rupture. It can fissure and crack. The body's response to any kind of injury is the little sticky elements of the blood, the platelets, rush in and try to seal it off. Those sticky platelets accumulate and form a clot, the clot occludes the artery, and in just a minute you can go from free flow of blood to the heart muscle to a sudden, total occlusion of that artery. How do you know it's coming? You don't. Everybody's heard the story of the person who had a perfect checkup and suddenly died three days later. This is the challenge that needs to be addressed because it accounts for a large portion of heart attacks.

"That's what causes most sudden deaths like that—the sudden catastrophic rupture of the thin cap of the atheromatous collection. The whole question is, how do you see this? With a conventional angiogram, even if it were done the day before on someone like the TV journalist Tim Russert, maybe 10% or 20% narrowing would have showed. The next day, he's dead. Conventional stress testing only shows areas where the artery is severely narrowed.

"With CT angiography, we can see these areas; not only the dye going through the artery, but we can see the bulky lipid-filled plaque hanging off the side of a major artery.

"Goldstein and Dixon are working to identify

high-risk people, even though nobody really knows yet how to treat them once they're identified. The opposing hypotheses of how to treat this are, first, to treat aggressively with cholesterol lowering medications. The second notion is that maybe we should cover this area up so it won't rupture ever, maybe by putting in a stent or a covered stent.

"This is the type of patient to whom we may give blood thinners. One of the reason that outcomes are so much better in coronary patients is the mainstay of very potent anti-platelet drugs. We have very innovative research going on at Beaumont to understand the natural history of these bulky, thin-capped plaques, and also to determine what to do once we have that information."

"Finally, an exciting area of big future growth is management of what we call structural heart disease: abnormal heart valves, holes in the heart, or other structural abnormalities. Some are genetic, some congenital, or just develop through life. Dr. George Hanzel is working with Dr. Cindy Grines and Dr. Rob Safian to develop this area of treatment with devices that can be delivered through a catheter.

"A normal heart valve may over time become a floppy, leaking valve, or it might get calcified and not work properly. This procedure uses the valve tissue that's already there, or a synthetic valve, pushing the old damaged valve out of the way and taking over.

"For holes in the heart, we have a variety of devices we send through the vein, through a catheter, that will expand, lock down, seal off a hole, and stay in place. Tissue grows over it and it's like there never was a hole.

"Another device seals off the mouth of the atrial appendage on the left side of the heart. A device is inserted through the vein, goes through the appendage, and opens up kind of like an umbrella, sealing off the mouth of the appendage. Tissue grows over it, and the patient no longer has to take blood thinners.

"Back to the valves, there's a device called a mitra-clip that will treat a big floppy mitral heart valve that's leaky because it flows back into the other chamber and doesn't form a nice seal. We can capture the two floppy edges of the leaflet, and the mitra-clip clips them together. When the valve tries to flow backward, the clip holds the integrity of the valve. This is all done with a catheter, inserted through the vein or artery.

"This is even better than laparoscopy, which makes a bigger hole. These devices are tiny enough to travel within the vascular system. The clip is about an eighth-of-an-inch wide and about half-an-inch long."

HISTORY IN THE MAKING

"A protocol we hope to be awarded is for a percutaneous aortic valve, which is a valve that goes into the position of the aortic valve, the main valve between the heart and the main artery that feeds the entire body. The aortic valve can get stiff and narrow and prevent blood flow. This device is delivered in a collapsed form, and once placed it opens up and pushes the calcium off to the side and opens that valve. There are leaflets inside this stent structure that prevent backward flow of the blood. Before Dr. O'Neill left, we were the first center in the United States to use a percutaneous aortic valve. That was an amazing technology. It was history in the making."

CINDY L. GRINES, M.D.

Professor, Internal Medicine, Oakland University William Beaumont
   School of Medicine
Vice-Chief of Academic Affairs, Program Director, Interventional
   Cardiology Fellowship, Beaumont, Royal Oak

"I've been at Beaumont 20 years,

and things have really changed in cardiology. Heart disease is still the number one killer, but the chance of dying of heart disease has plummeted and life expectancy is much higher. Mortality from heart disease has dropped dramatically. In large part that's due not only to prevention, but also the therapies we can now offer.

"The definition of 'cardiology' has expanded to something closer to 'cardiovascular medicine' because we're outside of the heart, doing peripheral vascular interventions in the carotid arteries in the neck, in the renal arteries, down in the legs, and so on.

"About 20% of all patients with heart attacks don't recognize the symptoms and don't seek medical attention until much later. And that's based on those who survived long enough to get an EKG, so a greater percentage are probably dying before they even think of seeing a doctor. Women have different types of symptoms than men and may not recognize that a heart attack is happening. They may not get the chest pressure or arm discomfort which is typical of men. Women may have back pain, pain between the shoulder blades, feel weak and dizzy or just get short of breath."

CARDIO "FIRSTS"

"There are a lot of 'firsts' in cardiology, and many of them happened here at Beaumont. We used the first rotablator, which is a high-speed drill to pierce heavily calcified coronary blockage. Beaumont was the first in the country to use gene therapy. We were the first to use medicated stents, the heparin-coated stents, in the midst of heart attack. We were the first to do percutaneous implants, meaning through a blood vessel, of an aortic valve; normally the valve would be installed through the chest. We were the first to do it through a blood vessel with a catheter.

"I came to Beaumont in July of 1990. Dr. William O'Neill was here, whom I knew from the University of Michigan. At the time, it was kind of scary to come here because this was just a community hospital, not very well known. When you're coming from the world of academia, you think you're going to fall off the edge of the Earth, never to be seen again. It turned out to be a good move, because at the time there was less bureaucracy here and we could do more."

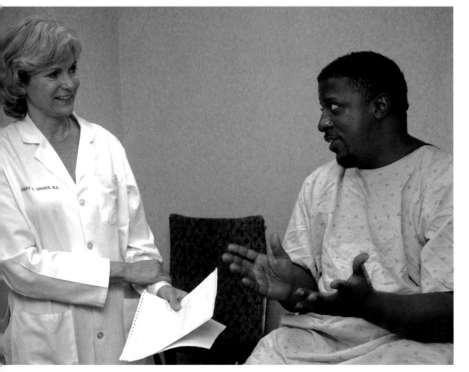

Dr. Grines making rounds on one of her patients.

BEAUMONT AGAINST THE WORLD

"Bill O'Neill and I did some of the first trials. These were called the PAMI trials—Primary Angioplasty and Myocardial Infarction. We were called cowboys and zealots and other unfavorable terms. The pharmaceutical industry was quite big at the time, a multi-billion dollar industry that was beating up on us, telling physicians in the area that we were committing malpractice. There was a big war being waged against us. We had no finances, no support, and were trying to fight back with this new idea. It was us against the rest of the world.

"We had twelve sites around the U. S. and in some other countries helping us. We randomized patients in the midst of heart attacks to receive either this primary angioplasty, which is the mechanical method of opening the blockage with a balloon, or the intravenous thrombolytic drug, which would dissolve the clot.

"So the twelve-center randomized trial showed that primary angioplasty was superior to thrombolytic therapy at reducing a combined end-point of death, recurrent heart attack, and stroke. We published it in 1993 in the New England Journal of Medicine. It really set the world on fire. We received vicious attacks throughout the entire decade. Subsequently other studies were done following in our footsteps, confirming our results. Then we performed what we call meta-analysis, where we pooled the data from all the trials, at that time about twenty-three trials comparing primary angioplasty to thrombolytic therapy and there again showing a highly significant reduction in mortality, reduction in the second heart attack, and reduction in stroke.

"Now it's a standard procedure around the world and has completely revolutionized the way heart attacks are managed."

NEW STANDARDS FOR ATTACKING HEART ATTACKS

"We have effectively changed the standard of practice. The next step is to figure out how we can improve upon this practice. After a primary angioplasty, there might be a certain number of patients who experience recurrent chest pain or might re-occlude the artery that we just opened up.

That's in large part because the balloon stretches the artery and might crack the wall of the atherosclerotic plaque, and there could be some elastic recoil as well as those cracks' falling into the artery, which might result in re-clotting.

"We then did a stent PAMI. We did an international trial in which we randomized 900 patients who received stents coated with heparin, which is a blood thinner, as opposed to the balloon alone. Again, at that time it was considered heresy to put a stent in the midst of a clot. These heart attacks are caused by atherosclerotic plaques that develop a clot in them, so there was some concern that putting a foreign body like a piece of metal would really be deleterious to the patient. But in this prospective randomized trial, we proved again that the patients did well and actually the stent served to scaffold the artery, propping it open for better blood flow, less formation of scar tissue, and less acute closure. That was a second revolution in how heart attacks are being treated.

"There are several other side studies we've done, but those two were the ones that changed the practice around the world. It's very gratifying to think that we've changed the practice of cardiology and saved lives."

CELLS AND GENES

"We're dabbling quite a lot into gene therapy. We've been using something called a 'fibroblast growth factor.' It's a gene that has been spliced out and then is put into an adenovirus, which is a cold virus. Cold viruses have a strong affinity for human cells and will infect very easily. This is an attenuated cold virus similar to a vaccine, alive but not necessarily going to cause a cold. When the cold virus attaches to the cell, it can release the fibroblast growth factor into the cell. We did studies in which we infused this into the coronary arteries of patients who had insufficient blood supply down their hearts. The purpose was to create angiogenesis, which is growth or birth of new blood vessels. These little capillaries grow around the blockage. Instead of one big fat bypass graft, there might be thirty little capillaries to do the job.

"We're looking at stem cells for better myocardial growth. The heart is composed of many different

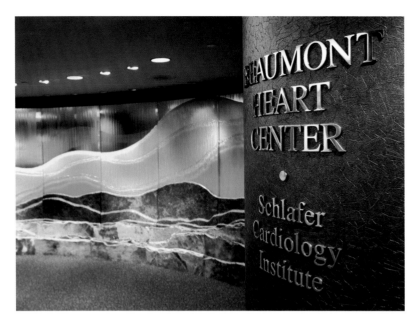

things. The heart muscle serves as a pump to send the blood out to the body, and after a heart attack there can be serious damage to that part of the heart muscle and it may never recover, so we're now treating that with stem cell infusion. The stem cells recognize there's inflammation and damage to that area, and they hone in on that area and attach, and basically redesign themselves. Stem cells can redesign themselves to be either muscle, blood vessel, or part of the electrical system.

"The study we're doing now uses a commercially available stem cell called a mesenchymal cell. The advantages are that it's available, and the study allows it to be infused into an IV. In the past, when we've been treating patients with stem cell, we would go in with an angioplasty during the acute myocardial infarction to open up and restore blood flow, then let that patient recover for three to five days. Then we would bring him back to the cath lab, go down into the same artery, inflate a balloon to occlude the blood flow to that heart attack area, then through the central opening in the balloon, and infuse those stem cells right there. We would actually be re-occluding the artery for a while. It's risky and expensive to do it that way, and is also painful if we use stem cells from the patient's own bone marrow instead of commercial cells.

"Preliminary results have shown that stem cells given intravenously actually do have some therapeutic benefit. We're evolving now to being less invasive by using the intravenous method and the commercially available cells instead of the patient's own cells. These things are experimental, but we're encouraged."

"We've been falling behind in this country with a lot of cutting-edge technology for a number of reasons. In Korea and South America, they don't have the restrictions we have here and can do whatever they want research-wise. The FDA has become way too restrictive. We can't do research the way we could in the past, partly because of those restrictions and because of the HIPAA requirements for patient confidentiality. It's become substantially more expensive and much slower. Very discouraging. It's demoralizing to investigators to be controlled too much. The type of research we were doing twenty years ago just can't be done in America anymore. Period."

CARDIOLOGY ON THE GO

"Today, technology is leaving the setting of the hospital and going into people's homes. We're moving toward having portable EKGs available all over the place, for instance in all EMS units so people can have pre-hospital electrocardiograms (ECG) and the hospital can prepare for what's coming.

"The paramedics are only called for about half of all heart attacks. The other half of the heart attacks drive themselves to the hospital. If portable EKG machines are available in public places, malls, boats, fairs and festivals, in emergency response vehicles, or even in homes, we can make a diagnosis on some patients and they may be able to chew aspirin or get immediate treatment from EMS responders.

"Simple things like having an automatic blood pressure cuff at home and checking blood pressure every day is an example of ordinary people's use of medical devices themselves. Some cuffs also show heart rate, so we use that when a patient is having palpitations and we're concerned he or she might have an arrhythmia. We have portable monitors people can wear that will automatically dial into a central station and send an alert.

"With so many new treatments and patients who monitor their own heart problems and overall health, cardiology has a bright future for saving lives and improving daily life for heart patients."

JOSEPH BASSETT, M.D.
Chief of Division of Cardiovascular Surgery, 1983–2007
Beaumont, Royal Oak

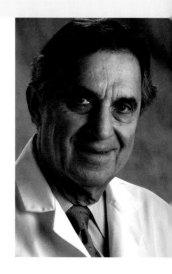

"I specialize in cardiac surgery.

I think I contributed a great deal to the services in heart surgery at Beaumont. They asked me to come here in 1979, prior to which I was working at other hospitals. I was appointed Chief of Cardiovascular Surgery in 1983, and was in that position for 24 years, until 2007, when I relinquished it. During my tenure, Beaumont placed eleventh in heart surgery as ranked by U. S. News and World Report.

"When I first started in practice in the early '70's, we did surgery for the correction of congenital heart disease. Most of the heart surgery at the time was for heart valve repair and replacement. At that time quite a few people had developed rheumatic fever in the past and came to us for valve repair. Rheumatic fever isn't a disease we hear about much, because it often came after strep throat, and nowadays people have treatment early, when they get a sore throat. Back in the old days, they didn't know much about it and anti-biotics weren't that good yet. We still see patients from third-world countries with valve damage secondary to rheumatic fever.

"Most of the progress came after the advent of coronary artery bypass. We took a vein from the leg and bypassed the blockage in the artery. As a matter of fact, some of the first ones I did were without the use of a heart-lung machine, which bypasses the heart and lungs during surgery and maintains blood oxygenation, flow and pressure. It is a blood pump with an oxygenator, so it circulates the blood and maintains tissue oxygenation. Today, it's hardly bigger than a basketball, and is mounted on a mobile frame. When I first started, the heart-lung were huge and took up a lot of space.

"Since coronary bypasses began, we have seen significant advances in heart surgery. Until a few years ago, we didn't attempt to repair a valve. We started doing that on a large scale about 20 years ago. If a mitral valve leaked, we would take it out and replace it with a mechanical valve or a pig valve. We've learned how to go in and repair the valve, cut out the parts that cause the leak, then sew the anulus and leaflets back together. The anulus is the outside ring of the valve. We've learned to reconstruct that by sewing in a prosthetic ring as a support structure.

"Also, since that time we've started using an intra-aortic balloon pump. It's not the same as an angioplasty, with which it is somes confused. An intra-aortic balloon pump has a balloon about seven inches long, and back in those days it was on a catheter as big around as a pencil. That would be threaded up the femoral artery after a cut-down. When the heart beats or contracts, the balloon collapses, making more room for the heart to pump into. When the heart relaxes to fill the other chambers, the balloon expands, giving a boost to the blood pressure. It's called 'counterpulsation.' The balloon is usually left in for two to three days, but it has been kept in for as long as three weeks. The procedure is still used, but it is much more refined now. Catheters are very fine, slightly larger than spaghetti.

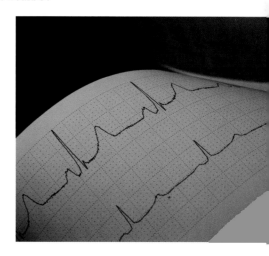

"A small opening in the skin over the femoral artery with a fine knife blade, probably two or three millimeters. A needle is then passed, followed by a guide wire and a sheath. The catheter is then passed through the sheath into the main aorta. These are the things that have really improved."

HEART SURGERY TODAY

"When I collaborated with Dr. William O'Neill, who was the Chief of Cardiology at that time, the two of us worked on a number of joint projects in cardiology and cardiac surgery. These were projects of a research nature and a number of publications occurred because of this research. He is one of the greatest cardiologist in the country. He left here to be Executive Dean of Clinical Affairs at Miami.

"I still perform bypasses and heart valve surgery. Most surgeons now use the mammary artery as well as veins from the leg. The left mammary artery runs under the breast bone on the left side. We attach that to the left anterior descending coronary artery, the one that runs in front of the heart. It's one of the main arteries and a very important one. We've found that the patency rate—the stay-open rate—is very much improved and those patients live longer. Internal mammary bypass patients live longer and feel better. This is well documented.

"There's been progress made with artificial hearts. If we have a patient who is not doing well and doesn't respond to the balloon pump, there are artificial hearts we can use. They're probably as big as a two-drawer file cabinet, and the ventricles are outside the body. There are some that can be outside the body, but most of these are to get the patient through a period of time, 'maintain' them for a while, until they can have a transplant.

"There is an artificial heart with batteries that are worn on a kind of vest and the patient can walk around.

"I've helped with some heart transplants, which are amazing. At Beaumont we did 20 to 25 heart transplants at least, and most had excellent outcomes. Some have been known to last 25 years, but most last between 7 and 15 years. There's a rejection problem, so transplantees have to be on anti-rejection drugs for probably their entire lives.

"The heart is an amazing organ. You're standing there with the heart in your hands, and it comes out, and there's a hollow cavity. Then you put the new heart in, from a person who has died, sew it together, give it a shock, and it starts pumping again. It has the intrinsic ability to beat by itself. The muscle beats because that's the way it's designed. It's electrical. No other muscle does that. The heart is quite a creation."

ON GOVERNMENT TAKE-OVER OF MEDICAL CARE

"It's not good. I've seen over the years how Medicare and Medicaid programs have gone. I think it's just more of the same things. It's not good for the patients because it's so inefficient. I'm afraid the goal is to push us all to government care. I've taken care of patients who are Canadians, who come to the United States to get medical care. Canadian doctors are told how many surgeries they can perform in a year and they're told how much money they can earn. People are not allowed to pay themselves for their own surgeries if they want to. They come here for surgery.

"Why should we live like that? If people have cancer, they should be free to have it taken out or mitigated. Heart patients should be able to have their surgeries."

MINIMALLY INVASIVE TRENDS

"The big buzz-words in surgery are 'minimally invasive.' It works in about 20% of cardiac surgery, usually for valve replacement or valve repair, not usually for coronary artery bypass. Most bypasses require two, three, four, or five bypass sites, and the back of the heart is hard to reach through a small incision. The aortic valve repair can be done through a small incision. I've done a few of those. These are all considered 'open-heart' surgery.

"We go right through the sternum, but we don't break it; we cut it with a small saw, like a small jig-saw. Then we use a rib-spreader, cut the pericardium, and do the heart surgery. If we go in from the side, we go in between the ribs. There's only a small skin incision on the outside, but inside there are larger incisions between the ribs.

"There's a desperate shortage of organs, which is really not necessary if people would be more willing to give up organs that are not being used anymore. There are some new mechanical support devices on the horizon for people who are in heart failure or need a transplant. We call it 'destination therapy.' These devices will keep people alive until transplants are available. We have to wait to see whether the government will allow us to use them."

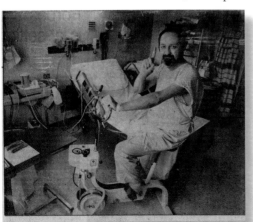

Beaumont's No. 1 heart transplant patient, Joseph Nadolsky, on his exercise bicycle

Transplant patient goes home with Beaumont's 1st new heart

By DIANA DILLABER
Of The Oakland Press

surgery performed July 31 by Jeffrey Altshuler, director of cardiac transplantation at Beaumont, said Colette Stimmell,

blood pressure, temperature and weight at home and visit Beaumont weekly for heart biopsies to check for signs of rejection, said

MARC SAKWA, M.D.

Professor of Surgery, Oakland University William Beaumont
School of Medicine

Chief, Division of Cardiovascular Surgery,
Beaumont, Royal Oak

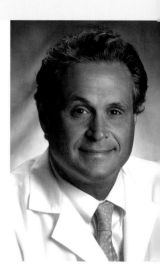

"I was actually born in Detroit,

and my father was a general surgeon, Chief at Sinai Hospital. When I came to Beaumont in 1987, the cardiac surgery program was up and running under the direction of Dr. Joe Bassett. At that time we were just doing the standard kind of valve replacements and by-pass surgery. I had special training in mitral valve repair and we started to do that procedure. We've probably done 3,000 repairs since then. We excise the frail portion of the mitral leaflet, put it back together, then install rings called angioplasty rings, which support the mitral valve.

"About two years ago, we started a new innovation—minimally invasive valve repair. In March of 2008, we did our first case, making about a 2 ½ to 3-inch incision on the right side of the chest. We're able to do the entire procedure, whether it is a repair or replacement of the mitral valve through that one incision. We make another small incision in the groin, expose the artery and vein, and use that for access to the heart/lung machine. We need to stop the heart or at least decompress the heart to do these procedures.

"The problem with valves is what we call myxomatous generation, where the valve gets thin and the structures deteriorate and cause rupturing. Myxomatous degeneration is the most common cause of what we call mitral insufficiency or mitral regurgitation.

"Other problems with valves include stenosis, meaning they get calcified and can't open, usually requiring valve replacement. The replacement valves are made out of pig heart valves, or pericardial valves made from the lining around a calf's heart. At Beaumont, we've always been on the forefront of putting in the latest and newest valves. In fact,

we participated in four or five trials now, one for a mechanical heart valve which is made out of titanium. That valve will last forever, but the patient has to be on Coumadin for that, to prevent clots. The valves made of tissue do not require blood thinners, but they only last ten or fifteen years.

"We participated in the Regent valve trial, which is a new design to the St. Jude mechanical heart valve, and we were the number-one implanters in the study, so there were lots of patients and data that came from Beaumont. We then participated in the Epic valve trial, which was a new pig valve, and participated in the Trifecta valve trial, which is not commercially available yet, but will be.

"We've evolved an aortic valve transplant technique here that is different from others. We're very aggressive in debriding the valve and the annulus. We also put our valves in a superannular position, a little higher than most people would in the aorta. We seem to get better hemodymic results than others and we have a lot of data to show that our results are different. I've been asked to speak about it and have been all around the world presenting it. There is a group in Germany doing this the same way we do, and they can reproduce the results. They're able to reproduce our results because they're implanting as we do. So we know we're doing something right."

"We were the first in the U.S. to implant a transcatheter valve just like a heart catheterization going through the groin. Cardiologists did that with our support. Now we're about to restart that program, not only going through the groin percutaneously, but also through the apex of the heart. We make a small incision on the left side of

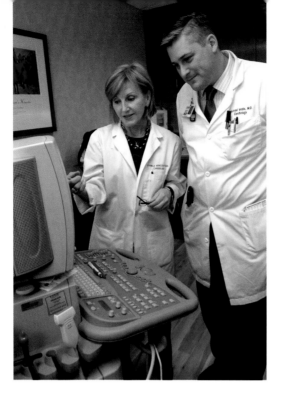

Pamela Marcovitz, M.D., Medical Director, Ministrelli Women's Heart Center and Michael Walls, M.D. discussing Echocardiography.

the chest, through the apex of the left ventricle, then make a little hole and insert the valve. This will be for sicker, higher-risk, or older patients. That program will be starting soon."

THE MINI HEART-LUNG MACHINE

"The actual heart-lung machine has changed very little in the past thirty years, until recently when people started to worry about how much fluid it takes to prime the machine and prepare for bypass. At Beaumont we were instrumental in redesigning the heart-lung machine into what's called a mini-circuit heart-lung machine. It's going to change the way people perform perfusion. We probably have the largest series in the world here for using a mini-heart-lung machine. It has reduced the blood transfusion requirements, reduced the time on the ventilator, and reduced post-operative bleeding. Most of the changes were in the circuit rather than the machine itself—the tubing. We changed it to about one-tenth the size."

MORE OR LESS?

"Now we're moving into minimally invasive coronary bypass surgery. This involves taking the vein from the leg and an artery from under the breast bone, and do it all with a three-inch incision on the left side of the chest. It's tricky. Patient selection is very important for that, and there aren't many centers doing it.

"Preventive medicine is definitely the big thing now. I think the reason coronary surgery has gone down is that coronary disease has gone down. People are much more conscious of their health. There is less smoking, less drinking, more exercise, and there are lipid-lowering drugs, cholesterol-controlling medications—all have made a huge difference. Perhaps the diseases will become problems later in people's lives. Our patients are older than ever before. I'm concerned somewhat about delaying surgical intervention because of stents and medications; it's possible that people are treated less invasively when they should be treated more invasively."

BARRY FRANKLIN, PHD

Professor of Internal Medicine and Biomedical Sciences,
Oakland University William Beaumont School of Medicine
Director of Cardiac Rehabilitation and Exercise Laboratories,
Beaumont, Royal Oak

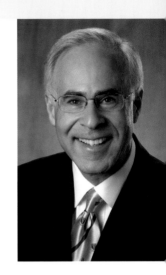

"I'm a Ph.D in Physiology, not an M.D.

I direct the Cardiac Rehabilitation program and the exercise laboratories here. I've been at Beaumont since 1985 and I love what I do. I do a lot of lecturing in my work, so I've visited the Mayo Clinic to give a talk, the Cleveland Clinic . . . I always leave those places saying, 'They don't have anything we don't have.' I think Beaumont is truly a gem and I consider myself fortunate to be here as a member of the medical staff."

"PUT US ON THE MAP"

"I work with patients who have heart problems—angioplasty, coronary bypass surgery, heart attack, and even heart transplants. In the rehab program, I've worked with a phenomenal team of nurses, physiologists, and support staff. We develop exercise programs that are safe and effective, evaluate our patients' cardiovascular fitness and function, identify coronary risk factors they may have, and work with them and their referring physicians on programs designed to facilitate comprhensive and cardiovascular risk reduction. I've been president of the American College of Sports Medicine and president of the American Association of Cardiovascular and Pulmonary Rehabilitation.

"Beaumont recognized long ago that if we're going to have a world-class cardiology program, with state-of-the-art labs and bypass surgery, then we need a place for rehab after interventional/surgical procedures, to reduce their risk for recurrent cardiovascular events or revascularization procedures. When they hired me, they said, 'Put us on the map. We want you out there. We want you speaking. We want you writing. We want you bringing in grants.'

"We have close to 500 publications now. Beaumont's rehab program is known world-wide.

In fact, if anyone asks what's the best heart rehab program in the nation, I'm confident we'd be listed in the top five. We publish a newsletter, do many media interviews, organize annual conferences on preventive cardiology, and do public relations community talks. Every time I've voiced an interest, Beaumont has said, 'Go ahead and do it.'"

CARDIOVASCULAR DISEASE

"In cardiovascular disease, there is no question that we've made great headway over the last two or three decades in making this generation healthier than the last. From 1980 to 2000, there was a 44% reduction in cardiovascular deaths. The cause is delineated beautifully in a recent New England Journal of Medicine article which said the improvement is partially related to current treatment for acute myocardial infarction. Here at Beaumont, we have one of the world's pioneers, Dr. Cindy Grines, who

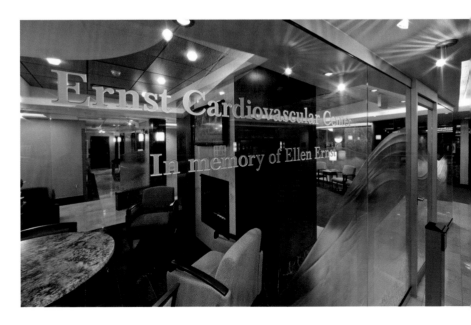

"From what I see, Beaumont has been a pioneering medical center. Our standards are very, very high. We're looking for people who are leaders, not followers."

pioneered angioplasty in an emergency setting, so if someone is having a heart attack and he or she gets to Beaumont, our interventional doctors can insert a catheter into the occluded coronary artery, which is about the size of cooked spaghetti. Today they can open up the artery and literally halt heart attacks in progress. But you have to get to the hospital quickly—generally within 90 minutes. Time is muscle!

"The major reduction in cardiovascular deaths is due to pharmacotherapies and getting people to stop smoking, start walking, and lose weight. Even small amounts of weight loss can have profound and favorable effects. Getting people to recognize that if they have a cholesterol concentration of 240, which is too high, they need to eat better, exercise more, and if that doesn't work, take their statin drugs. Statins work very well, without adverse effects for most people. Aspirin is also a wonder drug, cheap, and prevents initial and recurrent heart attacks. Lifestyle modification and pharmacotherapies can have huge effects on cardiovascular risk reduction.

"It's amazing to me how many people say, 'I'm not diabetic,' but when we take their blood sugar, it's 140 or higher. Some people are out there gaining ten, twenty, thirty pounds a year, and haven't had their blood sugar checked in years. They're diabetic and they don't know it! If we can tackle the major risk factors—stop smoking, get the cholesterol under 200, raise the good form of cholesterol (HDL), lower the bad (LDL), get the triglycerides down, treat and prevent diabetes, lower blood pressure, lose weight, and start exercising, the cardiovascular health of our nation would skyrocket.

"Why is this important? Because heart disease is the number one killer and crippler in our society. If I have my way, we're going to make most revascularization procedures obsolete. This hospital should have a world-class cardiology program and exciting, pioneering research going on, and we do.

"From what I see, Beaumont has been a pioneering medical center. Our standards are

very, very high. We're looking for people who are leaders, not followers. I've thoroughly enjoyed the opportunities here."

AN INTERESTING CASE

"One thing the health care community needs to do better is to provide hope and optimism to the patients we serve. We had a patient who was a 270-pound truck driver, 48 years old, and had just had a heart attack. I remember vividly sitting with this guy, asking questions like, 'How is your rehab program going?' and I'd get one-word answers. The interview was going nowhere. All of a sudden, he was crying.

"'Bill, what's wrong?' I asked.

"'Man, my life is over,' he said. 'I'm 48 and I had a heart attack!'

"I told him, 'I've seen your records. You had a right coronary occlusion. If you're going to pick an artery, pick the one on the right. It feeds the least amount of tissue. Your ejection fraction is still 50%, so you have normal pump function. You performed our stress test with no adverse signs or symtoms. I may be wrong, but based on everything I see here, I think you're going to be around many more years.'

"He said, 'You're crazy!'

"Well, you have the two best prognostic indicators. You have a good pump function and you're fit as a fiddle. I think you're going to do well.

"I got him to follow me to our rehab gymnasium and pointed out a man jogging on a treadmill. 'See that guy? He's been with us fifteen years. He had a heart attack just like yours. And that guy over there—he's been with us twenty-two years.'

"So the mind plays a major role in our destinies. I firmly believe we become what we think we will become. Medical personnel can set the stage and give people hope. I look at the chart to find information that is positive, to give the patient hope and optimism, to help him or her think, 'Hey, I'm one of those people who had a heart attack and will live to be 85 and do well. I'm not only going to survive heart disease, but I'm going to thrive with it!'"

18 Modern Marvels

KENNETH PETERS, M.D.

Professor and Chair of Urology, Oakland University
William Beaumont School of Medicine and
Beaumont, Royal Oak

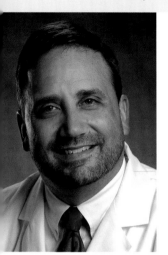

"Urology as a field is a surgical specialty,

but it has one of the more specialized sub-specialties, with a good mix of office patient care, surgery, innovative technology, and innovative research. Here at Beaumont we've been fortunate for years in that the Department of Urology has been strong as both a clinical and an academic department.

"There's nothing about urology that we don't cover, which provides a level of patient care above and beyond a general urologist, or anyone who has specific urological conditions that other centers or physicians don't handle. I've personally had patients come from as far away as Germany to see me for my specialty, which is pelvic pain, interstitial cystitis, and urinary incontinence.

"Before I took over as the Chairman of the Department of Urology, I was the Director of Research with Dr. Diokno as my chairman. We've done really innovative things at Beaumont that no one has done in the United States. For example, for 20 years we've been studying interstitial cystitis, a painful bladder disease associated with urgency and frequency. From the outset we've been involved with the National Institute of Health studies on new treatments for IC. Imagine feeling as if you have a horrible bladder infection, but there's no infection, so we can't give just medication to make it go away. It's a major problem. Patients really suffer, it affects their quality of life, and many can become disabled. It has been described since the 1800's, with no good treatment. Beaumont has been aggressive in studying this disease and has become known for diagnosis and treatment. We work for the National Institute of Health to help characterize this disease with something called the Interstitial Cystitis Database, and we're moving forward with new clinical trials.

INTERSTIM

"Beaumont has really been at the forefront of developing new techniques. We are one of the early adopters of Interstim, which is a pacemaker for the bladder. We make a tiny incision over the tail bone in a surgery that takes 45 minutes, and place an electrode near the nerves that go to the bladder. In these patients, the nerves are hyperactive. The patient has to urinate suddenly and can't control it. We test the Interstim outside of the patient's body for a couple of weeks by sending her or him home with a temporary pacemaker, and the patient keeps voiding diaries and pain scores and urge scores. About 85% to 90% of patients get at least a 50% improvement of symptoms by overriding the nerve signals the body was sending down the pathway.

"If it helps, we then implant it surgically two weeks later. It actually looks just like a heart pacemaker, but instead of putting it in the chest, we put it down by the lower butt cheek. It lasts four to five years with a battery, and has to be replaced eventually.

"There was a number of patients for whom this didn't work, so five or six years ago I did a study in which we compared placing the Interstim at what's called the sacral nerve, where it is FDA approved, to putting it at a different nerve, the pudendal nerve. The pudendal is yet another nerve that controls bladder function. There was some thought that the pudendal nerve might be in a better location, but there was nothing on the market to do that. We at Beaumont developed a pudendal nerve stimulation and actually did a clinical trial, published it, and compared one to the other where every patient got both. They didn't know which one they were

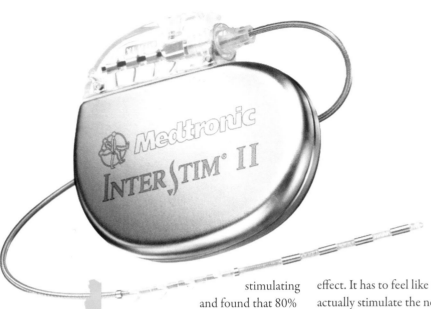

stimulating and found that 80% of patients did better with pudendal nerve stimulation. We've done over a hundred pudendal implants at Beaumont and are getting people from all over the country coming for this procedure. Both from a research standpoint and in clinical practice, this has really put us on the map as an innovator for managing over-active bladder and pelvic pain."

STEM CELL TRIAL FOR STRESS INCONTINENCE

"Stress incontinence is leaking that occurs because of coughing, sneezing or straining. It often plagues women after childbirth. Most of the time we either do physical therapy or surgery like a bladder suspension or sling. Although those work for many people, it doesn't work for everybody. So we brought Dr. Michael Chancellor, who is probably one of the top neuro-urologists in the country to Beaumont. He developed a technique using adult stem cells. A small biopsy is taken from a muscle in the leg, which is sent to Pittsburgh, where stem cells are created from the sample. Stem cells are the basic building blocks of the cell. No embryo, no controversy—just the patient's own muscle. About eight week's later, we get this vial, and right in the office we can inject these cells directly into the sphincter. We've treated forty patients so far as part of this research study. No one else in the United States has ever done a stem cell trial. Beaumont is the first.

"People have dabbled with tibial nerve stimulation to treat over-active bladder for years, but it never caught on because no one has been able to do a sham control trial. A sham, in this case, is a fake stimulation, used as a control to provide a placebo effect. It has to feel like the real thing, but can't actually stimulate the nerves. About three years ago, I developed a sham that would produce sensations of tibial nerve stimulation, and we just finished a 220-patient study that was a national trial. We're just publishing the results right now, showing that the tibial nerve stimulation is significantly better than a sham. We're hoping this data is going to help get us insurance reimbursement for this treatment as an alternative to surgery or fighting the side effects of medication that isn't working."

WE, ROBOT

"Beaumont has more surgeons trained in robotic urological surgery than any other hospital in the country. We have a big prospective data base and are looking at outcomes of robotic surgery. Surgeries that were big and invasive have become minimally invasive. Now we're taking on bladders robotically, taking out kidneys and correcting incontinence using the robot. It's a new tool in the last five or six years, and Beaumont has been on the forefront of developing a program with robots. These kinds of things really set Beaumont urology apart from other places."

FEMALE UROLOGY

"We have a high level of expertise in female urology. We publish lots of papers in peer-review journals and write book chapters. We are creating a center for female urological problems, because so many women suffer from incontinence, pelvic pain, vaginal pain, and sexual dysfunction. These problems are often not addressed because women feel embarrassed or just don't want to deal with them.

"If we had a center for female urology, we would have specialists in incontinence or pelvic pain, fellowship training in urology, and clinical and nurse practitioners who specialize in it. We would have integrated medicine—acupuncture, message therapy, and other alternative treatments to help manage complex problems.

"Patients with chronic pelvic pain often go to doctor after doctor, getting different medicines, but no one ever addresses the root of the problem. Beaumont has developed a physical therapy program with therapists who are specializing in pelvic floor therapy; it's called a myofascial release. If you imagine a twisted neck muscle that makes turning your neck hurt, and you're miserable, so you rub it and it breaks loose, or a massage loosens it. The pelvis is like a bowl. The wall of the bowl is made of muscle. In the bowl are the uterus, the vagina and the rectum. Those muscles are important for being able to urinate normally, defecate normally, and have normal sexual intercourse without pain. When those muscles are in spasm, there is urgency, frequency, retention, fecal disorders, and pelvic pain. We've worked with the National Institute of Health on clinical trials that show pelvic floor therapy with a trained therapist can be highly effective and eradicate any symptoms.

"We have patients who have been suffering for eight, ten years, and have gone to six, seven, eight doctors. We send them to physical therapy, the symptoms are markedly reduced, and they ask, 'Why didn't somebody do this for me before?'"

BOTOX—NOT JUST FOR WRINKLES

"We do botox injections for overactive bladder. Botox works for wrinkles because a wrinkle is a muscle spasm. The botox paralyzes the muscle, and the muscle relaxes. The bladder is a muscle. For people who have overactive bladder or urge incontinence, the bladder is in spasm. So we inject botox into the wall of the bladder, dotting the bladder with botox to cause the muscle to relax and no longer spasm.

"We have clinical trials going on right now at Beaumont and many other centers in the country."

NEW FRONTIERS FOR SPINA BIFIDA

"Right now we're getting international attention for something new and exciting. We started a research study at Beaumont, again the first in the country, to look at rerouting the nerves to restore voiding function, for example to help a child with spina bifida. Spina bifida is an inherited disorder in which the spine never really comes together at the tail bone. These kids typically can't pee, can't have normal bowel movements, and usually have to use catheters. They get infections and renal failure. The treatment has been medication to relax the bladder, and use catheters because the nerves never really developed down to the bladder and the bowel.

"So, in China there was a physician who started studying rerouting a nerve from the leg and connecting it to the nerve in the bladder. The concept is almost like a knee jerk—a reflex action. The brain doesn't have to be involved in a reflex; it just comes from the level of the spinal cord. This was initiated in a study in animals and people with spinal cord injuries—paralyzed patients—and then it moved on to patients with spina bifida. If the bladder can't get any nerve signals coming to it from the brain because either the nerves didn't develop or the brain can't send it down because of a spinal cord injury; so the brain can't communicate down below. Is there a way to create a reflex so this person can urinate again?

"Through an incision in the back, we can identify a nerve that goes to your leg, and separate part of that nerve, then identify the nerves that go to the bladder that don't function, then connect the leg nerve to the bladder nerve. Over about a year, those nerves can grow and now what was ennervating the leg is now ennervating the bladder. We can scratch the patient's leg, which sends an electric stimulation to the bladder, and he or she can urinate.

"No one had really done it outside of China. Dr. Diokno, Dr. Gonzolez, and I actually flew to China to see this. It was a remarkable concept with a high success rate. We wanted to make sure it was really happening and succeeding as we were told. We

DR. DIOKNO ON ARTIFICIAL URINARY SPHINCTER (AUS)

came back determined to study it. With some of the donated money we had through Mr. Ministrelli, we started a research protocol which was an incredible undertaking, incredibly expensive because it involved neurosurgery, hospital stays, MRI's, and lots of neurophysiological testing, then bladder testing. We treated nine people with spina bifida, mostly kids, and did the nerve rerouting, and we're almost at three years now. We found that seven of the nine kids developed the reflex, and when they scratch their legs, they can urinate. They can literally scratch their legs, take that act, and urinate.

"What happens in spina bifida is that the brain seems to figure out, since there is no cord injury, that the leg controls the bladder, and most of these kids do well. It's not 100%; it didn't fix everybody, but we have a number of kids now who can urinate, whereas before they had catheters. They couldn't have bowel movements, but now are completely off catheters. They're off medications, and urinating on their own.

"This has gotten us international attention. We're in the news over and over. We did this pilot trial and I just got a $2.3 million grant from the National Institute of Health to study this. We've brought in another site at Emory in Atlanta, so we'll have two sites, and right now we're working with Beaumont's coordinating center to create our database and case report forms. We're hoping in July (of 2010) or so to start operating on more kids. So Urology is a pretty exciting department, actually."

"Surprisingly, many patients suffering from urinary incontinence especially men who continue to suffer from continuous urinary leakage after prostate surgery or women who fail from bladder suspension/sling surgeries are not familiar with this implantable device that I have found very effective in correcting the incontinence problem. The AUS is also known as AMS (American Medical System) Sphincter 800 Urinary Prosthesis. It is a small fluid filled device that is totally implanted in the body to mimic the natural process of urinary control and urination. This device is made up of three parts, the cuff which is implanted to surround the urethra or bladder neck, the balloon that helps pressurize the cuff implanted in a space next to the urinary bladder and the pump that is implanted in the scrotal sac or the labia.

The device works with the cuff filled with fluid which gently squeezes the urethra closed to keep the urine in the bladder. To urinate, the cuff is opened by squeezing and releasing the pump bulb two or three times to move the fluid out of the cuff and into the balloon, thus emptying the cuff and allow the urethra or bladder neck to open and allow the urine to flow from the bladder.

Within a few minutes after urination, the fluid automatically flows back from the balloon to the cuff. When the cuff is full, it squeezes the urethra close and prevents leakage of urine.

The success rate of such an implant in controlling the leakage is over 90%. Some of the undesired outcomes include malfunction of the device, infection or erosion of the device into the tissue. If these events happen, repair, replacement, or removal may be needed.

I have implanted hundreds of these prostheses and I have been very gratified with the result.

I have been caring for a couple over the years who I both implanted the artificial urinary sphincter to manage their urinary incontinence. I mentioned this story because perhaps this couple may be the only couple who both have an AUS and both are very satisfied with the outcome. Although both have agreed to have their names released, I just mentioned their first names as they were quoted during an interview with both of them.

Donna A.: "I was desperate. Nothing was working.

Alfred A.: Having this procedure done has returned me to a normal life. I don't have to carry diapers everywhere any more. I had tried everything, but nothing worked with me.

Donna: "We'd go to movies and I'd have to stuff the diapers in my purse. We don't have to do that any longer."

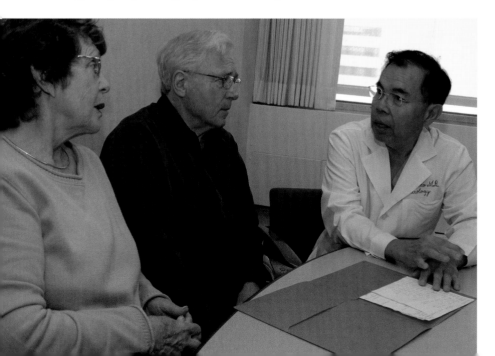

GEORGE WILLIAMS, M.D.

Professor and Chair of Ophthalmology, Oakland
University William Beaumont School of Medicine
and Beaumont, Royal Oak

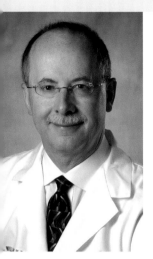

"I have been the Chairman of Ophthalmology

at Beaumont since 2001. I first came to Beaumont in 1988, recruited by my predecessor, Dr. Raymond Margherio. Dr. Margherio actually started the Ophthalmology Department at Beaumont. I was recruited by the large retinal group at Beaumont, Associated Retinal Consultants.

"I had been on the full-time faculty at the Medical College in Wisconsin, where I was a member of the retinal service; at that time, Medical College of Wisconsin was generally recognized as one of the premier academic retinal centers in the world. I had every intention of a life-long, full-time academic career.

"Then, Beaumont Hospital crossed my path. Dr. Margherio and Dr. Michael Trese suggested I see what was going on here. I recognized that they were able to do virtually everything I was able to do in academics, but in a private-practice model. They had an excellent fellowship and had managed to meld both a busy state-of-the-art clinical practice with basic research and clinical research, which is what I was doing in Milwaukee. Beaumont was already one of the premier private practice groups in the country. Coming here seemed to be something I needed to do.

"One of the big selling points was the strong support from the institution. Beaumont had made a commitment to provide us with state-of-the-art equipment whenever we needed it, provide support for research, which I needed to develop the retinal fellowship, and a state-of-the-art operating room for retinal surgery."

"To become a retinal surgeon, first you go to college for four years, then four years of medical school, four years of ophthalmology residency, and usually two years of retinal training. There's a lot of specialty care with ophthalmology. At Beaumont, we have fellowship-trained specialists who are nationally or internationally recognized leaders in all aspects of ophthalmology. We have surgeons who do corneal transplants, surgeons who specialize in plastic surgery around the eye, surgeons who specialize in glaucoma, and pediatric surgeons who specialize in children's eye diseases. We have one of the few programs in the country that has an ophthalmic pathologist—our Medical School Dean, Dr. Robert Folberg. He is one of a handful of people practicing in the world who are Board-certified in both pathology and ophthalmology."

WHEN IN ROME

"A retinal surgeon deals with diseases involving the retina, which is the back part of the eye, which actually senses light. Those diseases can range from retinal detachment to bleeding in the eye, to diseases such as macular degeneration, and our patients range from premature children to people over 100 years old. Beaumont is internationally known as a leader in the treatment of pediatric retinal disease. We have the largest pediatric retinal disease service in the world.

"We see babies from all over the world. Usually their trouble is caused by being premature, but there are other diseases that occur in children. Retinal disease in children is quite rare, so it would be unusual for most physicians to see these very often, but because of our international reputation we have extensive experience. In fact, our private retina group has an office in Rome for European patients. Our doctors leave on a Thursday, arrive in Rome on Friday, see patients all day Friday and Saturday, then take the next plane out and are back to work on Monday."

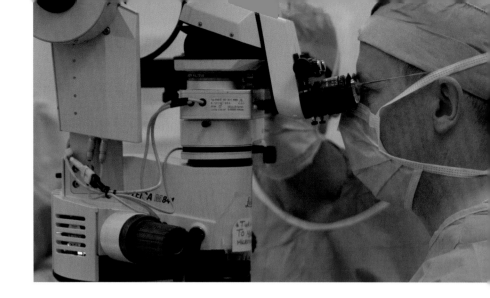

SEE INTO THE FUTURE

"We are directly involved with development of new technologies to implant a microchip seeing device that will allow people who are currently completely blind to see. We're privileged to be a part of that. We are collaborating with a group in Germany. We still don't have the device finalized, and as you might expect there have been technical glitches along the way, but it's exciting.

"We are also a leading center for clinical trials in other therapies for eye diseases, and the leading center in the world for a study of a new type of cell-based growth factor treatment that we think might have an application to patients with diseases like Usher's disease, which was what blinded Helen Keller.

"The common belief is that Helen Keller was blinded and deafened by a fever, but in fact she suffered from a genetic disease called Usher's Syndrome. It's a disease that affects both the cells of the ear and the cells of the eye. As a result, she became both deaf and blind. At Beaumont, we are developing new technologies which may benefit people with Usher's Syndrome and other genetic forms of blindness.

"Not only do we serve as a center for pediatric retinal disease, but the new techniques developed here at Beaumont have been adopted world-wide. Dr. Trese runs our pediatric retinal service; he is considered the leading pediatric retinal surgeon in the world.

"We're developing new treatments for macular degeneration, diabetic retinopathy, and our pediatric retinal service is leading an international trial on new treatments for retinopathy in premature babies.

The biggest advancements now are in the area of age-related macular degeneration, a disease that is very common in people beyond their mid-60's. It's a frustrating disease because it damages the central vision so people can no longer read or drive. Until a few years ago there was no good treatment for it, but new therapies have been developed. Our team at Beaumont participated in the development. It's a medication actually injected into the eyes. People naturally recoil when they hear about getting shots in the eyes, but it's very well-tolerated. We use such small needles that patients don't feel anything.

"We've made great progress in retinal detachment surgery. We have hundreds of patients come to us blind in one or both eyes, and we are able to operate and restore vision. We do it every day.

"With artificial seeing devices, genetic therapies, new drugs, and advanced surgeries, I believe there will come a day when we can prevent many more people from losing their vision. There is certainly hope on the horizon."

MICHAEL TRESE, M.D.

Professor of Ophthalmology, Oakland University

William Beaumont School of Medicine

Pediatric Vitreoretinal Specialist, Beaumont, Royal Oak

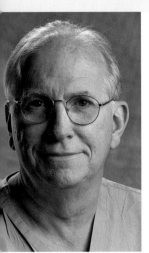

"Eye problems in infants and children

come from a spectrum of diseases. Some are caused by premature birth, some are genetic, and we see bad traumatic retinal detachments. I sub-specialize in pediatric vitreoretinal conditions. The back 4/5 of the eye is filled with vitreous gel. It's an interesting and a relatively young sub-specialty. Vitreous surgery only started in about the 1970's. The person customarily credited with its beginnings died on December 23, 2009. He's the person with whom I did my training: Robert Machemer.

"Originally I was from Michigan, moved away for nearly twenty years, doing training, and I came back to Michigan because I really do like Michigan and the Great Lakes. I became interested in vitreoretinal disease, doing training in things like detached retina, diabetes, and macular degeneration. But also, although it is much less common, I became very interested in retinal disease in children. When I moved back to Michigan, I started doing more surgeries, some difficult pediatric retinal detachments. One of the more common diseases we work with is something called retinopathy of prematurity, or ROP, which is a potentially blinding problem of prematurely born babies. It was actually first described in the 1950's.

"The first patient recognized to have ROP was a baby in Boston. The people in the nursery—the neonatologists and pediatricians—noticed that the baby's pupils were white. A couple of doctors went to examine this baby, one of whom was Everet Kinsey, who would end up working at Oakland University, very near Beaumont. They described the child as having retrolental fibroplasia. It's an old name. The lens is clear, but behind the lens an opaque membrane was present and that was actually the retina. The child had total retinal detachments. When I started working in this area, twenty or twenty-five years ago, the failure rates were extremely high.

"Many people made contributions to the treatment of this disease, and the failure rates now, with appropriate screening and early treatment, are closer to one to two percent. Enormous progress has been made."

"The retinal detachment is what blinds the child. We've done considerable work in retinal detachment surgery, and many of the techniques now widely used were developed here at Beaumont. Now we have eight dedicated pediatric anesthesiologists.

"We're very fortunate to be able to do surgery called a vitrectomy for 4-A retinopathy prematurity on a young child to cure retinal detachment. We take the vitreous out and take out scar tissue which is pulling on the retinal surface, and leave the lens in place. We developed that operation here, and it has made a huge difference in terms of care and prevention of blindness. If left alone, partial retinal detachment has about a 90% chance of going to total retinal detachment and blindness. With the surgery, the success rate is now 90%. It's an almost complete reversal.

"In a premature infant, the vitreous gel is a little different than in a term infant, but when we take it out, it gets replaced with fluid. The fluid is made in the front of the eye and fills the back of the eye, and the eye seems to tolerate that very well. Each one of those cases is extremely rewarding because you've really changed that child's entire life."

GENETICS

"We've also done work in other areas, some that are very clearly genetically controlled diseases. One of my partners, Dr. Tony Capone, another expert pediatric retinal surgeon, used to work at Emory University and joined us about ten years ago. Dr. Kimberly Drenser specializes in the pediatric retina. She does pediatric work and is also a geneticist. Dr. Drenser has set up a really quite extensive genetic lab with a database that is huge relative to some of these diseases, such as familial exodative vitreoretinopathy, congenital retinoschisis, persistent fetal vasculature syndrome (PFVS), or Norrie's disease. All these diseases have very clear genetic bases. In each, we've found some basic genetic pathway that contributes to disease formation. We've worked on developing both surgical solutions and medical drug therapy for some of these. We've been involved in several national randomized prospective trials that involved use of laser techniques, freezing techniques, retinal detachment repair, and we're currently in a study which we originated from here, which is looking at using some drugs with retinopathy prematurity.

"Here at Beaumont we've developed a fellowship program for all retinal vitreal surgery and medical retinal practice which is one of the finest in the country. We have fellows who come from every major university to train with us. People come from all over the world to observe. We currently have a fellow from Japan and one from Taiwan.

"We're a private practice and we've been associated with Beaumont since about 1978. We've spent a good deal of time working with the residency program. We've made enormous progress. I'm now a senior member of our group, and we have seventeen doctors across the state, with most being in southeastern Michigan.

"We have the largest pediatric retinal referral center in the world. It's something we've built since I came here in 1982. I have two other partners who do pediatric retinal work and I think we're the only place in the world that has three doctors doing pediatric retinal work."

WANTED: FUNDS FOR CHILDREN'S EYE RESEARCH

"We started an organization for pediatric retinal research because there just isn't enough money directed toward children's retinal research. Everybody wants to help children—you hear that all the time—but government funding and everything else are a little more directed toward people who vote. The children have no voice, no advocacy. We set up a group called ROPARD, which stands for 'ROP and Related Diseases, in conjunction with the Beaumont Foundation, which funds pediatric retinal research and now raises many hundreds of thousands of dollars a year. The group started off funding projects at the level of about $15,000 per year, and now has funded several six-figure projects. It's still hard to raise money, but it's very rewarding. It has led to some of the breakthoughs we've had in pediatric retinal diseases."

FUTURE VISION

"There's exciting progress on the horizon. We're working to discover the common biochemical features to many inherited retinal diseases. We think this particular work will yield drug therapy for these diseases, and some that might be applicable to advanced diabetic disease. That's very exciting. We've also improved screening techniques using digital imaging and software programs which we will hopefully implement at Royal Oak soon. We're actually using it at Beaumont, Troy. We have incredibly good success rates for ROP care over the past decade and a half. This software program should help other places achieve similar results and provide better care for children."

FERNANDO DIAZ, M.D., PHD

Professor and Chair of Neurosurgery, Oakland University

William Beaumont School of Medicine and

Beaumont, Royal Oak

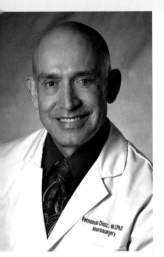

"I'm interested in putting together

a neuroscience center at Beaumont. I grew up in Mexico, came to the U.S. at 18 years of age, put myself through school by working nights and weekends, and went on for a general surgery residency and a neurosurgery residency. I have a Ph.D in neuroscience and my Master's is in business administration. I was the chair of neurosurgery at the Detroit Medical Center for fourteen years before coming to Beaumont, and I've been here three years.

"My interest is to put together a group of stars in the neurosciences who can make not only Detroit but Beaumont itself a destination for medicine in the entire United States. I see us competing with places like the Mayo Clinic, the Cleveland Clinic, University of Miami, University of California, and to get there we need the right people assembled, doing the right things. So far we've been able to recruit specialists with national and international reputations in head injuries, spine surgery, pediatric neurosurgery, and more.

"My area of interest has been stroke and aneurysms for the majority of my career. The new trend in neurosurgery to take care of these things mostly through tubes with stents and things like what the cardiologists use, so I've had to move away into what is called 'minimally invasive spine surgery,' and that is now the area I specialize in. Now we do big spine reconstructions through little openings.

"My next goal is to hire a Chief of Neurology. We don't have anybody in charge of neurology. We need to beef that up so we can put together a true neuroscience group. Currently we have a neurosurgery intensive care unit that takes care of patients with severe neurological problems. Twenty beds in the ICU are dedicated to neurosurgery. We have 65 beds on a regular floor dedicated to neurosurgery where we care for people who come out of the ICU, and eighteen of those beds and the balance are for people who are in different stages of going through the hospital and moving out. We are putting together a dedicated neuro-rehab unit within the same block of people so we can actually streamline care for the patients, simplify and optimize treatment plans so we can shorten the length of stay, and make them more comfortable and more directed toward getting better.

"We have fifteen dedicated providers who are nurse-practitioners and physician assistants (PAs). These are people who are dedicated to neurosurgery and who make the care of our patients easier and faster.

"We do approximately 2000 operations every year in neurosurgery, which is actually not very many. It's relatively middle-of-the-road in number. We're in the process of building up. We hope to build a relationship between all three Beaumont hospitals to have neurosurgery access at all three, with Royal Oak as the battleship, and services at Troy and Grosse Pointe, all integrated in a coordinated fashion so we don't duplicate services as we maximize care.

"We'll make 'boutique' areas of interest at all three hospitals, so there is something for each, and everyone will be excited, while we're also careful not to duplicate care."

A PAIN IN THE BACK

"As we all get older, the back begins to degenerate and decay, and if we take care of people the usual way, we can end up doing very large surgeries which sometimes are more harmful than the problem the patients have. Through the avenues of minimally invasive procedures, we can take care of these patients. Some of the people I care for personally have had back pain for many years and have gone from place to place and been told nothing could be done. Very often I'm able to fix their backs with relatively simple and small operations that get them back into activity. They come back smiling and very grateful because they're able to resume normal lives."

NEUROPATHY

"Neuropathy is damage to the nerves in certain parts of the body. There is a sensation of the nerve's 'falling asleep,' tingling, or a feeling of 'pins and needles.' Neuropathies are like headaches—a manifestation of many problems. It can be related to diabetes, which is one of the most common forms of neuropathy that cannot be prevented, but can be lessened with appropriate treatment of diabetes. It can also be seen with many toxins; lead can do that, arsenic, and some chemicals that are used in industry. Detoxifying agents can be used to help some people. Also being overweight can aggravate the problem, or bring on diabetes which relates to neuropathy."

THE FUTURE

"More than anything, we want to develop our state-of-the-art group and take care of neurological problems from cradle to grave. Many people have problems from childhood. We have three neurosurgeons who are pediatric-dedicated, working at Beaumont Children's Hospital, and we work with many specialists to take care of children. My idea of caring for people is to do it in 'multidisciplinary teams.' Those are groups of people from many branches of medicine who get together with a common purpose: making patients better. We do that well in pediatrics, in epilepsy surgery, very well

in cancer therapy, and with patients with spinal problems and pain. We want to expand it to include other disciplines.

"We do minimally invasive surgery through small openings, generally no bigger than an inch. Through these openings, we can remove spinal disks, remove tumors, straighten people up, or install hardware without damaging as much tissue as traditional surgery used to. We can use a camera or a microscope, or an endoscope.

"We will be able to be of great service and make great advances if we can establish the neuroscience center at Beaumont. That is the optimum goal."

HARRY N. HERKOWITZ, M.D.

Professor and Chair of Orthopaedic Surgery,
Oakland University William Beaumont School of Medicine
and Beaumont, Royal Oak

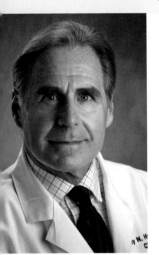

"I started here as a resident in 1974

in orthopaedic surgery, left for a year in 1979 to do a fellowship in spinal surgeries in Philadelphia, returned here in 1980 and practiced in my specialty, which since 1980 was spinal surgery, and in 1991 became Chairman of Orthopaedic Surgery. Beaumont's technological growth has dramatically changed how we practice. When I started, arthroscopy of the knee was just starting; now it's standard practice. That's just one example.

"We started with a program of ten orthopaedic surgeons, two operating rooms, two residents a year, and this dept has grown to one of the largest orthopaedic departments in the United States, and one of the busiest. We have forty-five fellowship-trained attending orthopaedic surgeons, twenty-five orthopaedic residents, and five fellows—two in spinal surgery, one in sports medicine, one in joint reconstruction, and one in pediatric surgery.

"We're also identified as one of the top orthopaedic hospitals in *U.S. News and World Report* year after year. The hospital and the department have received many awards. The orthopaedics department is respected nationally and internationally. Our joint replacement programs ranked in the top five nationally. Our spinal surgery section has an international reputation.

"We have a very active research program under the leadership of Kevin Baker, M.S. and Erin Baker, M.S., which has been developed over the past ten years, and this year at the American Academy of Orthopaedic Surgery we had the largest number of presentations in our department in history. We started with no research and evolved into a world-class research program. We have an outpatient center called the Beaumont Orthopaedic Center, which is located in the Medical Office Building, that functions as a full private office and provides training for residents and fellows for outpatient experience.

It's run by Mary Bass, the administrator there, and has a very dedicated staff. Orthopaedics has grown from a very tiny service to a very prominent service at Beaumont and has a national reputation.

"We have a very active sports medicine program here, with six fellowship-trained sports medicine doctors who provide comprehensive sports care, not only to high-performance professional athletes, but to weekend athletes and aging athletes who want to function as they did in their younger years.

"As years have gone by, the trend is that people are aging, but slower than in the past. They're more active into their later years. They don't accept limitations. We see this not only in sports, but in joint-replacement, spinal surgery, and other areas. Things that we may not have recommended ten years ago are now being done routinely for our aging population. For instance, hip and knee replacements. People in their late 80's for whom we would not have recommended joint-replacement are now getting those surgeries routinely because people in that age group are still very active and demand to be functionally active. Spinal reconstruction is being done for older-aged people whom twenty years ago I would've said was too much for them at that stage in their lives. I must also acknowledge our orthopaedic oncology service, the busiest in the state under the direction of Kim Les, M.D. Our level 1 trauma service provides state of the art care to our injured patients. We are one of the first hospitals in the tri-state area to do ankle replacement, under the direction of Paul Fortin, M.D. and Allen Grant, M.D."

I WANT TO HOLD YOUR HAND. AND YOUR DISKS

"There are many advancements in terms of hand surgery and restoring function. There are procedures to improve function and strength, mobility in the hand. There are agents that can be injected to try to restore cartilage, and these are being evaluated. We're moving toward having cartilage restoration, and also have regeneration of disks in the spine. We're involved in research here to produce a cell response that brings back degenerated disks to more normal disks. It changes the physiology to regenerate what the disk was when it was healthy. The research is fairly basic right now, but the future is bright. "

GO OUT AND LIFT SOMETHING

"Orthopaedics is the single most important specialty in terms of improving function for people as they age, for keeping flexibility, mobility, strength, and keeping joints going. In terms of prevention, we have always recommended that people should exercise regularly, eat a reasonable diet, maintain reasonable body weight, not smoke, and do the sensible things that lengthen quality of life. There's really nothing from the perspective of prevention that's fancier or more effective. It's much easier to take care of joints that have been maintained well than it is to restore function that has been compromised. If people follow the basics, they will maintain their joints in much better condition.

"Weight-lifting or resistance exercise will slow down the aging process in the bones. As we age, we lose our bone minerals. Weight-bearing exercise is important for bone strength and will slow down the natural process of bone loss."

BEAUMONT: A FAMILY BUSINESS

"People who work at Beaumont are wonderful. We have outstanding physicians here, but we also have to attribute much of our success to the nurses and the ancillary people who work here. Having been here a long time, I've seen second and third generations of families that work here. We're almost like a family, getting to know people on a first-name basis and having that family feeling that comes from being here a long time. The pride they take in doing a good job is unique in many ways. I've visited a lot of institutions in the country, and I don't often get the feeling I get here at Beaumont. One of the great things about this hospital is the people's pride and caring attitude. Nurses, nursing aides, secretaries, physician assistants, custodial people—everybody is always smiling and trying to improve. The community has grown up with Beaumont and they look at Beaumont as a second home."

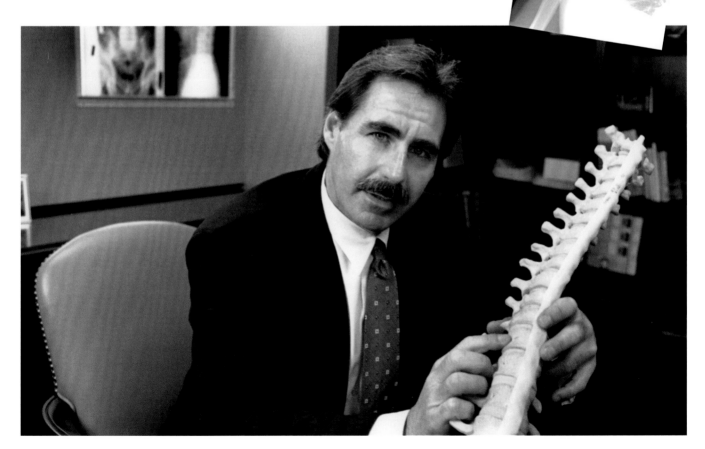

ROBERT WELSH, M.D.

Associate Professor of Surgery, Oakland University
 William Beaumont School of Medicine
Chief of Division of Thoracic Surgery
Vice-Chief of Surgical Services for Patient Safety,
 Quality and Outcomes
Beaumont, Royal Oak

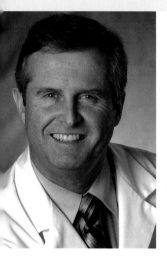

"My father, Gary Welsh, M.D., became

associated with this hospital back in the mid-1960's. He was recruited to Beaumont to do thoracic surgery and also to provide critical care, because they didn't have a critical care presence here at the time. Beaumont was only about ten years old. So he developed the Intensive Care Units here.

"He went on to wear quite a few hats here—a vice-chief of staff, director of medical education—and as I grew up in the area, I certainly was around Beaumont Hospital.

"During high school, I worked with a number of the surgeons at an animal research lab at the then-Pontiac State Hospital, where they were perfecting surgical techniques. I had good exposure to some of the senior surgeons at that time, when I was only sixteen or seventeen years old.

"I decided to pursue surgery and was really impressed with the program right here at Beaumont. One of the main reasons, which permeates the surgery department, was that they were here to train an individual, not to break him down and try to rebuild him. That's the way a lot of surgical programs were—they really destroyed you first, then tried to build you into what they wanted you to be. The difference at Beaumont was that they said, 'We can train you well, we'll give you a lot of clinical exposure, but we won't browbeat you while you're here. We'll be more nurturing.'

THE HEART (AND LUNG) OF IT ALL

"Cardio-thoracic surgery is surgery of all the organs in the chest as well as the chest wall. Heart, lungs, esophagus, rib cage, the middle part of the chest. At Beaumont, probably fostered by my father, it has been separated into cardiac surgery and general thoracic surgery. Doctors who do cardiac surgery will

do the heart and all the great vessels leading up to it, but they wouldn't do lung or esophageal surgery, and vice verse. We've kept it that way, allowing the doctors to become very specialized and expert in care of those patients.

HARD TO SWALLOW

"The feature we developed was esophageal surgery, which previously had been referred out. There was a very strong presence at the University of Michigan. With my training and emphasis in general thoracic surgery, which had a lot to do with esophageal surgery, I was able to demonstrate an expertise and as a result kept some of that work here. We treat cancers of the esophagus, benign motility of the esophagus, which is the esophagus failing to propel food in the way it's supposed to, and various other dismotilities of the esophagus. Sometimes the muscles or the nerve signals to the muscles don't work properly, so there are diseases such as achalasia, nutcracker esophagus, diffuse esophageal spasm, and others for which we might use surgery.

"We treat anti-reflux disease and hiatal hernias, and have come to emphasize minimally invasive approaches to these diseases. Through the '90's, we did most of our surgeries in an open fashion, until about seven years ago when Dr. Gary Chmielewski pioneered doing some minimally invasive lung resection at Beaumont, and I jumped on board with that. For lungs, we go in between the ribs with about a two-inch incision and take lobes out, as opposed to the nine-inch incisions of the past. In the mean time, I started doing some minimally invasive esophageal work, laparoscopic esophageal surgery, and we carried that on so that now we do almost every esophageal surgery laparoscopically, from anti-reflux to taking out cancers of the esophagus, and we do the same thing with cancer of the lung. We're still an unusual entity in that probably less than 15% to 20% of lobe-ectomies in the United States are done minimally invasively. When we started it was probably less than 10%, and esophagectomies are probably 3 to 5% minimally invasively, and we do that here also. When we remove the esophagus, we usually bring the stomach up in the chest."

THE KEYSTONE ICU PROJECT

"One of the major points in my career was to get involved with the Keystone ICU Project back in 2004. That project was promoted by Johns-Hopkins and also the Michigan Hospital and Health Care Association. They recruited almost all the hospitals in Michigan to collaborate and specifically work on using central-access catheters and bloodstream infections. We all agreed we would pursue certain basic, simple techniques in the insertion and care of those catheters. The result was a significant reduction in bloodstream infections, which is a huge consequence to patients.

"Because it was so successful, that collaboration has gone nation-wide and actually world-wide now. People will refer to the Michigan Keystone Project. I ended up being the physician-champion for Beaumont Hospital and the critical care units. It got me more involved in patient safety and quality, ultimately leading me to a patient safety fellowship, which I completed in 2007 or '08. As a result of that, I was given the position of Vice-President of Surgical Services. That centered my career around ensuring that the patients receive the care they should receive while not exposing them to potential harms, and while mitigating errors. We aggressively work to reduce the consequences the patient experiences from mistakes, while providing the highest quality of care the patient can receive."

BEAUMONT DOCTORS

"What makes 'a Beaumont doctor'? Safe care at the highest quality are things you hope your physician will aspire to achieve. You hope the physician will be an advocate for the patient on that path, to guide the patient to the best possible care in the most compassionate fashion. I've been involved in a variety of projects in the hospital, and one of the mottoes I've started to espouse is that we should care both *for* and *about* our patients. Unfortunately there are doctors around who only care for and

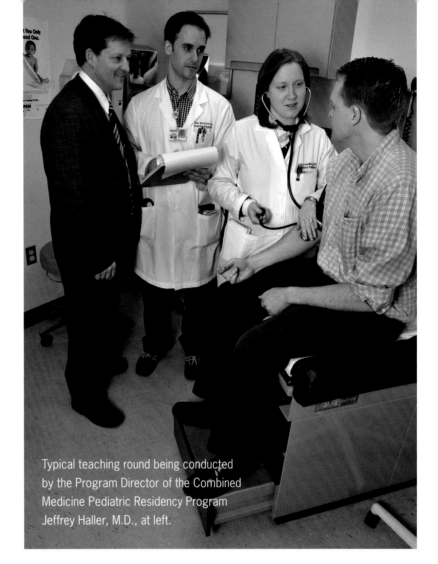

Typical teaching round being conducted by the Program Director of the Combined Medicine Pediatric Residency Program Jeffrey Haller, M.D., at left.

not *about*—every barrel has different kinds of apples in it. But this is what we hope is what being 'a Beaumont doctor' means. It's someone who recognizes his dedication to the patient. Being a Beaumont doctor means being inconvenienced. If you can't be inconvenienced, you shouldn't be here. I know that not every doctor holds those values, but I hope that Beaumont doctors hold them.

"As you become a Beaumont doctor, you begin gradually to reflect on what makes us special. Most of the doctors in the community here have gone to the same medical schools that we did, so why are we different? When you arrive here, the senior group of physicians leads you to understand the community within which we practice. We've had some great ones here in the surgical community . . . Dr. Arcari, Dr. Lucas, my father, and other surgeons who led us to understand what we should be providing. I think we hold ourselves to a certain standard. Guided by the senior doctors, young physicians begin to aspire to that standard."

The Other "C" Word: Cancer

The Walter and Marilyn Wolpin Comprehensive Breast Care Center is directed by Nayana Dekhne, M.D., a well-respected Beaumont breast surgeon. Beaumont Hospitals performs over 65,000 mammograms per year and treat nearly 1,000 new breast cancer patients each year.

FRANK VICINI, M.D.

Professor of Radiation Oncology and Internal Medicine,
Oakland University William Beaumont School of Medicine
Corporate Chief of Oncology Services, Beaumont Hospitals

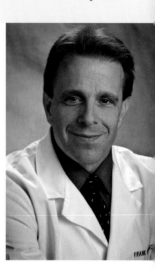

"Beaumont is an amazing place.

I don't know where to begin. During my third year of medical school (when you have to explore the type of medicine you want to practice) is when I stumbled upon radiation oncology. I applied to Beaumont's radiation oncology program, which at the time was a small community hospital program, not well known and nothing like what it is today. This was around 1984 about the same time Dr. Alvaro Martinez came here. I was part of the new group that Martinez brought in and one of the first residents to graduate through the new program. We went from a relatively unknown residency program to one of the top, if not the top, in the nation.

"We decided to make our program a premier academic center and expand the residency and fellowship training programs. Dr. Martinez and I also expanded the research base for radiation oncology. Twenty years later, we're known throughout the world.

"Dr. Martinez focused on research and education and brought in some key individuals; we hired the right physics personnel around 1992. We brought in all the key leaders early on, while they were just starting their careers. Alvaro has a knack for finding 'diamonds in the rough.'

"Beaumont gave him the support he needed to bring in the right people for physics—one of them is now the head of physics in Toronto, another at Thomas Jefferson University, and the third is the head of physics at Johns Hopkins—they are now at the premier academic programs in the nation. Remarkably they were all at Beaumont at the same time. They put together a research program that became one of the top in the nation and developed cutting-edge techniques to treat cancer with radiation that we still use today, like placing a CT

scanner on the linear accelerator. Alvaro tells that great story where he and one of the physicists had gone to a meeting at the Ritz-Carlton in Dearborn and accidentally walked into the wrong room where engineers were talking about finding cracks in engine blocks. There was an automobile engine hanging in the front of the room, rotating. Alvaro saw it and got the idea of rotating a CT scanner around a patient for targeting purposes. That single day really changed how things were performed in our specialty, and ultimately provided the funding to do more research which just keeps building on itself even today.

"We expanded into different areas—breast cancer, prostate cancer—these things grow like snowballs. You bring in the right people, they keep writing and producing and publishing—now I'm the principle investigator on a national trial for breast cancer . . . it's one of those nice things, all built on an initial vision and has been a tremendous success story. Clinical expertise, research experience, and an educational focus—we're proud of what we've done. I've been head of Oncology for seven years now. I've tried to take some of what we did in radiation oncology and translate it into the other areas of oncology.

"In 2003, Dr. Ron Irwin, who was the predecessor to Dr. Diokno as CMO, was the Corporate Chief of Oncology Services. He was a musculoskeletal oncology surgeon. We were sitting in the cafeteria and out of the blue he said, 'Do you want to be the Chief of Oncology?'

"I laughed and said, 'Oh, sure. When do I start?'

"But he was serious. A day later, I went back and said, 'You know, you have to validate this position. You can't just anoint somebody to do it.'

"He said, 'Well, that's how I'm doing it. You have

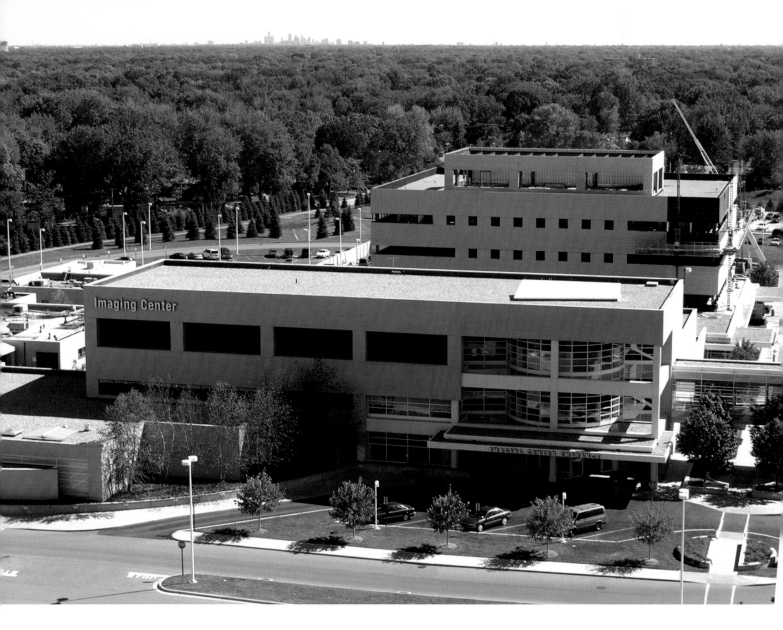

Imaging Center

The Imaging Center is the brain child of Jalil Farah, M.D., former Chair of the Department of Radiology. It houses the Breast Imaging Center under the leadership of Murray Rebner, M.D., a national leader in his field.

24 hours to decide.'

"It was really an old-school way of doing things. Find the person you want, and put him in place. I didn't really have any ambition to run a large cancer program, but ultimately I felt I could have a greater impact on patient care, so I took the offer."

IT'S LONELY AT THE TOP

"Suddenly I was a magnet for problems and my responsibilities tripled. We've moved up the ladder in the community with respect to our credibility as an excellent oncology program in the state. "

CCOPS AND CYCLOTRONS

"In 2002 we became a 'CCOP'—a Community Clinical Oncology Program. It's a grant that one gets from the National Cancer Institute to help

perform cancer clinical trials. Our goal, now that we're starting a medical school, is to move up in terms of our NCI cancer center designation. We want to become a 'Cancer Center.' It's actually a defined term. It says you're up there with the premier programs.

"All the components of a major cancer center are coming together. Since we're experts in radiation oncology, one of the newer technologies available is the use of Protons, a very expensive technology to treat cancers. The radiation beam is generated from a cyclotron. There are only five centers in the nation that have this. We spent about a year and a half studying protons and wanted to bring them to Beaumont since we were true experts in physics and that's what is needed to make them successful. Unfortunately, it's very expensive. To put together a center would cost about $160 million dollars.

"We think of individual types of cancers, like lung cancer, as a disease entity for which we're providing coordinated care, and even going 'upstream' into the areas of cancer prevention, genetics, and screening."

THE YOUNGEST SURVIVOR OF THE WRECK OF THE ANDREA DORIA

"I was in the womb in 1956. My parents had come to America to escape poverty after the WWII. My mother had gone back to San Marino to visit her mother. San Marino is the oldest free republic in the world, seated in the Appenine Mountains, completely surrounded by Italy. It's the oldest sovereign state in the world, founded in the year 301, and has the oldest constitution still in effect, and that makes it the world's oldest constitutional republic.

"My mother was on her way back to the United States, and was six months pregnant with me, sailing on an Italian liner called the *S. S. Andrea Doria*. She had my older sister with her, who was three years old. The ship was tooling along in the fog close to Nantucket Island when—*boom*. We collided with another ship, the *Stockholm*, whose icebreaker prow slammed right into the starboard side of the Andrea Doria.

"Within thirty minutes, the order came to abandon ship. My mother was terrified, of course, my sister just wandering around, everybody going crazy. Well, a gentleman came along and helped get my sister and my mother into the life boat.

"They never saw that man again. My father had taken a train to New York and when he got to the pier somebody asked him where he was going. He said he was going to meet the *Andrea Doria*, and was told it sank with no survivors. So there he was, wandering around the dock, stunned.

"Last year was the 50th anniversary of the sinking of the *Andrea Doria*. On Long Island, there was a reunion for the survivors. I dragged my 85-year-old mom and my sister out there, along with my own kids. There were presentations during the day, and an evening banquet. It was Sunday night, my mother didn't want to go, the kids were getting impatient—well, there was assigned seating at tables with other people, and finally we sat down next to an older couple. I started talking to the man next to me. He asked me whether I was a survivor, and I said, 'Kind of . . . my mother was pregnant with me. She was there with my sister . . . '

"He asked, 'Was your sister three years old at the time? I helped get a little girl and her mom into a boat.'

"I said, 'I think you saved my life!'

"There were a couple hundred people at the banquet, so it was a wild stroke of luck. What are the odds that he would still be alive? What are the odds that he would even come to the reunion? What are the odds that he would be sitting next to me? It was unreal!

"He had never talked about that in all these years. His wife was there, and even she didn't know about it. They had gotten married that year the ship sank.

"It was fascinating to talk to Frank. He felt bad because my mom and my sister were the only ones who didn't have life jackets. The ship was listing over at a very steep angle. He left his own mother, scrambled up this tilted deck and back into the ship to find life jackets for my mom and sister. As he's leaving, the water started coming in. He barely got out himself.

"It's an amazing story . . . and that's why I'm 'Frank Andrea Vicini.'"

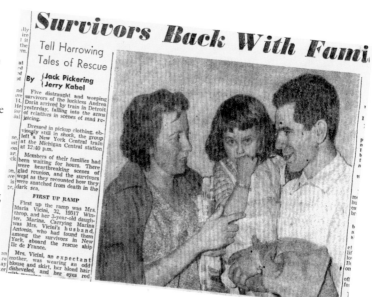

RONALD IRWIN, M.D.
Chief Medical Officer, Beaumont Hospitals,
2002–2006

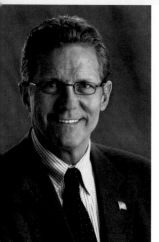

"Orthopaedic oncology is the treatment

of tumors of the musculoskeletal system. I deal with sarcomas rather than carcinomas, which involve organs like breast, prostate, GI tract, etc. I take care of childhood and adult sarcomas and I take care of all the metastatic disease, which is organ cancers that go to bone, and most of them do. Every one of those have a certain percentage of metastasizing, usually to the lungs or liver, and that is what kills them—the lung or liver disease, not the bone cancer.

"When I started doing this thirty years ago, osteosarcoma victims had a 20% chance of surviving, so 80% died, and now it's almost the other way around. Less than 1% of all cancers are in the bone, and less than 1% of all cancers are sarcomas. There are about 2000 osteo-sarcomas in the United States every year, and about 6000 soft tissue sarcomas.

"I was born in Detroit, went to the University of Michigan for undergrad and med school, planning to be an obstetrician. I hadn't even heard of Beaumont until my mother-in-law told me about it. I found it was very nice and I matched with Beaumont, which means the medical student picks the hospital and the hospitals do the same, and if the choices match, the student goes there. There were plenty of people telling me I was crazy to go to a community hospital instead of a university.

"I had orthopaedics during the second to last month of my rotating internship, and I loved it. I also fell in love with oncology, and with pathology, looking at X-rays of tumors and what they look like on slides, and thought it was fascinating. I took care of some cancer patients and I loved the way cancer patients are. They smell the flowers better, they notice things better because they have limited time.

"My chief, Dr. Stanko Stanisavljevic, did as much to advance Beaumont's image as anyone. He came from Yugoslavia and practiced at Henry Ford Hospital. He became an international expert in dysplasia of the hip in infants. He came to Beaumont with an idea to start a residency in orthopaedics and everybody thought he was crazy, but he started it in 1972. He did all the teaching initially, and built a tremendous program for about twenty years. It was the first private-practice orthopaedic residency in the country, and I took heat for taking my orthopaedic training at Beaumont instead of Wayne State or Michigan or somewhere else, but I had a sense it would be good. I went away for two years in the Navy and while I was gone the program matured. Stanko let me go to the Mayo Clinic my senior year of residency and I became the first orthopaedic oncology fellow there for the last six months of my five-year training program. At Mayo I learned to do big horrendous amputations—hind-quarter amputations, fore-quarter amputations—but the most important thing I learned was how to talk to people with cancer.

"When I came back, Stanko said, 'I want you to just do tumors.' I protested, but he was right. I had just spent 5 years learning how to 'do' all orthopaedics from fractures to surgery—and tumors are a very small piece, but you don't establish a reputation as the go-to doctor by doing everything. Ten years later I went to Harvard to learn how to do the fancy things we had started doing in those ten years, like limb salvage—saving limbs with cancer instead of cutting them off, or taking the pelvis out without losing the leg.

"I came back and changed my shingle to musculoskeletal tumor surgery *only*. Again, everybody thought I was crazy. I said no to all the carpal-tunnels, bunions, and other surgeries, and aimed at the people who were going to Mayo or Cleveland Clinic. I went all over the state doing talks on what we could do at Beaumont and doctors started sending their bone tumor patients to me. Eventually it worked out, and Beaumont ended up being the place to go for bone tumors, taking care of about 30% of the musculoskeletal in the state. After about ten years they finally hired a few people to do this at Ford and U of M, and I took on a partner.

"While this was going on, I was evolving toward medical administration and was very interested in that. I was elected president of the medical staff in 1990 and was re-elected four times for two-year terms. They asked me to head the cancer

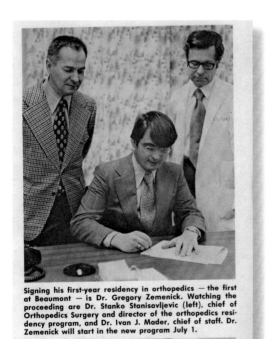

Signing his first-year residency in orthopedics — the first at Beaumont — is Dr. Gregory Zemenick. Watching the proceeding are Dr. Stanko Stanisavljevic (left), chief of Orthopedics Surgery and director of the orthopedics residency program, and Dr. Ivan J. Mader, chief of staff. Dr. Zemenick will start in the new program July 1.

program, and that's when I became an employee of the hospital, as Associate Medical Director and Corporate Director of Oncology Programs in 1998. We had two hospitals, Royal Oak and Troy, each with a cancer program with different reports, running independently; I replaced them into an Oncology Integrated Network and started a Clinical Trials program through a CCOP. I ended up replacing Dr. Robert Reid as the Chief Medical Officer in 2002, and I was only 56 at the time. Things were getting complicated as Beaumont turned from a hospital into a big corporation. I hated the constant meetings and could never get over being more of a surgeon than an administrator. Ultimately I went back to my first loves: teaching and patient care."

"I stepped down as CMO in 2006, but didn't like what had become of my practice. Things weren't as I'd left them. McLaren Health System recruited me to become Director of Orthopaedic Oncology and I became Associate Director, Great Lakes Cancer Instititue in 2007, so I teach throughout the McLaren Health system, seven hospitals, and see patients and do my surgery at Mt.Clemens Regional Medical Center.

"I was at Beaumont from 1971 to 2007, except for two years in the Navy and two fellowships. The orthopaedic program has taken off. Dr. Harry Herkowitz took over for Dr. Stanko and has done a magnificent job building that program".

GARY CHMIELEWSKI, M.D.

Associate Professor of Surgery, Oakland University William
Beaumont School of Medicine

Principal Investigator, The Cancer Community Oncology
Program (CCOP), Beaumont Hospitals

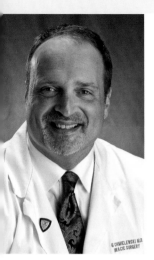

"I'm a thoracic surgeon, and about

85% of my practice is cancer-related. We also do non-cancer surgeries like reflux disease, hernia repairs, collapsed lung treatments for benign diseases, but if you're in thoracic surgery, most of your work will be oncology-related. I wouldn't consider myself a super-star, but I'm certainly in a place that promotes its doctors' interests.

"We're a four-man group in our thoracic surgery practice. We do minimally invasive surgery, and probably do things that hardly anybody else in the area is doing. It's almost unheard of to have a four-man thoracic group in a university setting. Beaumont has always supported us with promoting our robotic surgery, minimally invasive lobectomies and esophagectomies, so it's been the kind of environment where we're helped to do whatever we think is right for our patients.

"I've developed a research interest fairly late in my career, which is unusual. I'm 48 and usually if you're going to be a researcher and an academic, you do it earlier. Beaumont has been great for nourishing this interest. I have an interest in Barrett's esophagus, which is a pre-cancerous condition of the esophagus, and there's a new procedure called radio frequency ablation, which can get rid of the Barrett's tissue so the cancer risk is lessened and we can head off esophageal cancer before it develops. Two years ago I took training in radio frequency ablation and when I got back here, I thought, 'I can do this myself,' or 'I can develop a program here at Beaumont and do this in a multi-disciplinary fashion.'"

"I wrote out my plan to involve gastroenterologists, a dedicated pathologist, the Cancer Clinical Trials Office, the Biobank, and molecular biologists at local universities. Beaumont supported me. When I was trying to get started, Tom Brisse, the hospital administrator at Troy, said, 'If you can't get funding, let me know and I'll pay for the equipment out of my personal stipend.' That's the kind of place this is. Tom saw that this was going to be a great thing for patients, and started me on the path. Now we have the only program in Michigan for this which is a multi-disciplinary program. It has been very successful.

"Along those lines, I went to Dr. David Decker, who is one of the oncologists who started the Cancer Clinical Trials Office (CCTO) and was the principal investigator for our Cancer Community Oncology Program (CCOP). He single-handedly put this program together. Because of it, we have a stronger cancer program and bring clinical trials from the national scene to the local area. About ten years ago, I went to Dave and said, 'I want to join the American College of Surgeons Oncology Group.' It's a research group that brings clinical trials to patients, but I didn't know how to join because I didn't know what I needed. Dave said, 'Imagine that! A surgeon who wants to do research!'

"Dave provided the nursing support, guidance, and everything I needed. Since then I've been very active in ACSOG, and because of that I'm the only thoracic surgeon in private practice who is on the ACSOG Thoracic Committee. All the others are heads of university programs. My practice and the thoracic program at Beaumont have benefited because of this.

"We just received our five-year grant renewal of $4.8 million."

"So once again I was in a system that supported me in trying to be better. I'm now the Principle Investigator for the CCOP. It's a great opportunity to improve the scope of our oncology services to the community."

CCOP

"The Cancer Community Oncology Program is a fabulous mechanism, started in 1983 by the National Cancer Institute. They saw a lot of research going on, but it wasn't getting down to the rank and file of physicians and their patients. This is a way that the government-facilitated research and clinical trials with busy community doctors so new cancer treatments and preventative measures get down to patients all over the country. Right now there are 50 Community Clinical Oncology Programs, and Beaumont's is one of the most active. We just received our five-year grant renewal of $4.8 million.

"Our participation in the CCOP process benefits the patients because they get exposed to new treatments. It benefits the hospital and the physicians. There's a dialogue going between myself and the oncologists, in e-mail, reading, talking to other clinicians at the national meetings, about what's happening in cancer care. It keeps us thinking about always improving, doing things better for our patients.

"This is a huge opportunity for the hospitals' oncology program and a humbling experience to be able to lead this. I have a lot of help, with Joyce Nancarrow-Tull, RN, our administrator working with 27 Clinical Research Associates to care for patients and guard the integrity of the data and promote patient safety in clinical trials. The Beaumong CCOP makes our cancer program much stronger."

MY FIRST LOVE

"I did five years of general surgery, then went into cardiac thoracic, which is three more years of training. Over those three years, you're trained in general thoracic surgery, adult cardiac surgery, and pediatric heart surgery. Everybody who goes through that wants to be a pediatric heart surgeon. There's an old saying—'If you're a surgeon, you think you're a god. If you're a pediatric heart surgeon, you *are* a god.'

"I have the common sense to know that we already have more pediatric heart surgeons in the world than jobs available for them. After six months of wanting to be a pediatric heart surgeon, I made the decision early on to switch to general thoracic surgery, because it was what initially attracted me to the specialty. So I decided to specialize in general thoracic before it was the 'cool' thing to do. I'm glad I made that decision. I love what I do and I'm excited about the surgery and research end of things. I work with three great thoracic surgeons—Drs. Robert Welsh, Sang Kim, and Michael Coello. Collectively we're doing things that very few centers in the country are doing right now. I look forward to working with my partners and Beaumont to make our practice a premier thoracic program."

PREM KHILANANI, M.D.

Professor, Department of Medicine, Oakland University William
    Beaumont School of Medicine
Chief, Division of Hematology and Oncology, Beaumont, Troy

"I wanted Beaumont to be a shining light."

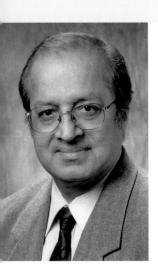

"I went to medical school in India,

hoping to come to the U.S. for higher education. I came to America, planning to go into cardiology. But soon I got a call from India telling me my sister was ill. I hurried back to Bombay and was told my sister was in the operating room. The surgeon invited me to scrub in, and showed me that my sister's abdomen was peppered with cancer. My head reeled. How could this happen? As I prepared to tell my mother and father, I decided to go into oncology.

"That's the way I started—not as a career, but as a mission. I would establish a cancer center at Beaumont, Troy. Which I did.

"I have been the Chairman of Hematology and Oncology at Beaumont, Troy since its inception in 1977. I was invited to start the cancer program. At that time, Troy was a small community hospital in the boondocks.

"Determined that Troy would succeed, we assured doctors that we could take care of patients. We established a good surgical department and also started giving chemotherapy. In the course of time, I convinced the hospital that we needed radiation oncology and radiation therapy. I showed them the statistics. There were many patients we could treat who were instead going to surrounding hospitals. We needed specialized breast cancer surgeons, colo-rectal surgeons, urologists dealing with the prostate, thoracic surgeons for lung cancer, head and neck surgeons—we needed to treat all these specialized cancers.

"Once we established the radiation oncology, we then had a multi-disciplinary approach to cancer. We have started a one-stop approach. We gather a patient and his family to sit with a pathologist, a radiologist, radiation oncologist, a surgeon; the patient and his family can hear the options, ask questions, give their opinions and be involved."

THE TUMOR REGISTRY

"We started the Tumor Registry. This is a documentation of all the cancer patients, divided into sub-types, and we follow it five, ten, fifteen years, documenting the treatments—radiation, surgery, chemotherapy. Then we can also compare with national statistics, and whether we are following established guidelines that become standard."

MAJOR BREAKTHROUGHS

"The major breakthroughs have been in early detection. With mammography, we can pick up cancer that is as small as an onion seed. If we were to examine a patient by hand, we could never detect something that small, but with mammography, MRI, ultrasound, we can. Under ultrasound-guided treatment, we can insert a needle and hit the little spot. Whatever comes out with the needle, we can analyze. It's called 'ultrasound-guided biopsy.' When we pick up a cancer that early, then treat it with a multidisciplinary approach—the earlier we detect, the more we get cured patients."

"I wouldn't give you the idea that everybody will be cured. There are still brain cancer, pancreatic cancer, melanoma, and others that are resistant and can be devastating. But there is great advancement in prevention and early detection. If you get your

CARL LAUTER, M.D. ON CANCER
AND INFECTIOUS DISEASE

"On the clinical level, the relationship between infectious disease and cancer patients is that cancer patients have such a low defense against infection. On a research level, there's much more to it. We're studying mechanisms of how people get cancer, and some of those that have to do with cancer development also have to do with infection. There are certain germs that will lead to cancer.

"For instance, one of the leading causes of liver cancer in Asia used to be Hepatitis B—a virus infection of the liver. With the introduction of the Hepatitis B vaccine, Hepatitis B has been nearly eliminated in places like Hong Kong and other parts of Asia, and as a result, liver cancer rates have plunged. That's a good example of prevention—an infection has prevented cancer.

"A case in the United States which is on the news all the time is the human papilloma virus. It's responsible for 98% of cervical cancer in women. It's a viral infection that is sexually transmitted. We now have an HPV vaccine which should be 90% effective in preventing cervical cancer if we can get the parents to vaccinate all their boys and girls. Boys can't get it, but they can transmit the germ. The germ goes back and forth.

"And there are other examples, but those are the two most well-known."

colonoscopy in a timely fashion, you don't get colon cancer. If you do get it, we have surgery, chemotherapy, and good radiation.

"For breast cancer, we are developing genetic testing for predisposition, so we can watch the patient and the daughters for certain abnormalities. In the management of lymphomas, we can give the patient systemic chemotherapy and get him into remission. If the patient needs a transplant, we can give a transplant. Every patient is a movie for me. The ups and downs . . . every patient's life."

THE MARROW BANK

"In the case of lymphoma leukemia, we need a bone marrow donor. If we don't have one, we have to search the Marrow Bank. With one patient, we did a world-wide search and found a donor in Paris. The patient's family was taking up a collection to get $40,000 to fly the donor from Paris and set him up in a hotel. Then somebody had a better idea. We scheduled the patient's marrow transplantation for Monday morning, and on Sunday evening marrow was taken from the donor in Paris. It was frozen and flown overnight to the transplantation unit. This is possible because of the world-wide Marrow Bank.

"One patient was a policeman, 25 years old, married, two beautiful daughters. He came to the ER for a flu, and his blood counts were low. It turned out to be acute leukemia. I treated him with chemotherapy to wipe out the old bone marrow. He went into remission and needed a marrow transplant. This kind of patient has to be in the hospital round

the clock. The police department said they would have to let him go because they couldn't continue to pay a policeman who was not on the job. I approached the Police Chief and said, 'This is a young man. Give us a chance to cure him. Let us give him the transplant.'

" While I was talking to the Chief, the other policemen overheard. They had a meeting and told the Chief, 'Don't give us vacation time. Pool it, and whatever is needed in time off, give it to him.'

"That's what they did. Luckily, his sister was a match for marrow, and now he's back to work. Whenever I check, his marrow is normal. But he has an XY gene. So I tease him that he is a girl now."

CANCER AND PREGNANCY

"There are more problems with ladies who become pregnant while on chemotherapy, or who are pregnant and then develop cancer. The treatment has to be a compromise. For a non-pregnant woman with breast cancer, ideally we do a CT-scan, but we can't do that with a pregnant lady, nor can we do radiation. But a biopsy can be done. We have learned that we should avoid chemotherapy in the first trimester. It's dangerous. The third trimester is safe, the second—if absolutely necessary.

"It's a sad situation for everybody—mom, dad, and the doctor. You worry day and night. Am I doing the right thing? I hope I'm not doing damage to the baby . . . if I cut down treatment to protect the baby, am I harming the mother? How does a doctor sleep? Every day is a story."

ALVARO MARTINEZ, M.D.

Professor and Chair of Radiation Oncology, Oakland
University William Beaumont School of Medicine and
Beaumont Hospitals

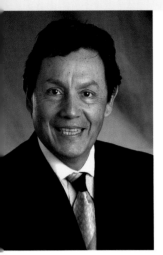

"The concept of adaptive oncology

is the following—the CT, the MRI are diagnostic tools originally designed to diagnose cardio-vascular diseases or orthopaedic problems, but not for cancer diagnosis. The concept of the adaptive oncology image center is to take these tools that were not specifically designed for oncological diagnosis, for intra-treatment evaluation, and for post-treatment assessment in the follow-up of effectiveness, or the ability to diagnose an early recurrence, when it's likely we can still give the patient a second chance.

"So we're purchasing these tools, meaning the PET/CT, the Three-T MRI (Three-Testlar, the unit of very high frequency). The concept is that we get these machines and modify them by removing what is not important for oncology, and enhance what is important. It's similar to adjusting a metal detector to detect only gold, or some other specific metal, and ignore others. Eventually every oncology unit in the world will be purchasing an 'oncology suite,' with a collection of machines specifically adjusted to detect certain kinds of cancers.

"What happens today to patients is that they have to go to one facility to have PET/CT, go to another facility for MR (MRI), and another facility for other treatment, and so on. We are designing an oncology suite, so the patient can go to just one facility and get everything he needs. It's a tremendous convenience to the patient, but in addition to that, the suite will give a specific diagnosis for a specific oncology problem. It will work for all the cancers, but it is only for oncology. For brain cancer, and head and neck cancer, the Three-T MR is an ideal tool. For cancer of the cervix or the lung, the PET/CT is ideal. They're different tools because there are different kinds of cancers and we need to look for different things biologically.

Now we're going to have an imaging center with tools that are specifically designed for oncology, and have the greatest convenience for the patient."

CANCER AS A CHRONIC DISEASE

"Now, think about the cancer process as a chronic disease, like diabetes. We don't cure diabetes, but we treat diabetes. Think about most cancers as chronic diseases. We have to have some diagnostic tools to diagnose how early or now extensive the cancer is, regardless of whether it's brain cancer, breast cancer, prostate cancer, lung cancer—doesn't matter. The concept is the same. We need to know how early or late it is, because the treatment options are different. That's called staging. We need to develop a specific tool for staging of the cancer. Then we have to develop specific tools to assess or to evaluate the treatment's effectiveness. That's called intra-treatment evaluation. As we give the patient chemo, we should be able to evaluate whether the chemo is working or not. If it's not working, why should I keep treating the patient?

"Equally important, if I'm giving the treatment for eight weeks, I would like to know by week number two whether it's working. Why continue if it's not doing any good? So part of this concept is where the word 'adaptive' comes from—we will adapt the treatment to the patient's specific needs. Is he responding or not responding? Do we need to move to surgery instead of radiation, or more radiation instead of surgery? We can adapt, instead of using the same treatments for everybody. That's the whole concept of what we're trying to do that is unique—the adaptive oncology image suite.

"Nobody else has this idea in the world. This is it. But we don't have the tools to do intra-treatment

242

> "At Beaumont, we have gradually developed what I consider one of the prominent programs nationally and internationally in radiation oncology."

evaluation. We're going to need not only the pieces of equipment that I mentioned—the PET/CT, the Three-T MR—we also need the equivalent machines for the laboratory. We need a Micro-Pet and Micro-MR to use on small animals. We already have those machines in my research laboratory. Here at Beaumont in the Research Institute, I have nearly 9000 square feet of space where I have the laboratory. We also have a small animal radiator that simulates the radiator for humans, so we have the duplication of the human system in the animal system.

"There are two sources of animal cancer. One is naturally occuring tumors in animals. If you have a pet, and your pet develops cancer, the vet can tell you to come to the Beaumont center because we have a comparative oncology unit. We can practice on naturally occuring cancers, help the pet, which we find through the veterinarians.

"The other source develops in mice that are genetically engineered to develop certain cancers, or genetically mutated species that we can use to study the biology of tumors.

"These are the components of the basic research. So why do we need Micro-MR or Micro-PET? It's because we have to develop the tools on the micro level before we go into humans. That's the 'integration' of cancer research and treatment. All of these are diagnostic tools. They are not treatment tools. Once we can follow the multi-cancer cell because we have a specifically designed device to follow that cell, then we can start thinking about tracking and attacking that cells. Cancers move all the time."

THE RIBBONS ARE WORKING

"There has been wonderful progress lately. There are rallies and marches against cancer, and yet the public in general doesn't know how well the fund-raising and philanthropy are working. For instance, with breast cancer we seldom remove breasts anymore. The pink ribbons are working. And the blue ribbons, also, for prostate cancer. Radical prostatectomy, in my opinion is more mutilating than radical mastectomy because in the radical prostatectomy the patient may lose erectile function; sexual function is gone totally.

"Today, as an alternative to radical prostatectomy, we do brachytherapy. This is a Greek word, 'brachy,' which means 'a short distance.' 'Therapy' means 'treatment.' Brachytherapy is placing needles inside the prostate, then through the needles we deliver radioactive material. We take the needles out, and the radioactive pellet remains inside the prostate and cures the cancer, and the prostate remains inside the patient. He has low risk of losing erectile function and incontinence, and it is an out-patient procedure.

"We at Beaumont have been the pioneers in brachytherapy for prostate cancer. So that is good news for the prostate cancer patient."

ORGAN PRESERVATION

"The concept we're moving toward is organ preservation. Instead of removing the breast, we remove the lump, preserve and radiate the breast. Instead of removing the prostate, we do brachytherapy. We can do it once, or twice, based on the stage of the disease. If it's very early, we can do it with one. If it's advanced, we can do two or three. Cancer genetics is helping us find cancers early, because we can trace it in a family line.

'Brachytherapy is also ideal for working on children, because we don't have to do radiation from the outside, which does some damage while the children are growing. Children develop leukemias, lymphomas, tumors of the soft tissues, which is called carcoma, they develop brain tumors that are fairly aggressive."

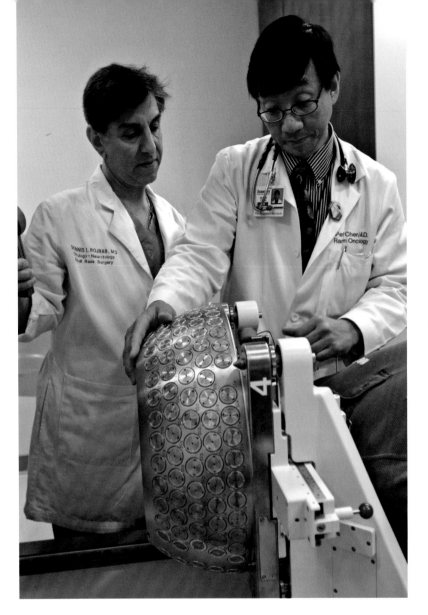

Dennis Bojrab, M.D. Otolaryngologist, and Peter Chen, M.D., Radiation Oncologist, inspecting the Gamma Knife, a highly specialized machine to treat lesions in the brain using focused beam of 203 small cobalt sources.

THE GAMMA KNIFE

"The Gamma Knife is a specialized machine to treat intracranial lesions. We can treat tumors with benign processes—for example, there is something called neuralgia of the facial nerve that produces pain, so we can treat that with the Gamma Knife and it's extremely successful. The Gamma Knife is a focused beam of 203 small cobalt sources, and they all have access to little holes and bring the radiation to a pinpoint area, where they intersect. The point is to move the tumor around until it is exactly where we need it to be. That's called stereotaxis. That's what the neurosurgeons do. Based on that coordinated system of stereotaxis, we can aim that very focused radiation beam on that small tumor in the brain, or in the nerve. It's a specifically designed tool to treat intracranial tumors, but we are limited by the size of the tumor. If it's bigger than three centimeters, we can't treat it, because we cannot give that much radiation without hurting the brain. We can get away with it if the area is detected early and is small."

THE FUTURE: TARGETED THERAPY

"We are designing tools that let us see the big gross things. Once we have that, we can enhance the tools to let us look at the microscopic level. That's what we're doing in the laboratory, but in medicine everything takes years and takes money. The ability to treat these cancers on the cellular level is probably ten years from now. We are working toward targeted therapy, which is to tag radioactive material and send it directly to the tumor, irradiating only the tumor. It is the future of chemotherapy and radiation therapy."

MIKE KILLIAN ON BREAST CANCER

"My wife comes from a family of six sisters. Their mother had breast cancer. Her three oldest sisters not only had breast cancer, but each had primary site bilateral breast cancer, some years apart. That's two episodes of breast cancer, one in each breast. There's a genetic link. There has to be.

"My wife was very vigilant about all this, and did all the mammograms and careful follow-up. She read in a magazine that breast MRI was the way to go for screening women at high risk, so she decided she wanted one. That was June a few years back.

"She got her MRI, but it was positive. They found something. She needed surgery. They call it a partial mastectomy now; it used to be called a lumpectomy. On a Thursday in July the doctor who ran our breast care center said, 'I can do it Monday.'

"By Friday, it was clear. The sentinal node was clear and no spread was found. The cancer was very early and very small. She is the poster child for early detection, for taking care of yourself and paying attention."

RADIATION and CHEMOTHERAPY

For follow up treatment, the doctors told me several things: "Radiation is most often an external beam shot at the spot of the cancer to make sure any microscopic cells with cancer that might be in there are killed.

"The other treatment is chemotherapy—exactly what it sounds: chemicals. Studies have been done on breast cancer that if the sentinal node is involved, we know the cancer has spread and that she needs systemic chemotherapy. If the sentinel node is not involved, the cancer may not have spread. If we look at the tissue and there's a margin, a clean margin all around, we presume that the cancer hasn't spread. In cases where the cancer has not spread, they do DNA tests on the cancer itself, and they're able to determine which cancers are high-risk or low-risk for recurrence. If a patient happens to have high-risk, then she gets chemotherapy. Jeff Margolis, my wife's medical oncologist, said he wouldn't have believed that she would need chemo, but this specialized test revealed that the cancer was high-risk for recurrence.

"By this time, my wife had already gotten the message that she was cured. The doctor told her there was good news and bad news. The bad news was that she needed chemotherapy. The good news was that the cancer grows in the presence of estrogen, and she could be treated with estrogen blockers. If she went through chemo, we could reduce her risk for new cancer from something like 20% down to less than 10%.

"She is on an estrogen blocker called Femora, and she had chemo and the radiation. She's cured, but she has to stay on the Femora. There's the chance she'll get another cancer, so she gets a test every six months, either a digital mammogram or an MRI. The doctors do a fabulous job. She has even had a genetic test done. The genetic oncologist, Dana Zakalik, has done a wonderful job, and we know know that my wife doesn't have the BRCA 1 or 2 gene. She does have another gene that is a lower-level risk. If a woman has the BRCA 1 or 2 gene, we were told, she's not only susceptible to breast cancer, but also to ovarian cancer. My wife and her sisters are now in the King Study out of the University of Washington in Seattle, to find out what possible groupings of genes might lead to breast cancer in a family.

"All these things fit together. I am very happy that Beaumont has a Breast Care Center, and a Genetics Program, and such good physicians."

20 THE OAKLAND UNIVERSITY WILLIAM BEAUMONT SCHOOL OF MEDICINE

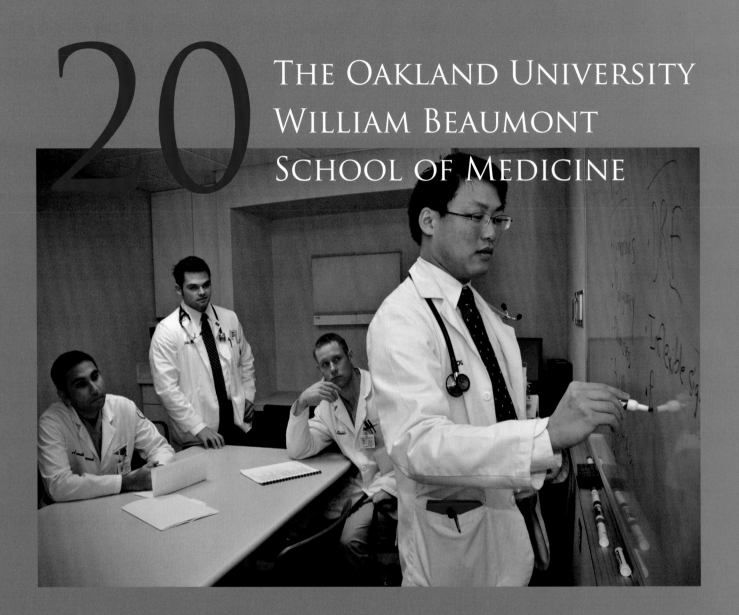

KEN MYERS ON THE MEDICAL SCHOOL

"Our long-range plan assumed that one day, as our educational programs continued to develop, we might end up with a branch of one of the great Michigan medical schools on our campus. These medical schools are excellent, but they already had their established ways of doing things. The plan of a joint venture with Oakland University may be better for Beaumont because we have the chance to start a new medical school, with everything fresh and new.

"Oakland University is a world-class university. We've had long-time affiliations with them in nursing and technical areas of research, so this is a very important piece of Beaumont's future."

ROBERT FOLBERG, M.D.

Founding Dean, Oakland University William Beaumont
School of Medicine

"What clearly sets our medical school apart

is that we provide an opportunity for students to get out of the traditional scholarship of medicine and get into something broader. Beaumont has great clinical facilities, and that's well known, but what might not be known is that, first, we have a problem of a general shortage of physicians around the country. Michigan will be short more than 4000 physicians in the next ten years if we don't do something about this. We're going to generate more physicians, but the school starts with 50 students in its charter class, and increases by 25 students per year until it plateaus at 125. If we were only about numbers, we would've projected a class size much higher than 125.

"So it's more than just about numbers for us. It's about the type of physician we're trying to generate. We should say straight out that this is not a medical school that is dedicated to a particular theme. There are medical schools which, for very good reasons, have declared that they have an emphasis on primary care. We have an outstanding school in the state, Michigan State University, that does that very well. We could have declared that we were interested in rural health care, and there are some schools in the state where that is done very well. We could have declared that we're interested in turning out medical students who are clinician-scientists or primarily scientists, where they expect the students to go into careers of research, and there are medical schools who do that very well also, and that's great.

"We envision ourselves as a school where we permit the students to identify their interests and their potentials. If a student comes in with interests and experience that clearly indicates that he would be an outstanding scientist, we'll support him or her. Some may declare that they really want to treat patients in a clinical setting. Others will come in for second careers. Some will have grown up as migrant farm workers. The school isn't 'themed.'

"The leadership of this school—myself and the associate deans—have experience in medical education collectively exceeding 170 years. We all have some background in education. Some of us are researchers, some are specialized in student affairs, curriculum, academic management, or other aspects, but almost everyone in the leadership of the school are educators. Of the founding leadership of this school, 70% are first-generation college graduates, the first college-educated people in their families. Roughly 50% of the school leadership are women.

"So our philosophy is that the school has no bias as to whom we accept or what the students individual goals may be. Certainly we're extremely inclusive. Students can come into this medical school and discover their personal interests and potentials. How can we help them? That's one challenge.

"How can we direct students to opportunities where the need is greatest? For instance, we may need 4000 physicians in the next ten years, but we may not need many more sports medicine specialists or cosmetic surgeons. There may be a great need for other specialties. We hope students will go into the areas of greatest public need. Obviously we would like to pick out the best and the brightest and encourage them to do residencies at Beaumont.

DR. FELTEN ON THE MEDICAL SCHOOL

"We can decide how we want to build our medical school. Many of the medical schools are financial black holes because they bring in all these basic scientists, come to find out that 80% of them don't want to teach, and view teaching as a disgusting requirement. They have a 'let's get this over with' attitude, and think that teaching is something you do if you can't get grants.

"We've had Beaumont faculty, even our research faculty from the Research Institute, becoming actively engaged in medical school course work and instruction, and again our administration has been very supportive. We're bringing this into existence as a medical school with an extraordinary infrastructure and a phenomenal base.

"One of the things we're seeking that I really like, Dr. Folberg's idea, supported by our administration, is that they want to foster master teachers—people who are truly the best. The reason the instruction in basic science is so good is that they have master teachers. You'll have your entire physiology course taught by maybe two people, and they're both masterfully good teachers, and they're there because they want to teach, not because they're scrambling to maintain their research grants and they spend 99% of their time in the research lab and you can only see them on their way to and from the airport for the next conference, and you'll never see them after a lecture because they're on their way to the next lab meeting. That's not a way to educate medical students.

"The way to educate medical students is to truly engage them with the faculty, just like what happens in a clinical setting. We want to bring that to the basic sciences setting."

About 60% of medical students will land within a hundred miles of the area where they do their residencies. We have an interest in continuing the tradition of the Beaumont doctor."

THE CAPSTONE COURSE

"We have the Capstone course. It runs for four years, and starts with an instructional phase. Every student has to do a project before he or she leaves. For some, that will be doing basic research, in a myriad of fields. Or it could be something different. Rather than saying, 'Do a project,' our student will spend six weeks getting formal instruction from the medical librarians who teach in the medical school. They will learn medical information literacy. They will learn how the information is organized, how to mine it, how to extract it, about conflict of interest in publishing, drug companies, and so on. They will learn an approach toward the electronic medical records not so much in terms of how to use it, because they'll get that in clinical situations, but to learn to ask questions like, 'What are the outcomes of the ways I'm practicing medicine and how does that stack up against others in my area throughout the country? What can I continue to learn about

the way I practice just from the way I do things?' All this comes to our passion about preparing. Knowledge isn't enough for physicians. There must be competency—but we expect our students to go for beyond competency—we expect them to excel."

BREAKING TRADITIONS

"The next segment of the course is fabulous, being taught and organized by one of the Beaumont physicians. It is an introduction to the clinical trial. It goes for about eight weeks. They learn how to organize a clinical trial, how to ask interesting questions and develop a trial. What are the ethics of clinical trials? What are the oversight mechanisms? They get to rotate through research labs and all this time they think about projects they might want to do.

"Here's where we break from tradition. We ask students to think about what they can do not only inside the hospital and the lab, but outside. For example, medical students could interact with mass media to get populations to change their own behaviors. Could a student run a targeted campaign about getting children vaccinated? Could a medical student get interested in health care policy, perhaps do an internship in Lansing? Could a student team up with federal legislators, maybe follow them to watch how legislation goes through Congress? Perhaps a student could assist in opening a clinic in a distressed area or for a targeted ethnic group. This is in harmony with Beaumont's mission to assist the surrounding community while advancing medicine.

"If a student selects a project that is of high scientific impact or high social impact in his or her first three years, we intend to reward the student with extra scholarship money in the fourth year. Students will be invested with the community and more likely to stay in the area.

"Students must be good communicators and be self-motivated life-long learners. How can we do that? Well, it has to be practiced. Fewer than 50% of instruction contact with faculty will occur in the lecture hall. Most of it occurs in small groups, with adequate preparation. For instance, Dr. David Felten is the Director of the Beaumont Research Institute and the Associate Dean for Research for the medical school. He is a world-class educator in the area of neurosciences and has published a textbook that's widely used in that area. David could be in a lecture area, discussing the organization of the spinal cord. Then we could have students break up into teams, and each could address a problem presented to them or different problems. The reason we break them into teams is that they need to learn how to be in a team, how to be a member of a team, how to communicate within a team, and to be present, because you just don't skip a session. You don't skip a session of rounds or in the operating room, and you don't skip a session in medical school. That's professionalism.

"Then the teams assemble as larger teams, and they begin to teach each other. That's what doctors do.

"A course called the Art and Practice of Medicine will couple with a course called Medical Humanities and Bio-Ethics. Students will begin to think about things that they need to know other than procedures. There are focus groups coming in from the community, teaching us about sensitivities students need in order to become competent

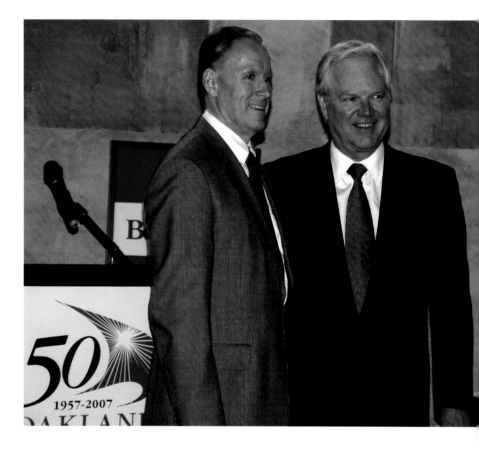

physicians. How do we deal with different social groups? How do we deal with the visually impaired? The hearing impaired? People from other cultures?

"We also have a course called the Promotion and Maintenance of Health, talking about how physicians can promote the health of the communities they serve, not necessarily just treating disease. It really is powerful.

"The curriculum is structured in such a way that we focus on the quality of the education. This school is also set apart because we don't have multiple basic science departments. You won't find a department of anatomy or cell biology, a department of pharmacology, departments of physiology, physiology, micro-biology, as you do in many established schools. Increasingly the National Institute of Health wants research done in what they call trans-disciplinary mode. So we have developed a basic science department that recruits scientists into programs rather than departments."

President Gary Russi of Oakland University and CEO Ken Matzick of Beaumont Hospitals during the announcement of the new Oakland University William Beaumont School of Medicine on July 31, 2008.

THE BEAUMONT CULTURE IN THE MEDICAL SCHOOL

"We have a vision and have designed the school to be pliable because we know things will change. We are preoccupied with culture, not in the terms of fine arts, but the working environment of the school. We recruit our faculty very carefully, because they are role models for our students and how we want our students to behave when they become physicians. If they're in an environment that's all about numbers, we want our students to know that nothing is really all about numbers. We want them to be treated individually just as we want them to treat their patients, because to the individual patient, that visit from the doctor is the most important event of the day, or the month, or the year, or maybe even the lifetime, depending on the diagnosis And it doesn't have to be a disease. 'Congratulations, you're expecting your first child.'

"We spend a lot of time creating a culture, because we know that twenty, thirty years from now, the things we've put into place will change, but we want the affiliative, affirmative culture to remain steady, and for the school to be one of the premier places to come to become a physician, a physician educator, a physician scientist, or a scientist. That's an outstanding legacy."

Oakland University Provost Virinder Moudgil, Ph.D assisting an undergraduate student into analyzing tumor suppressor proteins extracted from breast cancer cells.

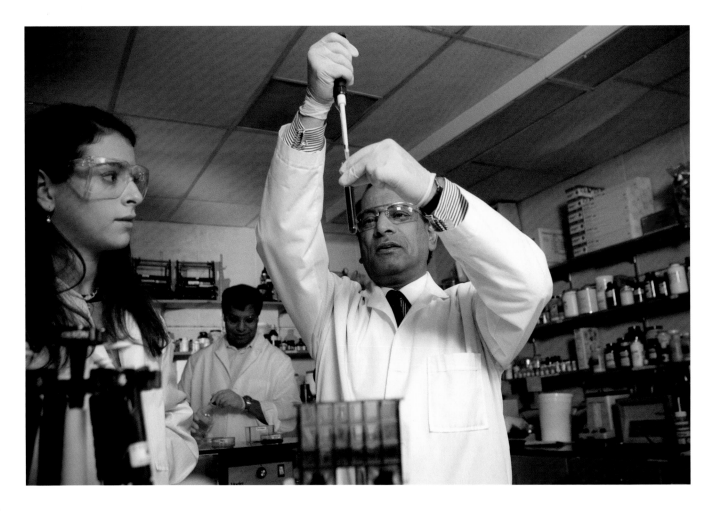

DR. FRANKLIN AND DR. WILLIAMS ON THE MEDICAL SCHOOL

Franklin: "It's very exciting to be working on the medical school. Although there are certain challenges with finances and keeping our regular program and teaching in the medical school, it shows a pioneering vision on Dr. Diokno's part, as well as Ken Matzick, and Gene Michelski. Granted, we're in tough economic times and we may be a bit overextended, but these guys have done one heck of a job in a very tough environment. I applaud where Beaumont has gone and where it's going, and I think the long-term future is going to be very bright."

Williams: "I'm the head of the Department of Ophthalmology for the new medical school. We teach eye doctors and eye surgeons now in a residency program, and hopefully we'll be bringing some of our medical students into our training program. We have a very active clinical education program right now under the direction of Dr. Musich. We have one of the largest non-university-based clinical graduate education programs in the country.

"I think one of the things that should be emphasized is the unique model we have at Beaumont with the blending of private practice culture with world-class academic medicine. There are few places that have been able to do that as successfully as we have. That's going to be an increasing challenge for us going forward. The integration of the medical school into our private practice culture, I expect, will have some rough water, but the opportunity is great to combine those two types of cultures and make it unique. Beaumont is an amazing institution and we've been successful for a long time. Now the challenge is to continue that success."

Typical morning teaching rounds headed by Robert Begle, M.D., Medical Director, Medical Intensive Care Unit and Director, Sleep Laboratory for Beaumont Hospital-Royal Oak.

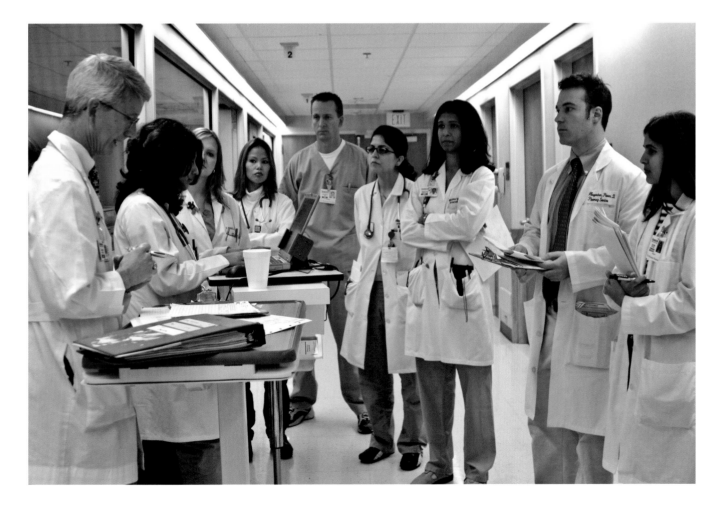

21 THE FUTURE

Artist's conception of how the skyline at Thirteen and Woodward might look like in the future.

DR. DIOKNO ON BEAUMONT'S FUTURE

"Our big vision is to have a medical school faculty building at the corner of Thirteen Mile Road and Woodward Avenue, in the area where there is now a strip mall. It will be a multi-story building for all the offices of the faculty. All of the professors will have their offices there and they can see patients or students.

"There could also be some classrooms and an auditorium. There could also be perhaps a small hotel for people coming from all over the country, and a shopping complex so we do not totally eliminate the convenience of stores and restaurants. That will be the Oakland University William Beaumont School of Medicine Faculty Building.

"Another thing we're looking at is a sports medicine complex. We are striving to have a new emergency medicine pavillion, right at the north part of the main hospital. It will be the third incarnation of the ER. The original ER was replaced by an expanded emergency area, and now there will be a new one, but that requires a lot of money. These are the new accomplishments toward which we are working for Beaumont's future of service to the community and the world."

Beaumont Genetic Services: "This is new technology. This is the present and the future."

DANA ZAKALIK, M.D.

Professor of Internal Medicine, Oakland University William
Beaumont School of Medicine
Corporate Director of Cancer Genetics, Beaumont Hospital

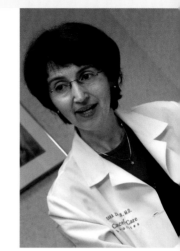

"I helped start the Cancer Genetics Program

at Beaumont out of a need to provide cancer genetic services to our patient population once several very important genes were identified that predispose men and women to cancer. In the mid-1990's there was the identification of two genes that significantly predispose women to breast cancer. Women's risk goes up ten-fold. They have almost an 85% to 90% chance of getting breast cancer and also ovarian cancer, as well as other cancers. Medical science has been hunting for those genes for a number of years. Once they were identified, commercial testing became available for patients.

"We in medical oncology have always known that breast cancer runs in families, some with the mother, sister and daughter all having breast cancer. We suspected for a long time that there is a gene, so now we've identified it, and in the late '90's testing became available to all physicians. Now doctors must take accurate family histories to find out whether an aunt or uncle or someone else had cancer, so we can recognize the red flags in family history and do the appropriate testing.

"Like all genetic testing for predisposition for diseases, the patient needs genetic counseling. To do this in state-of-the-art correct fashion, the doctor has to see these patients, take extensive family history, provide pre-test counseling, and only with informed consent can a person draw a patient's blood for the gene test."

"So here's Beaumont, an institution of 1000 beds that didn't have this service. I felt there was a need and started putting the pieces together brick by brick, for a cancer genetics program. I and other visionary individuals at Beaumont were able to get the hospital to allow us to do this. It wasn't easy. The administration allowed us to have space and a genetic counselor, and I went out single-handedly giving talks all over the campus about cancer genetics. I talked to residents, staff, and the

public to raise awareness and the fact that we now have these genes. If you have a family history of cancer, the genetic testing should be automatic.

"The genes are called BRCA 1 and 2. When I first started, many physicians didn't even know what they were, or that they were hereditary cancer-predisposition genes. Now there are thousands of articles, but back in the '90's that wasn't so. Physicians who had gone to great medical schools hadn't heard of the genetic association between breast cancer and ovarian cancer. They didn't know that males could pass breast cancer or ovarian cancer through a male lineage.

"This is new technology. This is the present a nd future."

"MARKED"

"There were many misconceptions about genetic testing, like people were afraid of it or thought they'd never get health insurance, or that they'd be dropped from their insurance or their premiums would go up. In some ethnic populations, having a gene that predisposes you for cancer can leave you a 'marked person.' We engaged in an educational campaign to get the public to stop being scared and to combat those fears of ignorance."

BUILDING A CANCER GENETICS PROGRAM

"My vision for Beaumont is to build a premier clinical genetics program, but also involve education and research, because genetics lends itself to research. There is not much known about it and it offers tremendous, ample room for research and contributions in research areas.

"We began seeing and counseling patients. I was doing the counseling with a nurse whom we trained, but we knew that the complexity of genetics and risk management really required a Master's Degree. In September of 2005 I hired a genetic counselor to work with me, the physician.

"We got so busy that we had to add a second counselor in '08. We've grown about 30% in volume every single year. That's how positive a reaction we've had from referring doctors and the public. People are now recognizing the importance of genetics.

"Predisposition is an important part of what we do. We see young women, some very young, who are walking around with ten times the risk for breast cancer, ovarian cancer, six times the risk for pancreatic cancer, and a family history of male breast cancer, or whose mother died at 35 years old. Male breast cancer in the family should be a red flag for predisposition.

"In addition to BRCA, there are other cancer-predisposition genes. There is a colon cancer gene that predisposes people to an 80% chance of getting colon cancer. We're seeing more patients referred to us who have very young-onset, which is the hallmark of all these genetic syndromes where there's cancer somewhere in the family.

"When I see a family like this, I start taking very careful family history. Is there any other cancer, and does it fit either of these syndromes? The colon or breast can have pancreatic cancer in it.

"Not all cancers can be easily reduced to a single gene. It just so happens that breast and ovarian cancer have their own syndrome—that's BRCA 1 or 2. The colon has it own, called Lynch Syndrome. That's the colon, but also uterine cancer and pancreatic. Henry Lynch is still alive and practicing, the father of colon cancer genetics. There are more rare cancer predisposition syndromes out there which we're seeing as our program gets bigger."

USING GENETICS IN CANCER PREVENTION

"Ultimately, the whole goal is prevention of cancer. There's no point in identifying these genes if we can't do anything about it. Once we identify these people, we make recommendations about various preventative strategies, ranging from increased surveillance and screening, like breast MRI or more frequent colonoscopies, to preventive surgery. Many women with the BRCA gene are choosing bilateral mastectomies with reconstruction. It sounds drastic, but when you're faced with an 80% chance of getting breast cancer, a lot of these women don't want to bother with MRI's because MRI's are not 100% guaranteed to discover breast cancer. Many are educated women and understand that folks who haven't read as much as they have sometimes get angry when they hear me talk about preventive surgery. How could we think of this?

"A majority of these women are fairly sophisticated, especially the ones who have seen their mothers or aunts die. I see many young girls who say, 'My mom died when I was twelve and I watched it happen. I want to be tested so I can be proactive and do the proper prevention and never get cancer.'

"Ovarian cancer is very hard to detect because there is no good screening test. These BRCA patients have anywhere from a 25- to 45% risk of getting ovarian cancer in their lives by the time they're seventy years old. We tell them to remove the ovaries because the same two genes, BRCA 1 and 2, predispose women to breast and/or ovarian cancer. It's a huge discovery."

ONE GRANDMOTHER

"We have a fascinating family in which the grandmother had ovarian and breast cancer. She had one cancer, ovarian, at a young age, then breast cancer, then it came back. She went through our program. She was gene-positive. That grandmother lived long enough to tell her family that if anything happened to her as a result of her cancer, her dying wish was for her family to do fund-raising and raise awareness about genetics, and to pay for testing for others. It turned out that two of her daughters had ovarian cancer, so this whole family had the genetic propensity. The family showed up at our clinic with a beautiful poster with a photo of the grandmother, with a pink ribbon and the testimonial from the grandmother about what had happened to her.

"She hoped for her granddaughters that testing would prevent their having the fate she did. They were young—eighteen, nineteen-year-old girls. So this family contacted Fox Health Beat. When the granddaughters came in for testing, it was filmed as a story on Fox News.

"The Fox people wanted to cover the result live. On the air, I announced that they both had the gene. It was a very touching story."

"We've built a very successful program that is making a difference for patient and for me as a medical oncologist. I was used to treating cancer after it happened, and sometimes after it had metastasized, sadly. To be able to identify high-risk people and do something before they even get the cancer is, for me, very rewarding on a personal level."

Beaumont's Multi-organ Transplant Services: "I want to turn this place into a top-notch center where any sort of organ or multiple-organ disease can be cared for . . . ."

ALAN KOFFRON, M.D.

Professor and Interim Chair of Surgery, Oakland
  University William Beaumont School of Medicine
  and Beaumont Hospitals
Chief, Division of Multi-organ Transplants, Beaumont,
Royal Oak

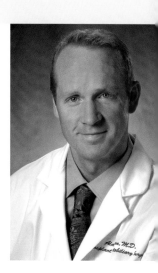

"I'm an archetypal Iowa boy. I did most

of my medical training in Iowa and got the bug for organ transplants at the Transplant Division at the University of Iowa. I was fascinated by the way medical science can look at a body part and figure out a way to graft it to another body. I went to Chicago and was a transplant surgeon for over a decade at Northwestern University on Michigan Avenue.

"Beaumont asked me to come and speak about minimally invasive liver surgery, which I helped pioneer. Briefly, to take out a liver tumor, it usually takes a huge side-to-side incision. We developed a way to do it laparoscopically. You might ask how we take out a whole organ or a big part of it through a little incision; we actually liquify it in an impermeable bag and remove it with suction. This turns a three-week hospital stay with eight weeks' recovery into an overnight stay, or sometimes even an outpatient experience. I came here to discuss that innovation, and met Dr. Diokno and others, and immediately thought this place was very different from what I had experienced before.

"When I came to Beaumont, a behemoth of a place, I noticed that people were very appreciative and supportive if someone did something innovative or particularly helpful. I haven't looked back. It's a place where people really care that they make a difference in someone else's life. The leadership of Beaumont tells us to make a difference, and makes us feel as if we do."

"Part of my charge to come here was to bring liver surgery here and reinvigorate the transplant division to be multi-organ. They promised me a lot to do that. They have been enormously supportive, and we're rising slowly. We invigorated kidney

transplants, then liver transplants came on the scene. The indications for transplantation broadened and the different diseases we can successfully treat with transplantation has broadened with it, not only just with one organ, but kidney and liver, or liver-kidney-pancreas, or liver-kidney-pancreas-intestine. It may seem rather Frankensteinian and more difficult, but carefully done and in the selected patient, transplantation can be quite substantial.

"We have a good hold on the organ-rejection problem, with medications getting better every year. For example, liver rejection is nothing but a nuisance. Only two out of ten people have a rejection attempt, and we call it an 'attempt' because ninety-five out of a hundred times, we can get it back in equipoise by adjusting with medications to calm down the person's immune system. The only reason we lose organs nowadays is when somebody stops taking care of himself, not because we can't control it.

"One of the big innovations—and we're part of the research for this—is finding better medications. It would be nice if a transplant patient could take a pill maybe once a month, and just live happily with whatever body part he or she happened to need during life. And it will come."

A CRITICAL NEED FOR ORGANS

"When she was six, my daughter said, 'Dad, you don't have enough organs.'

"I said, 'I know.'"

She said, 'Well, if you'd be willing to accept one, why wouldn't you be willing to give one?'

"That was pretty insightful, I thought."

CHILDREN AND TRANSPLANTS

"Can we transplant adult organs into children? Yes, a portion of them. For example, the liver. The usual circumstance is that we have a very young child who is going into liver failure. That's where organ shortage is even more severe. There are adults dying and donating their organs, but those organs are huge and can't possibly be crammed into a child. There are very few little organs around.

"We're burying thousands of viable organs every day, organs that are desperately needed. People are squeamish about donating the organs of their loved-ones who have died, but oddly everybody wants to receive a transplant if the choice is that or the abyss."

LIVE-ORGAN TRANSPLANT

"In the late '90's, more people were getting transplanted for more indications, but the organ supply plateaued and stayed static. That's when live-organ transplant began—taking an organ or part of one from a living person to save another person. We took it to the next stage and tried to do it through band-aid type surgery. Here at Beaumont we've done laparoscopic kidney transplants. The problem with doing it is that we don't want to damage the organ to put it in. Plus, the actual implantation—sewing the organ in—in a confined space takes longer and the organ is without a blood supply, so it has to be chilled so it doesn't degenerate.

"Whenever I consider doing a minimally invasive procedure, the first thing I think of is the risk-to-benefit ratio. If I'm going to risk the patient's life or health by trying to improve something else, I have to come to a reasonable conclusion. Patients needing transplants are at the ends of their roads, so continuing on with a scar is not much of a decision. But for someone who is otherwise healthy, we can do it without a scar and a long recovery."

"There are several places—Cambridge and others—who have done genetic engineering and have made strides in changing the way pig organs are recognized by the human immune system to prevent immediate destruction. Instead of the organs now being rejected within seconds, it's gone

to minutes, and now hours. It'll be interesting to see how far science can go to change one organism to get spare parts for another. The better we educate people to give up their organs when they don't need them anymore, the less we'll have to change another organism from which to borrow organs."

"Every Wednesday we take a kidney out of somebody with band-aid surgery and put it in the recipient of his or her choice. The donor has two kidneys and only needs one. We evaluate the donor to be sure he's healthy enough, and evaluate the recipient to make sure the kidney will work. The kidney is about the size of a fist, but once we stop the blood supply in a certain sequence, it shrinks about thirty percent. Now I'm dealing with a plum-sized organ instead of a fist-sized one, and I can remove it through a small opening. A belly button is full of wrinkles and folds, and if I open it using an S-shaped incision that can be stretched, the kidney can be slid out, and then the 'S' is put back into shape, and there's no visible incision. The donor can go to the beach and not have a scar showing.

"In the 'old days,' donation meant a three-month recovery and people would say, 'I'd love to donate, but I'll lose my job and my house . . . ' Now we can do this with a couple of band-aids, you're back to work in a week, and you're wearing a 'Hero' badge.

"I'm in the business of making somebody with end-stage organ disease better, and we can do that in a way that makes their relatives and friends more likely to say, 'Yes, I'll do it.'"

"We just started something called 'electroporation,' where we place a needle in a tumor and in a hundredth of a second the tumor is killed. The liver tissue grows back in. In some cases, the patient doesn't even need surgery to remove a tumor. He hiccups a little in his sleep, wakes up, and the next scan shows the tumor is no longer there. Instead of leaving a scar, the procedure allows the tumor to die in a way that the normal liver grows in behind it. The liver is privileged in that it does that. The more experience we have with the liver, the more we modify techniques to the spinal cord, heart, or brain tumors without the bystander death of tissue from the treatment.

AN INGENIOUS ORGAN

"From adult to adult, 50% to 60% of the liver is taken from the donor. Both livers will grow back to full size within a few weeks. It's the only organ that grows back. There's research now trying to determine how that occurs. Maybe someday we can use regeneration for spinal cords or other parts. That's why I gravitate toward the liver. The liver is stupid in one way—it doesn't reject—and smart in another way—it regenerates continually. We estimate that the human liver could run for about three hundred years if we didn't die earlier than that or injure it in some way. Over the years I've transplanted 80-year-old livers into young people. That's the only organ that doesn't have a mileage limit.

"Unfortunately, liver cancers don't cause pain. These cancers can grow to the size of eggplants and don't present symptoms until they start pushing on something else. Fortunately, Beaumont is very good at screening. If somebody has a medical condition—hepatitis or Wilson's disease—that might lead to liver cancer, they screen appropriately. For example, about eight out of a hundred people per year with Hepatitis C will develop a cancer. Check them when they get their yearly cholesterol check, and we can catch a cancer while it's still pre-malignant. Beaumont is phenomenal about doing ultrasounds every six or twelve months and noticing a cancer when it's small and can be treated with radio waves or removed with a band-aid surgery, so it doesn't reach a point where the patient needs a transplant. Beaumont allowed me to start a liver tumor clinic that's focused on gathering those people who should be screened. Between me and my three colleagues here, we do more of this type of surgery than anybody in the world so far.

"The liver is a kind of catcher's mitt for the whole body. Eighty percent of the cancers in the liver are from somewhere else. As the cells break free and percolate through the blood, the liver catches them. That's why the liver can be susceptible to all these cancers. If we can remove the cancer, the liver grows back. If the cancer is of the liver itself—there are three or four cancers that originate in the liver—we can replace the liver, which of course cures the cancer.

"You can tell I like the liver. It's an ingenious little organ."

BEAUMONT'S PASSION

"I left a top-five transplant center to come to Beaumont. The passion here for medicine allows more potential than any other place I've ever been. The physical plant is spectacular. The people who populate it allow us to grow and expand and innovate as much as possible. They don't stop and say, 'Well, we've never done that here.' Here they say, 'If you give me a good story and there's passion behind it, do whatever you can do.'

"I want to turn this place into a top-notch center where any sort of organ or multiple-organ disease can be cared for, in the right setting to allow people to go on until such time where we can fix whatever genetic trouble occurred. I jovially say we're in the used-parts business."

THE FUTURE

"I hope that science will progress to the point where animals can be changed a little bit so they bear organs we can put in humans and the human immune system doesn't mind. If you come to me in forty years and say, 'I have a liver problem,' I'll say, 'Let's go downstairs and you can pick one off the shelf.' And you'll go to the operating room, and instead of having surgeons, you'll have something more like a device that allows us to non-invasively implant the organ into you, and I give you a medication that from that moment on allows your immune system to tolerate the foreign material.

"I can anticipate this because I know that Beaumont will invest in something that's promising and then allow us to advance as far as advances can be made."

JAMES GRANT, M.D.
Professor and Chair of Anesthesiology, Oakland University William
Beaumont School of Medicine and Beaumont Hospitals

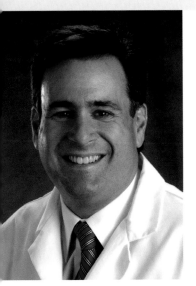

Beaumont's Ambulatory Surgical Services: "Convenience, delivery of high quality safe care in a cost effective manner will drive many more services into stratigically located ambulatory centers."

"As our patient's needs continue to grow,

they have increasing desires to have Beaumont services closer to their home. In 2004, Beaumont began the development of our first ambulatory surgical center (ASC) in Macomb Township, Michigan. Although ASC's were very common throughout the country, their growth was somewhat slower in Michigan largely because of a very complex regulatory environment, but because of a strong partnership between Beaumont and its private physicians, we were able to successfully launch the North Macomb ASC in 2007, with a second facility serving Western suburbs opening in West Bloomfield just 18 months later."

"Free-standing same-day surgery centers were made possible largely because of the great innovations in the anesthetic agents used both during operations and after the procedure. Probably one of the most dramatic changes was when propofol (brand name: Diprivan) was released in the United States. Propofol allows the patient a very smooth awakening, feeling less groggy and with significant decreases in nausea and vomiting. Before propofol's release, the major anesthetic induction agent was sodium pentothal, which although a good drug, has significant nauseating effects and left the patients with lingering sedation. Nausea and vomiting, once seen as a leading reason for unplanned admission after surgery, has become a thing of the past. Also, newer inhalational agents like sevoflurane and desflurane have enabled the anesthesia team to deliver safer anesthesia which also readies patients for a quick discharge from the facility."

"One of the services that has seen a great increase in ambulatory surgical centers is orthopaedic surgery. This has been made largely possibly by the introduction of perineural catheters inserted under ultrasound guidance by the anesthesiologist. Pain control, a very common reason for both planned and unanticipated admissions, has significantly been diminished by the introduction of this new approach to post operative care. Now, instead of oral drugs that go throughout the body and effect daily living, we are able to send patients home, with infusion devices that deliver local anesthetic directly to the nerves allowing a clear sensorium. This new modality in post operative care has clearly allowed patients to return home and return to their normal activities in a fraction of the time they previously experienced."

DR. DIOKNO ON AMBULATORY SURGICAL CENTERS

Thomas R. O'Donovan, Ph.D. wrote the sentinel work on ambulatory surgical centers in 1976 and was perhaps the catalyst to the proliferation of same-day surgery performed either within the hospital setting or in a free standing facility.

With the increasing competition and improvements in anesthetics and techniques there was resurgence in the early 60's to expand ambulatory surgery. Another contributing factor is the concept that early ambulation is superior to prolonged inactivity as documented by Beaumont surgeon Paul T. Lahti, M.D.

Thomas's son, Patrick O'Donovan, Vice President for Planning for Beaumont Hospitals commented on the work of his father and how it influenced the direction of his own career.

"His influence and example for me was indescribable. I graduated Michigan State in 1982—the depths of one of the worst recessions ever. When I decided to pursue health care administration as a career, he encouraged me to get a Masters Degree, and I graduated from University of Michigan in 1984. He told me the best hospital to work for in Michigan was Beaumont, and I was fortunate to secure an internship followed by an administrative residency under the direction of David Ladd, from whom I also learned a great deal as my career got started. I've been in Planning ever since and my dad was right—Beaumont *is* an outstanding place to work!"

Quality and Safety that is cost-effective: "Value-Based Medicine will be front and center for all that we do at Beaumont now and in the future."

SAMUEL FLANDERS, M.D.

Associate Professor of Pediatrics, Oakland University William Beaumont School of Medicine

Senior Vice President and Chief Quality and Safety Officer, Beaumont Hospitals

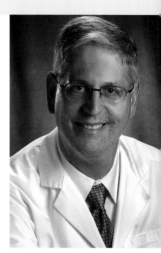

"My responsibility is oversight of

the quality and safety of the whole Beaumont system, the hospitals as well as the ambulatory facilities. Hospitals all across the country are looking at how effectively heart attacks, heart failure, pneumonia, and so on, are being treated, preventing infections in surgical patients, and other complications. A big part of my job is to figure out reliable ways to make those results good for our patients.

"Hospitals don't have the greatest safety record. We're not on a par with the airline industry or nuclear power, but we work every day to get to those ideals. If we look at the risk of death from various activities ranging from commercial air travel with its extremely small chance of death all the way to bungee jumping, one of the most dangerous activities is being admitted to a hospital, in terms of a whole variety of risks of problems and of medications, because we administer thousands of them. We give half a million doses a month just in the Beaumont, Royal Oak hospital. Each has to be the right dose at the right time to the right patient. That's a lot of complexity to manage. There are falls, infection—the list goes on, so our job is to try to install systems that will guarantee that bad things don't happen. We have to make the right things happen for every patient."

SPEAK UP IF YOU SEE A PROBLEM

"Another advancement is called 'a safety culture.' This is something the aviation industry worked very hard to cultivate. A co-pilot will speak up if he or she sees that the captain is about to make a mistake. We work very hard to get that culture ingrained into the medical field. Everyone should feel comfortable speaking up if he sees something that's about to go wrong, even if a surgeon or other esteemed professional is about to do something wrong. It's a well-documented factor in health care, where someone in the operating room is pretty sure

the doctors are about to, for instance, operate on the wrong leg; a medical student or a brand-new nurse might not speak up to a doctor who's been working for 30 years, but anybody can make a mistake. We want everyone to feel free to speak up.

"A check list for the operating room is a huge improvement. The list is run down point by point, to make sure we have the right patient, know what's supposed to happen, whether there are any medical concerns like needing blood to be available—it's like a pre-flight check list a pilot uses before take-off. The surgical team stops what they're doing before the cutting begins, and answers all the questions until everybody is satisfied, and the operation proceeds. In Michigan, that project is called 'Keystone.' One of our surgeons here, Dr. Rob Welsh, is one of the people who helped found the Keystone Project.'

"I'm amazed at how much Beaumont's physicians and nurses already know about patient safety and how far along they were before they even had anybody in my position. I'm not coming to fix a broken system, because the system here was already very good and the level of knowledge among the staff, while not universal, is much more than I'm used to. For instance, Dr. Welsh has formal training in patient safety. He completed a patient safety fellowship, and there's another surgeon at Beaumont, Troy, Dr. Jim Lynch, who did the same thing—took time out from his schedule to travel for training. That's unusual. Usually you don't see physicians doing that sort of thing, but these are practicing doctors who thought it was the right thing to do, so they got involved and moved the hospital along the curve.

"Another striking thing here is that we've recently enrolled ourselves in some benchmark databases that allow us to compare our results against other hospitals in the country, including big-name institutions. When we look at our mortality rates here, they are exemplary among hospitals that are rated with at least 750 beds, of which there are about twenty in this big database. We're at the top of the list on the good side—we are essentially tied for Number One. I was pleased that right out of the box we ranked so highly."

KAIZEN

"In health care, we plan everything to the last degree. Sometimes we have to do that—having an OR set up to do brain surgery with everything in place. But for most things we do, we can experiment and gradually improve—delivery of medication from the pharmacy to the floor, delivery of blood, and so on. The key is to not look for the big improvements, don't look to save two hours, but shave one or two seconds or minutes off the time. Practices like this in factories have shown that if the people are trained to recognize opportunities and capture one second or two, there will be much more improvement than trying to hit a home run every time. They might make ten changes a day, ten very small changes, and at the next work station they're doing the same thing, and over time it adds up. Focus on taking a little bit of waste out of the system every single day, and the money takes care of itself.

"We're applying these techniques to health care, which makes a hospital more nimble, faster, and able to change quickly. We started with one nursing department right here at Royal Oak, actually sending the nursing unit manager and some of the staff to a factory for training in how to do this. This process is called 'Kaizen,' a Japanese word which means 'gradual, continuous improvement.' It's the philosophy that they will never sit still. To use a baseball analogy, it's that they will try to hit singles all day, every day. Americans try to hit home runs all the time. That takes longer, and you're constantly planning, planning, planning to hit a home run. If you fail, you're back to planning, planning, planning—committees, meetings, and wasting time."

ONE SMALL IMPROVEMENT, OR TWO, OR THREE . . .

"The nursing staff discovered they had a problem with the devices we put on patients' legs to prevent blood clots after surgery. The device is hooked to a pump that squeezes the legs, milking the vein, so the blood doesn't sit around and form a clot. Well, the patient might have to go to the bathroom, so the nurses must disconnect the machine and sometimes it wasn't getting re-connected when the patient got back to bed. They came up with a simple system of putting a little sticker on the outside of the room if the patient has the device, then every time a nurse goes into the room, the device can be checked to make sure it's hooked up. They went from a low score to over 90%. Simple, devised by the front-line people, making a huge difference for patients.

"If you're a nurse and five times a day you have to walk down to the end of the hall to get a pill cutter because the cutter is missing from the room where you work most of the time, you're wasting time and energy. This was a real example. I saw that happen, and now we have pill cutters anchored to the walls in every medication room. Those are the seconds that add up and let a nurse spend more time at the bedside of the patient.

"Now we're reaching out to suppliers. For instance, we found that drugs were not being delivered in a timely fashion from the pharmacy to the nursing units, which slowed the nurses down as they tried to call the pharmacy and clear up miscommunication.

"We're also working on patient transportation, because patients have to be moved all over for tests. A number of us spent time following the transportation workers around, because you can't understand somebody else's job by hearing about it. We followed for two days, saw the barriers, and now are working to reduce road blocks, the wait for elevators—for example they have to wait for special elevators, but the regular staff uses these elevators just for getting around, so we're asking the staff to use the public elevators unless they're transporting a patient or a piece of equipment."

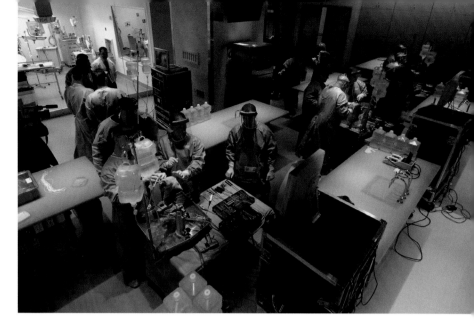

"Sometimes there was a problem finding a stretcher. There wasn't a standard place, so the staff had to search multiple floors to find one. We're creating three locations with a plan to keep stretchers supplied to those areas, like grocery cart corrals.

"None of these are rocket science, but they add up. When we first started this, we discovered that only about 26% of the time was the nurse doing value-added work with the patient. The other 74% was spent waiting, walking, or hunting for things. A patient wouldn't want to pay for any of that, but it was necessary to do the work. Supplies were running out, dressings were supposed to be in the rooms that weren't there, and there was no system to make sure those things were replenished when they got low. Now we have a system for that. Our nursing time with patients is up to 62% now. The nurses spend more time with the patients, who are safer by definition, because things are less likely to fail. Everything is happening more reliably."

"EXCUSE ME, BUT I THOUGHT WE WERE DOING THE *LEFT* LEG TODAY."

"We do tell our doctors to check their egos at the door. Everybody needs to be accountable for surveillance. If we have a junior nurse in the operating room and a senior doctor is about to operate on the wrong leg, we want that junior nurse to feel absolutely comfortable speaking up and saying, 'Excuse me, but I thought we were doing the *left* leg today.'

"That's a safety culture. It's not easy because it's not the way health care is taught. The intensity of the job of a trauma surgeon or a heart surgeon is such that things can go wrong in a heartbeat and we don't want people having a committee meeting while a patient is bleeding to death. They need to act decisively, but the same mindset that makes them good doctors can interfere with the ability to listen to a subordinate. The challenge is that we don't want to undo their training. We don't want to waste the guy who's trying to stop the bleeding from an aorta and make him wishy-washy about giving orders. He must rely on himself and his immediate team, but we want to teach these skills so that people will feel comfortable speaking up."

THE SURGICAL CHECK LIST

Beaumont's Simulation Laboratory

"With the new medical school, we're going to do very well because this method will be baked right in. We're starting with our residents now, getting them involved with patient safety so they don't grow up to have egos so big that they won't listen to their teams. One excellent solution is the surgical check list. No matter how many times a pilot has flown a plane, he still goes through the pre-flight check list with his co-pilot. We have a check list in the operating room and we do the same thing. We have a check list in the ICU for certain things related to the central lines that we put in people, which can get infected and possibly kill or injure a patient. There are certain medications we put in them and certain things that have to be done every day, and somebody has to figure out whether the patient still needs the central line. Using check lists, even though they're so simple and obvious, can save lives."

"I've been delighted by the receptiveness of the senior administration here and all the administrators and doctors to trying this change of habit. They're been very open to this. There are many more physicians involved in the administration of the hospital than in most hospitals. This was a great move for me. I'm excited to be here."

Center for Simulation and Team Dynamics Education and Research: "The future is here but more to come."

It was, and is still, the deadliest plane crash in the history of manned flight. On March 27, 1977, in heavy fog at Los Rodeos Airport on the island of Tenerife in the Canary Islands, 583 people were killed when two Boeing 747 passenger planes collided on the runway. KLM Flight 4805 was taking off and Pan Am Flight 1736 was taxiing. The KLM plane was off the ground when it struck the spine of the Pan Am plane, tearing it open and igniting a fireball. Both planes were destroyed. Only 61 people survived.

Causes of the crash were manifold. The blinding fog prevented the tower or the planes from seeing each other. The airport was congested with planes. Both 747s had been diverted to Los Rodeos; the airport was not constructed to accommodate such big craft. The taxiing process on runways offered limited space, forcing taxiing on the runways themselves rather than only in taxiing areas. Finally, the communications were sloppy and non-standard. The disaster put a focus on the last, but certainly not the least, element: how human beings communicate in a team environment, and how inarticulate communications can result in tragedy.

John Nance, a Network Aviation Analyst on the PBS NOVA documentary "The Deadliest Plane Crash," said, "Ultimately, the reason that the KLM aircraft began rolling down that fog-shrouded runway was this was a team, but it wasn't allowed to operate like a team. So one man made a mistake and that mistake stuck."

Everybody who watches movies has heard the familiar order-response sequence used aboard ships and submarines. First comes the order from the commanding officer: "Helm, two-seven-zero." Then the response: "Two-seven-zero, aye." It's a compass order, to turn the ship to the west. The person saying "aye" is receiving the order. He acknowledges that he heard it, and the repeat helps make sure the commander gave the order correctly and offers a redeemable moment if the order was misspoken.

The airline and shipping industries have identified this problem and tried to figure out how to teach team dynamics, to take a really good look at communication and how it applies to risk management. How can these things be taught and practiced, with distractions built in to the training sequence?

The answer was simple: simulation. This means actually practicing scripted scenarios with possible disasters incorporated into them, like interactive games, and develop procedures to counter each distraction or miscommunication before a little thing turns into a big mess that can't be turned around.

The idea is simple. Execution is not. Simulation is complex, technical, time-consuming and expensive. As in these other high-risk industries, health care has discovered that large percentage of problems are not caused by obvious incompetence or technical failings, but by the elements of how people work together and the frailties of teams, even teams of brilliant experts.

HEALTH CARE'S BRAVE NEW SIMULATED WORLD

An Emergency Room might get a call from an ambulance about an auto accident. A nurse and a resident take the call. Suddenly there's a swarm of ER personnel, including trauma nurses, charge nurses, surgery residents, ER residents, anesthesiologists. Who's going to be in charge? Is it a Level 1 or Level 2 trauma? And, by the way, everybody's dressed alike. It's not as though the senior neurologist wears a hat displaying his title and experience. The nurses and doctors may not know each other, or if they do, they might not recognize who's behind the mask.

What if the patient is bleeding? The procedure to get blood in hospitals is complicated, and complexity flirts with danger. If the blood doesn't arrive quickly, nurse after nurse calls the blood bank, and there's only one tech in the blood bank. "Where's the blood? Did we call for blood?" is asked over and over again by the docs, but nobody directly answers, even though there might be five nurses trying to get blood.

Now there's a surgeon here. Is he or she in

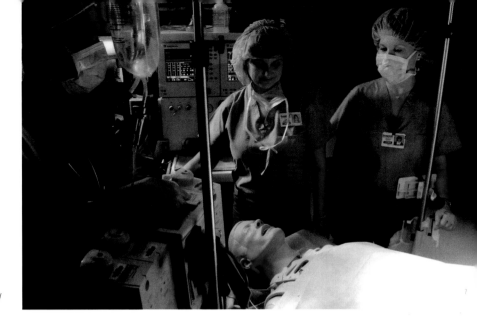

charge? That surgeon may be legendary in his field, a famous doctor with decades of experience. Does a 24-year-old nurse dare speak up if something is about to go wrong? The doctor hasn't said a word to anybody. What is the protocol here? Important minutes are being lost…

Good thing it's only a simulation, right?

Beaumont's leadership recognized that this new method of training and teasing out problems is very important, and that it is neither easy nor cheap. Could a huge, complex organization use the methods of simulation to make it more efficient, more cost-effective, and better for its patients?

Yes. Beaumont now has a Center of Excellence for Simulation Education and Research, and is planning on expanding the simulation laboratory with more virtual-reality simulators right in the midst of the hospital, very close to the operational environment. Studies are being developed in crew management and training scenarios that expose the function of a team and what a health care team really is. The scenarios are integrated in such a way that professionals act as they would if the situation were real. There are high-tech mannequins hooked up to wireless simulators, and each mannequin is remotely controlled by a technician off to the side. The mannequin talks, breathes, has heart sounds and a pulse, symptoms, and even bleeds.

Beaumont also has an infant simulator mannequin, and a pediatric scenario in which a baby is brought into the ER. Anything can be done with the mannequin that can happen to a real baby. Is the young ER doc in charge, or is the pediatric intensive care nurse with twenty years' experience in charge?

To plug this hole in heath care teams, Beaumont uses the position of "Care Coordinator," like a sergeant or officer of the watch, which creates one-stop shopping. The Care Coordinator stands back and writes everything down. If a doctor asks, "Where's the blood?" it's the Care Coordinator's responsibility to find out, and no one else's. The Care Coordinator knows the doctors and the nurses, so they don't necessarily have to know each other.

The ER is quieter now, more calm. Chaos and uncertainty are greatly reduced, and good outcomes increased. Beaumont is gradually working this concept through all its departments.

THE MEDICAL SCHOOL: A CLEAN SLATE

In the past, part of the problem of team dynamics has been that senior personnel are imposing to others, and often don't display a welcome to challenge or corrections. In short, they're intimidating. Doctors, especially, are venerated in their fields, making others hesitate to speak up. With the opening of Oakland University William Beaumont Medical School, a brand new school with no ingrained bad habits, team dynamics and cross-disciplinary skills will be addressed every day, as will a sense of respect from the top down rather than only from the bottom up. The practice of team dynamics will be integrated further back in the education process, for doctors and also nurses, who are the doctor's constant allies. Using simulations to improve safety, culture and outcomes, this new-age concept of care will swiftly improve delivery of health care at almost every level, for the real world.

JOHN TU, M.D.

Assistant Professor of Internal Medicine, Oakland University
William Beaumont School of Medicine
Vice-President and Chief Informatics Officer, Beaumont Hospitals

Electronic Medical Records (EMR):
"Changing health care forever."

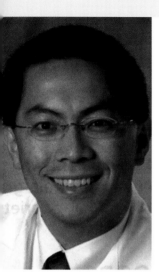

"Medical informatics is the technology

of integrating and enhancing the use of computer technology in medicine. I'm an internal medicine physician by training and did a couple of years of medical informatics, and decided to pursue that field. I came to Beaumont two years ago, when Beaumont created this opportunity and I jumped on it.

"I was born in Taiwan and came to the U.S. when I was 13. My undergrad studies were in electrical engineering, and then I decided to go to medical school at the University of Illinois, then did residency training at Massachusetts General Hospital for medical informatics."

A HYBRID WORLD

"Most places today, including Beaumont, hire more people to manually collect all the data, and there is more and more demand for more data to be collected, and more for our nurses and physicians to have to remember. Imagine if you're a lawyer in trial court, and you're forced to type up everything yourself, without a transcriber helping you. That's the amount of work load we're asking of our clinicians. Those are things a computer does very well. Our goal is to minimize those tremendous efforts. It not only controls costs, but also frees people to do what they should be doing—better patient care in more critical areas, versus doing mundane chart reviews.

"That's what I'm here to help Beaumont accomplish. Besides patient care, Beaumont also has an academic agenda: research and education. Typically, hospital electronic health record information systems' foremost focus is on clinicians, nurses, and patients. We want to include the residents, fellows, and medical students. Usually, education and research are on the back burner because there aren't enough resources to integrate those areas. One of my key initiatives is to integrate those areas so we can incorporate the discoveries and research into our EMR system.

"Here, we're using the EPIC system. There

are several vendors, so physicians may encounter differences in the way the systems work if they travel between hospitals. Eventually, two or three good systems will become the standard. It's a big change for physicians, but we have training programs to teach them how to use EMR systems. One of our design principles is to standardize as much as possible.

"For example, we design a heart failure order set, a set of things we're normally supposed to do when we're taking care of a patient with heart failure, including multiple tests, different medications, and so on. There might be three physicians from three hospitals who are reviewing these order sets, so the sets need to agree. We have to force integration, get people to talk to each other and figure out which standard they want to use, and break down some of the communication barriers as well as cultural barriers. Many physicians have strong personalities, so standardization often depends on who is in the room doing the negotiating. At the Royal Oak hospital we have innovations coming from various specialties, like cardiology or imaging, creating some of the newest ways to do things. We'll have a meeting with them and create order sets to support their patient care with the new innovation. Then we make it available to Troy and Grosse Pointe. It's much easier for me to get a group of physicians to agree within Royal Oak than to get agreement at three hospitals at once. I'm working with my IT colleagues to get everyone in the Beaumont system to sit down in the same room and agree.

"Working with all these physicians is very rewarding and one of the reasons I came to Beaumont. Working with docs from three hospitals is something unique, so I'm enjoying it because I love a challenge. Not only must I know how to apply the technology and informatics, but I'm building relationships as we urge the physicians to buy into the system and make a success for our customers.

We can push, but not too hard."

INFO-NURSES

"Nurses are easier to work with, partly because they're all employees and they understand a hierarchical structure where someone can say, 'This is the system we're using.' They're more amenable to learning new systems, and they like having a system that shows them everything they need to see—what the doctor said, which medication to use, the patient's history—it's all right in front of them.

"There are two approaches to implementing systems like these. One is the big-bang approach, where everybody suddenly stops what's been done for the past twenty years and has to learn a new way. In general that doesn't work for a huge organization like this. We're using a phased fashion, moving a group to 30% functionality, then maybe six months later adding another 40%. Maybe 20% more later. Each group comes up at different rates. For example, about a year ago nurses at Royal Oak and Troy were doing things 100% on paper. We switched to 20% EPIC. So they're documenting vital signs, blood pressures, heart rate, respiratory rate, allergies and medications, and simple assessments of the patient's condition on EPIC.

"It's a challenge because we live in a hybrid world, 20% electronic, 80% paper, still struggling back and forth. Just this past weekend we crossed a major goal line, and our nurses are now doing 80% in the electronic system. But the physicians are not. We want to get the nurses there first, because they will be our backups when the physicians go 'live' with electronics."

WIRED DOCS

"With the coming of our medical school, we intend to integrate into the curriculum the training for these electronic changes, so our young doctors come out already knowing them. I'm part of the faculty at the medical school. We'll be teaching what we call the 'Capstone' course on informatics. The students will be exposed to things like decision support—why something is done, what some alternatives might be, and how to improve care of the patient.

"I'll be exposing the students to the ways the system can help them, but also training them on actually using the system. In the past, I've seen the newer residents using shorthand and abbreviations for texting, then type in their progress notes using the same shorthand, not using proper spellings or punctuation. That's not professional. It could be misunderstood. It's not good for patient care.

"Students and residents will constantly challenge us, push us forward. When we're teaching residents, we have to be sharp on our clinical judgments and we're forced to keep up on things."

"Most physicians know what they were trained to do in medical school and residency programs. Sometimes that learning slows down, even if they go through continuing medical education. They know how to treat their patients, but with all these new things changing rapidly, no sane person can keep up. It's not possible to take care of patients today with just paper, so we're going to accelerate our method of learning, the way we treat our patients in terms of innovative processes. When somebody does something new, maybe sticks a catheter into a coronary artery or some place it's not supposed to go, and it works, it won't be five or ten years before that gets into practice. The electronic systems will shorten the vetting periods and growing pains of new practices. Physicians will have to make those calls, but the system will be well-established to provide that basic set of standards so people know what's out there.

"For instance, our imaging department is very aggressive in using imaging study for immune diseases they're treating. Doing research protocols, we can help them recruit patients using our system. Today, they'll make announcements and everybody has to remember which patient has which condition—is this patient A, B, C, or D, and does he have X, Y, or Z? Do you think most physicians remember? Not really. So they hire lots of research nurses who flip through endless paper charts and determine who meets the criteria. All that can be animated through EPIC. That's going to get us more test subjects, quicker results, and improvement in care."

NO MORE PAPER CHARTS

"Beaumont is just beginning that phase of our journey—our 'Operational Infrastructure'—so people can start taking care of their patients without paper charts. There are certain system flags and clinical decision support built into the system. We build in very precise rules that say, 'If A,B, and C occur, do X, Y, and Z.'

"It's a monumental task. The next ten years there will be leaps and bounds of advancement. I'm in the right place at the right time. My journey here to Beaumont was not planned, but opportunity fell in my lap. I thought I would be at Chicago forever, but suddenly this came along out of no where. I said, 'Honey, do you want to move to Michigan?'"

KEN MATZICK and DR. JOHNSON ON ELECTRONIC MEDICAL RECORDS

Matzick: "Doctors are making more use of Electronic Medical Records. We're in the fifth year of a $100 million investment in an Electronic Medical Record system. We've installed the 'front and back ends'—registration, scheduling, billing, clinical, emergency room, pharmacy—and we're about to tackle the big one: in-patient clinical records and electronic order entry by physicians.

"There are tremendous safety benefits and efficiency is gained. Things won't be ordered twice unnecessarily, you get instant reporting, much less error, and many benefits. There is some disruption for physicians, who have learned to write in illegible handwriting which takes hours to figure out and lends itself to errors—they won't be able to do that anymore.

"Anyway, our hospital-based physicians and those who work for us are on the EPIC system, the core clinical record system. Because the system was invented in a physician's office, it's designed for the office setting, and doctors can fairly easily adapt their offices to use it. The concept evolved from there to serve hospital needs.

"It's extremely valuable to have one patient record that is universally available to all the care-givers and is updated simultaneously with treatment. Everybody gets the information as soon as it's available and can access the record and find out what the other medical person did and what needs to happen next. We can reconcile what kind of medicines the patient is on. As you can imagine, it's very good in the emergency room.

"A module we're very excited about is called 'myBeaumontChart,' with which the patient has access to his or her own medical records and can make updates. You can also have access to your elderly relative's charts and of course your children's. The new system allows you to manage that using a web browser, even hundreds or thousands of miles away. When Electronic Medical Records are integrated into our lives, the incidents of medical mistakes will plummet."

Johnson: "Of any industry in the United States, the one that has the greatest deficit in information technology is health care. Medical care is way behind the cutting edge. Where is the information in the doctor's office linked to the patient's room, or the ER? We absolutely have to have electronic medical records—EMRs. The patient shows up in the ER, had a CAT scan a week ago at some facility, but the ER can't get the report, so they order another CAT scan. That's inefficient, time-consuming, and costly.

"Now, Beaumont has invested in the EPIC Information System out of Madison, Wisconsin. They only take on large health care systems. It's a big project and very capital-intensive, and a big change for doctors. We implemented it in our ambulatory care network in Grosse Pointe for three months; their productivity dropped slightly just from learning the system, but after three months they actually were up a bit. Doctors are, obviously very scientifically based, need information, and need it up-to-date."

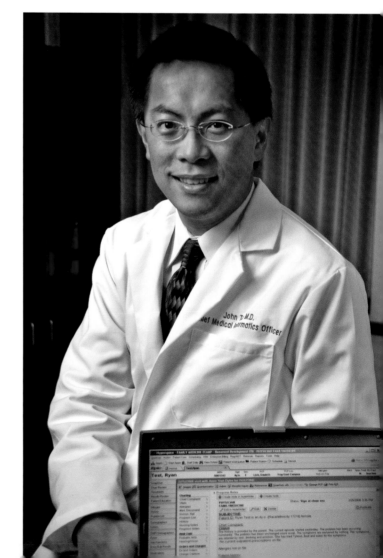

John Tu. M.D. our first Vice President of Medical Informatics is instrumental in helping Beaumont implement electronic medical records.

Electronic Medical Records (EMR):

"Another way we're changing health care from a Beaumont perspective is giving every patient access to his/her own electronic medical record. It's called "myBeaumontChart.""

SUBRA SRIPADA
Senior Vice President and Chief Information Officer

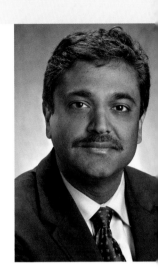

"I am one of the new entries to this

management group. Many have been here a long time, so I bring some outside experience. In the past decade I've been a consultant in the health care field, both in technology and in business, in national and international consulting. I've done considerable work related to health care and planning for the future, developing strategies and actions. I've been in Michigan for the last 25 years, but I'm originally from India, and grew up there. I actually have a B.A. in mechanical engineering and a Master's in industrial and systems engineering.

"I'm not a typical information officer, the kind who grows through the Intelligence Tech field. Organizations are investing a ton of money into technology, and what I've found is that most boards and leadership teams don't understand enough about IT to be able to bring it into the strategic dialogue. Therefore it sits in the back room until somebody says, 'Oh, you need another fifteen million?' It's constant tension.

"So when Gene Michalski (CEO as of 2010) offered me the chance to come back into health care, I was looking for an opportunity in which I could make a huge difference and be part of the changing landscape. The fact that we have a CEO change, a directional change, and health care reform, we find ourselves building a strong brand name on excellence of care, based on outcomes and based on the physicians who are here. The secret sauce of Beaumont physicians is the caring and the competence. It's follow-through and skill in terms of what they bring to each patient.

"As we become bigger and bigger, turning into an academic center, we want to be sure in these changing times that we arm the medical staff with right technology to continue to differentiate Beaumont from others. For instance, what a doctor used to have to imagine and diagnose is now in a 3-D color image right in front of him. The technology is at such a point that there are ways to greatly limit the amount of radiation to which patients are subjected, using pinpoint X-rays.

"The advances in technology allow non-invasive surgeries. I played golf with somebody who is a Beaumont patient. He said he chose Beaumont because of the technology they were able to show him. They took out his kidney over the weekend, and he was playing golf in less than a week."

BITS AND BYTES AND EMRS

"Technology is not just computers and bits and bytes. It is the overall delivery of care, the continuity of care. And how do we enable all of that? How do we put information into the hands of the physician who is making the decisions at the right time? That's my job.

"One of the first pieces of medical writing I did was on Electronic Medical Records (EMRs). It's fabulous and fun and inevitable, but it comes with challenges. EMRs mean ultimately eliminating paper from the medical process, from the doctor/nurse/patient/treatment interaction. Everything is done with computers—computers in the patient's room, hand-held computers in the doctor's hands. We just went live with a major implementation with part of the EMR, called Computerized Physicians' Order Entry. There is no paper. They are placing orders electronically. When a doctor sees a patient, whatever the diagnosis is and whatever is being prescribed—lab orders, X-rays, etc.—all goes into he computer.

"The computer, then, is smart enough to kick back questions to that physician. It might ask that based on the medical record, are you sure this patient has this history, or that this medication might interact with another medication that has a certain active ingredient. This question pops up, and the doctor doesn't have to keep all this in his head, or fish for paper records, or call his staff before knowing

KEN MYERS ON THE FUTURE

"A hundred years ago the average lifespan was 49 years. Most people didn't live long enough to get a chronic disease. Medicare had just started back in 1966 when I first came here, and there was a saying: 'People over 65 require twice as much health care, twice as often as those under 65.'

"And that was true. People are living longer now, and better health care is a significant factor. Also, people are taking better care of themselves and being active longer. People are living longer, but the elderly are requiring more health care. It has been estimated that people over 85 require maybe four times as much health care, four times as often. Babies and children are not dying at the rates they did before the '50's and '60's. Younger and younger premature babies are being saved. There have been huge strides in pediatric cancer, to a point where most children now survive instead of the other way around. Because of these factors, there will be an increasing demand for health care in the future.

"Over time, hospitals are going to become intensive care facilities. You'll have to be really sick to be admitted to a hospital. Many medical problems will be handled in ambulatory or home care settings. More and more surgery will be done outside the hospital. Even now quite a bit of surgery is done in doctors' offices and ambulatory care facilities.

"Moving procedures out of the hospital setting means lower costs, patients' going home sooner, and more efficiency. Technology has been advancing to allow physicians to do things in ambulatory care settings that once could only be done in hospitals."

what to do with this particular patient's symptoms. Are you sure you want to order another X-ray? The patient had one seventy-two hours ago. Here are the results. This lab test is valid for six months and the patient just had one at the last visit. It also eliminates the penmanship problems. So the EMR is a smart animal.

"Also, if your doctor happens to be out of town, maybe in Hong Kong, New York, or Hawaii, and you have a question, you can call his office, the office can contact the doctor, and on his EMR the doctor can see your medical history and doesn't have to go from memory or tell you to wait until he comes back.

"For this, we need partnerships with physicians. It's a dialogue. Many physicians say, 'I didn't go to school for all this stuff. I'm used to just throwing it at my secretary and letting her handle it.'

"One way to solve this is to bring the nurses along first. It's a management-change issue. Doctors have a lot on their minds, many patients, and the number of patients they can see in a day is their main concern. We can give them the best technology in the world, but if it reduces the number of patients they see, they're going to fight it. Typically the physician comes to the hospital in the morning, goes on rounds, sees patients, tries to keep information in his head or write it down, can't find a way to write it down, and is reduced to scribbling something on a bit of paper, throws it on a desk, and moves on. Now I'm asking them to type something. So to whom do they turn?

"Nurses and secretaries. So we started in the ER, because that's our front door. About 60% of our admissions come through the ER. We looked at all three emergency centers and made them completely electronic as of October of 2009. The next February, we took all of our nurses and made all the nursing documentation electronic. Between February and June, they had enough time to mature their use of the system and become experts. Some of them became super-users.

"Then we went live with doctors. Now, when the docs come along, the nurses are right there and know what do to. All of our employed doctors will be using EPIC, our information system, in their offices. They'll use iPads, iPhones, laptops, and some will use a computer on wheels, which walks around with them. EPIC told us this is the smoothest implementation they've seen anywhere.

"Another way we're changing health care from a Beaumont perspective is giving every patient access to his/her own electronic medical record. It's called 'myBeaumontChart.' We have about six hundred patients on the pilot program. The patients will be able to receive his results, make appointments, have secure messages, ask questions, and the doctor can respond in a reasonable time."

THE FUTURE

"There is going to be massive change. This book is really about what has been done in the past fifty years. The last part, about the future of Beaumont, is really a preface for the next fifty years."

William Beaumont Hospital
Board of Directors and Trustees

Beaumont Voices

A

Federico Arcari, M.D. 20, 57, 103, 149, 160, 167

B

Harold Barker, M.D. 55
Joseph Bassett, M.D. 211
Dr. William Beaumont 33
Kay Beauregard, R.N., M.S.A. 77
Stanley M. Berry, M.D. 170
Lorraine Boudreau 68
Thomas M. Brisse 106, 192
Nancy Bruske 98

C

Dean Caputo, R.N. 80
Diane Carey 12
Margaret Casey 181, 189
Susan Catto, M.D. 144
Shane M. Cerone 69
Gary Chmielewski, M.D. 238
Betty Chu, M.D. 172
Christine Comstock, M.D. 124

D

Fernando Diaz, M.D., Ph.D. 226
Ananias C. Diokno, M.D., F.A.C.S. 9, 17, 27, 75, 130, 171, 192, 221, 252

E

Luke Elliott, M.D. 155

F

David Felten, M.D., Ph.D. 174, 176, 248
Samuel Flanders, M.D. 259
Robert Folberg, M.D. 247
David Forst, M.D. 107
Barry Franklin, Ph.D. 215, 251

G

Val Gokenbach, D.M., R.N., R.W.J.F. 78
James Grant, M.D. 99, 258
Cindy L. Grines, M.D. 208

H

David Haines, M.D. 205
Dorothy Hanna, R.N. 74
Richard Herbert, D.O. 73, 108
Harry N. Herkowitz, M.D. 228
Dennis Herrick 58
Donna Hoban, M.D. 18, 153, 161
Roger Howard, M.D. 110
Greg Howells, M.D. 162

I

Khalid Imam, M.D. 140
Ronald Irwin, M.D. 236

J

A. Neil Johnson, M.D. 94, 266

K

Prem Khilanani, M.D. 101, 102, 240
Michael Klllian 15, 245
Alan Koffron, M.D. 255
Mark Kolins, M.D. 29
Ernest Krug III, M.Div, M.D. 146
Ruben Kurnetz, M.D. 47

"AN ETERNAL LIGHTHOUSE"

It was opaque darkness,
Neither the moon nor the stars
Yet yonder twinkling and flickering liveliness,
And now a silhouette of a hospital . . .
A power outage, yet a luminescence.
What is the source of the light?
Operators diligently working by day and night.

Nurses tending to patients,
Docs talking to families,
Professors teaching their residents,
The students imbibing the experience,
All silently seated in the auditorium.
Where is the source of the light?
The light is in learning and knowledge.

The C-section done in a timely fashion,
The CPR concludes with heart ticking,
Patient in ICU, extubated, with lungs breathing,
Patient walks again with new knee joint.
Where is the light?
It's in the smiles, laughter and success.

Petri dish with cultures responding to drugs,
Operations done remotely with robots,
Patients participating in clinical trials,
Publications galore in international journals.
Where is the light?
In futuristic technology and applications.

All in all, it's still one family
With hugs, kisses and smiles,
Sometimes tears, many times joy.
More patients come by word of mouth.
Where is the light?
In success, empathy, and connection.

Prem V. Khilanani, M.D.

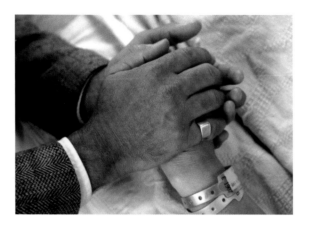

"*Beaumont has very much focused on the little things in life, so that every employee becomes a patient advocate who knows that every patient is a fragile person. Even the person who carries the trays is reminded every day that we're here for the patients, to be friendly, to smile, to be cordial, to leave our own problems at home and concentrate on the patients. Things have changed and we've gone high-tech, but we want to maintain what we've always had, and that's 'high-touch.'*"

DONNA HOBAN, M.D.
Beaumont, Grosse Pointe